Bone Health and Osteoporosis

A Report of the Surgeon General

2004

U.S. DEPARTMENT OF HEALTH AND HUMAN SERVICES
Public Health Service
Office of the Surgeon General
Rockville, MD

National Library of Medicine Cataloging in Publication

Bone health and osteoporosis : a report of the Surgeon
    General. - Rockville, Md. : U.S. Dept. of Health and
    Human Services, Public Health Service, Office of
    the Surgeon General ; Washington, D.C. : For sale
    by the Supt. of Docs., U.S. G.P.O., 2004.
    p.436
    Includes index.

    1. Bone Diseases - prevention & control. 2. Bone
Diseases - etiology. 3. Osteoporosis - prevention &
control. 4. Bone and Bones - physiology. 5. Health
Promotion - methods. 6. United States. I. United
States. Public Health Service. Office of the Surgeon
General.

    WE 225 B71259 2004

This publication is available on the
World Wide Web at
http://www.surgeongeneral.gov/library

For sale by the Superintendent of Documents, U.S.
Government Printing Office, Washington, D.C. 20402.

Use of trade names is for identification only and does
not constitute endorsement by the U.S. Department of
Health and Human Services.

Suggested Citation

U.S. Department of Health and Human Services. *Bone
Health and Osteoporosis: A Report of the Surgeon
General.* Rockville, MD: U.S. Department of Health
and Human Services, Office of the Surgeon General, 2004.

Message From Tommy G. Thompson
Secretary of the U.S. Department of Health and Human Services

This first-ever Surgeon General's Report on bone health and osteoporosis illustrates the large burden that bone disease places on our Nation and its citizens. Like other chronic diseases that disproportionately affect the elderly, the prevalence of bone disease and fractures is projected to increase markedly as the population ages. If these predictions come true, bone disease and fractures will have a tremendous negative impact on the future well-being of Americans. But as this report makes clear, they need not come true: by working together we can change the picture of aging in America. Osteoporosis, fractures, and other chronic diseases no longer should be thought of as an inevitable part of growing old. By focusing on prevention and lifestyle changes, including physical activity and nutrition, as well as early diagnosis and appropriate treatment, Americans can avoid much of the damaging impact of bone disease and other chronic diseases.

In recognition of the importance of promoting bone health and preventing fractures, President George W. Bush has declared 2002–2011 as the *Decade of the Bone and Joint.* With this designation, the United States has joined with other nations throughout the world in committing resources to accelerate progress in a variety of areas related to the musculoskeletal system, including bone disease and arthritis.

As a part of its *Healthy People 2010* initiative, the U.S. Department of Health and Human Services (HHS) has developed an important goal for Americans—to increase the quality and years of healthy life. Our hope is that Americans can *live long and live well.* Unfortunately, fractures—the most common and devastating consequence of bone disease—frequently make it difficult and sometimes impossible for people to realize this goal.

HHS is committed to developing a wide array of creative and innovative approaches that can help make the goal of living long and living well a reality for Americans. Several programs of particular relevance to bone health include:

- *The National Institutes of Health's Osteoporosis and Related Bone Diseases ~ National Resource Center.* The National Resource Center provides timely information for health professionals, patients, and the public on osteoporosis, Paget's disease of bone, osteogenesis imperfecta, and other metabolic bone diseases.
- *The National Bone Health Campaign.* Targeted at 9- to 12-year-old girls and their parents, this campaign uses Web sites and other activities to promote nutritional choices and physical activities that benefit bone health.

- ***Steps to a HealthierUS Initiative.*** HHS launched this initiative in 2003 to advance the President's goal of helping Americans live longer, better, and healthier lives. At the heart of this program lies both personal responsibility for the choices Americans make and social responsibility to ensure that policymakers support programs that foster healthy behaviors and prevent disease.
- ***VERB*$_{TM}$. *It's what you do.*** This national, multicultural, social marketing campaign encourages young people ages 9–13 to be physically active every day as a means of promoting overall health, including bone health.

This Surgeon General's Report brings together for the first time the scientific evidence related to the prevention, assessment, diagnosis, and treatment of bone disease. More importantly, it provides a framework for moving forward. The report will be another effective tool in educating Americans about how they can promote bone health throughout their lives. I appreciate the efforts of Surgeon General Richard H. Carmona and the many scientists and researchers who contributed to the development of this report.

Preface

From the Surgeon General,
U.S. Department of Health and Human Services

As Surgeon General, my primary role is to provide the American people with the best scientific information available on how to improve health and reduce the risk of illness and injury. This first-ever Surgeon General's Report on bone health and osteoporosis provides much needed information on bone health, an often overlooked aspect of physical health. This report follows in the tradition of previous Surgeon Generals' reports by identifying the relevant scientific data, rigorously evaluating and summarizing the evidence, and determining conclusions.

A healthy skeletal system with strong bones is essential to overall health and quality of life. Yet, today, far too many Americans suffer from bone disease and fractures, much of which could be prevented. An estimated 10 million Americans over age 50 have osteoporosis (the most common bone disease), while another 34 million are at risk. Each year an estimated 1.5 million people suffer an osteoporotic-related fracture, an event that often leads to a downward spiral in physical and mental health. In fact, 20 percent of senior citizens who suffer a hip fracture die within 1 year. One out of every two women over 50 will have an osteoporosis-related fracture in their lifetime, with risk of fracture increasing with age. Due primarily to the aging of the population and the previous lack of focus on bone health, the number of hip fractures in the United States could double or even triple by the year 2020.

However, the evidence in this report is clear: Hope is not lost. Over the past several decades, scientists have learned a significant amount about the prevention, diagnosis, and treatment of bone disease. Our next and most critical step is to transfer this knowledge from the research laboratories to the general population.

One of my priorities is to promote disease prevention by helping Americans take actions to make themselves and their families healthier. The good news is that regarding bone health, these steps are clear—with appropriate nutrition and physical activity throughout life, individuals can significantly reduce the risk of bone disease and fractures. Health professionals can also make significant improvements in our Nation's bone health by proactively assessing, diagnosing, and treating at-risk patients and then helping them apply this scientific knowledge in their everyday lives.

However, individuals and health professionals acting alone will not make a long-term difference. This brings us to the primary message of this report: A coordinated public health approach that brings together a variety of public and private sector stakeholders in a collaborative effort is the most promising strategy for improving the bone health of Americans. This report calls for the development of a national action plan to achieve improved bone health, and it highlights the unique and valuable perspectives that key stakeholders can bring to this effort. While government ought to be a part of the plan's development, leadership must be shared among the many public, private, nonprofit, academic, and scientific stakeholders.

Over the past 2 years, I have worked to improve the health literacy of Americans; that is, to ensure that individuals can access, understand, and use health-related information and services to make appropriate health decisions. To that end, a short, easy-to-read companion piece to this report has been developed. Available in English and Spanish, this *People's Piece* takes the best scientific information available in this report and provides Americans with important, practical information on how they can improve their own bone health.

I am encouraged by the participation of so many people and organizations in developing this report, and I would like to thank them for their willingness and eagerness to assist us in gathering the best scientific information available. I am confident that their passion will be a catalyst for action. Working together, we can take real steps to improve the bone health status of Americans. Our reward for this effort will be to prove the forecasters wrong—instead of seeing ever-increasing numbers of individuals suffering from the agony of bone disease and fractures, we will see the day when fewer and fewer Americans bear this burden.

Richard H. Carmona, M.D., M.P.H., FACS
Surgeon General

Acknowledgments

This report was prepared by the U. S. Department of Health and Human Services under the general direction of the Office of the Surgeon General.

Richard H. Carmona, M.D., M.P.H., F.A.C.S., Surgeon General, U.S. Public Health Service, Office of the Surgeon General, Office of the Secretary, Washington, D.C.

Christina Beato, M.D., Acting Assistant Secretary for Health, Office of the Secretary, Washington, D.C.

Arthur Lawrence, Ph.D., R.Ph., Assistant Surgeon General, U.S. Public Health Service, Deputy Assistant Secretary for Health (Operations), Office of Public Health and Science, Office of the Secretary, Washington, D.C.

Kenneth Moritsugu, M.D., M.P.H., Deputy Surgeon General, U.S. Public Health Service, Office of the Surgeon General, Office of the Secretary, Washington, D.C.

Allan S. Noonan, M.D., M.P.H., CAPT, U.S. Public Health Service, Scientific Editor, Surgeon General's Report, Office of the Surgeon General, Office of the Secretary, Washington, D.C.

Stephen I. Katz, M.D., Ph. D., Director, National Institute of Arthritis and Musculoskeletal and Skin Diseases, National Institutes of Health, Bethesda, Maryland.

The editors of the report were

Joan A. McGowan, Ph.D., Senior Scientific Editor, Surgeon General's Report, Director, Musculoskeletal Diseases Branch, Extramural Program, National Institute of Arthritis and Musculoskeletal and Skin Diseases, National Institutes of Health, Bethesda, Maryland.

Lawrence G. Raisz, M.D., Scientific Editor, Surgeon General's Report, Board of Trustees Distinguished Professor of Medicine, Interim Director, Musculoskeletal Institute, Division of Endocrinology and Metabolism, University of Connecticut Health Center, Farmington, Connecticut.

Allan S. Noonan, M.D., M.P.H., CAPT, U.S. Public Health Service, Scientific Editor, Surgeon General's Report, Office of the Surgeon General, Office of the Secretary, Washington, D.C.

Ann L. Elderkin, P.A., Managing Editor and Project Director, Surgeon General's Report, Health Systems Research, Inc., Washington, D.C.

The scientific writer was

Larry S. Stepnick, M.B.A., Scientific Writer, The Severyn Group, Inc., Ashburn, Virginia.

Coordinating authors were

Deborah T. Gold, Ph.D., Associate Professor, Departments of Psychiatry and Behavioral Sciences, Sociology and Psychology: Social and Health Sciences, Duke University Medical Center, Durham, North Carolina.

Susan L. Greenspan, M.D., Professor of Medicine, University of Pittsburgh, Pittsburgh, Pennsylvania.

Anne Looker, Ph.D., Senior Research Epidemiologist, Health Examination Statistics, National Center for Health Statistics, Centers for Disease control and Prevention, Hyattsville, Maryland.

L. Joseph Melton, III, M.D., Eisenberg Professor, Department of Health Sciences Research, Mayo Clinic and Foundation, Rochester, Minnesota.

Lynne Wilcox, M.D., M.P.H., CAPT, U.S. Public Health Service, Editor-in-Chief, Preventing Chronic Disease, National Center for Chronic Disease Prevention and Health Promotion, Centers for Disease Control and Prevention, Atlanta, Georgia.

Deborah E. Sellmeyer, M.D., Assistant Professor of Medicine, Director, University of Calfornia San Francisco / Mt. Zion Osteoporosis Center, San Francisco, California.

David Reuben, M.D., Professor of Medicine, Division of Geriatrics, David Geffen School of Medicine, University of California at Los Angeles, Los Angeles, California.

Contributing authors were

Laura Bachrach, M.D., Pediatrics Department, Stanford University Medical Center, Stanford, Connecticut.

Douglas Bauer, M.D., Associate Professor of Clinical Medicine, University of California, San Francisco, San Francisco, California.

John P. Bilezikian, M.D., Professor of Medicine and Pharmacology, College of Physicians and Surgeons, New York, New York.

Dennis Black, Ph.D., Professor, Department of Epidemiology and Biostatistics, University of California, San Francisco, San Francisco, California.

Jane Cauley, Dr.P.H., Associate Professor, Department of Epidemiology, University of Pittsburgh, Pittsburgh, Pennsylvania.

Jan A. Christensen, M.S.W., J.D., Manager, Diabetes, Kidney and other Chronic Diseases, Chronic Disease and Injury Control, Michigan Department of Community Health, Lansing, Michigan.

Carolyn Crandall, M.D., F.A.C.P., Associate Professor of Medicine, Iris Cantor-UCLA Women's Health Center, University of California at Los Angeles, David Geffen School of Medicine, Los Angeles, California.

Steven R. Cummings, M.D. University of California, San Francisco, San Francisco, California.

Denise Cyzman, M.S., R.D., Senior Project Coordinator, Health Promotion and Disease Prevention, Osteoporosis, and Other Chronic Conditions, Michigan Public Health Institute, Okemos, Michigan.

Susan Davidson, M.S., R.D., Consultant, Germantown, Maryland.

Bess Dawson-Hughes, M.D., Professor of Medicine, Metabolism Lab, Tufts University, U.S.D.A. Human Research Center on Aging, Boston, Massachusetts.

Deborah A. Galuska, Ph.D., M.P.H., Epidemiologist, Division of Nutrition and Physical Activity, Centers for Disease Control and Prevention, Atlanta, Georgia.

Gail Greendale, M.D., Professor of Medicine and Opbstetrics-Gynecology, University of California at Los Angeles, David Geffen School of Medicine, Los Angeles, California.

Robert P. Heaney, M.D., F.A.C. P., F.A.C.N., John A. Creighton University Professor, Professor of Medicine, Department of Medicine, Creighton University, Omaha, Nebraska.

Gregory Heath, D.H.Sc., M.P.H., Division of Nutrition and Physical Activity, National Center for Chronic Disease Prevention and Health Promotion, Centers for Disease Control and Prevention, Atlanta, Georgia.

Ann Hewitt, Ph.D., C.H.E.S., Assistant Director, Master in Healthcare Administration Program, Seton Hall University, Center for Public Service, Mendham, New Jersey.

David P. Hopkins, M.D., M.P.H., Staff Scientist, Health Promotion and Chronic Disease Program, Oregon Department of Human Services, Portland, Oregon.

Anne M. Kenny, M.D., Assistant Professor, University of Connecticut Center on Aging, Farmington, Connecticut.

Sundeep Khosla, M.D., Professor of Medicine, Department of Endocrinology, Mayo Clinic and Foundation, Rochester, Minnesota.

Douglas P. Kiel, M.D., M.P.H., Director of Medical Research, Research and Training Institute, Hebrew Rehabilitation Center for the Aged, Boston, Massachusetts.

Anne Klibanski, M.D., Chief, Neuroendocrine Unit, Massachusetts General Hospital, Neuroendocrine Unit, Boston, Massachusetts.

Nancy E. Lane, M.D., Associate Professor, Division of Rheumatology, University of California at San Francisco, San Francisco, California.

Craig B. Langman, M.D., Isaac A. Abt, MD Professor of Kidney Diseases, Feinberg School of Medicine, Northwestern University, Chicago, IL. Head, Division of Kidney Diseases, Children's Memorial Medical Center, Chicago, Illinois.

Peggy Lassanske, President, Elder Floridians Foundation, Tallahassee, Florida.

Meryl LeBoff, M.D., Director, Endocrine-Hypertension Division, Skeletal Health and Osteoporosis, Brigham and Women's Health, Boston, Massachusetts.

Karen Lim, Acting Executive Director, National Asian Women's Health Organization, San Francisco, California.

Geraldine Mackenzie, Supervisor, New Jersey Department of Health and Senior Services, Older Adult Health and Wellness, Trenton, New Jersey.

Catherine MacLean, M.D., Ph.D., Assistant Professor of Medicine, Division of Rheumatology, University of California at Los Angeles School of Medicine, Los Angeles, California.

John McGrath, Ph.D., Chief, Public Information and Communications Branch, National Institute of Child Health and Human Development, National Institutes of Health, Bethesda, Maryland.

Heather McKay, Ph.D., Associate Professor, School of Human Kinetics, University of British Columbia, Vancouver, British Columbia, Canada.

Paul Miller, M.D., F.A.C.P., Clinical Professor of Medicine, University of Colorado Health Sciences Center, Denver, Colorado. Medical Director, Colorado Center for Bone Research, Lakewood, Colorado.

Heidi D. Nelson, M.D., M.P.H., Investigator and Associate Director, Clinical Prevention Center, Oregon Health Sciences University, Portland, Oregon.

Eric S. Orwoll, M.D., Professor of Medicine, Program Director, General Clinical Research Center, Associate Dean for Clinical Research, Assistant Vice President for Research, Oregon Health and Science University, Portland, Oregon.

Rebecca Payne, M.P.H., Public Health Analyst, Nutrition and Physical Activity Communication Team, Centers for Disease Control and Prevention, Atlanta, Georgia.

Munro Peacock, M.D., Professor of Medicine, General Clinical Research Center, Indiana University Medical Center, Indianapolis, Indiana.

B. Lawrence Riggs, M.D., Distinguished Investigator, May Foundation, Purvis and Roberta Tabor Professor of Medical Research, Mayo Medical School, Division of Endocrinology, Mayo Clinic and Foundation, Rochester, Minnesota.

G. David Roodman, M.D., Ph.D., Professor of Medicine, Division of Hematology/Oncology, School of Medicine, University of Pittsburgh, Pittsburgh, Pennsylvania.

Clifford Rosen, M.D., Chief of Medicine, Maine Center for Osteoporosis Research, St. Joseph Hospital, Bangor, Maine.

Elizabeth Shane, M.D., Professor of Clinical Medicine, College of Physicians and Surgeons, Department of Medicine, Columbia University, New York, New York.

Kathy Shipp, P.T., Ph.D., Assistant Research Professor, Physical Therapy, Community and Family Medicine, Duke University Medical Center, Durham, North Carolina.

Ethel S. Siris, M.D., Madeline C. Stabile Professor of Clinical Medicine, Endocrinology Division, Columbia University and Columbia Presbyterian Medical Center, Harkness Pavilion, New York, New York.

MaryFran Sowers, Ph.D., Professor, Department of Epidemiology, University of Michigan, Ann Arbor, Michigan.

Anna N. Tosteson, Sc.D., Professor, Departments of Medicine and Community and Family Medicine, Dartmouth Medical School, Lebanon, New Hampshire.

Nelson Watts, M.D., Director, Bone Health and Osteoporosis Center, University of Cincinnati, Cincinnati, Ohio.

Connie M. Weaver, Ph.D., Distinguished Professor, Department Head, Foods and Nutrition, Purdue University, West Lafayette, Indiana.

Michael F. White, Consultant, Michael F. White and Associates, Women's Health Council, Association of State and Territorial Directors of Chronic Disease Programs, Alexandria, Virginia.

Michael P. Whyte, M.D., Professor of Medicine, Pediatrics, and Genetics, Bone and Mineral Diseases, Department of Medicine, Barnes-Jewish Hospital at Washington University School of Medicine, St. Louis, Missouri.

Joseph D. Zuckerman, M.D., Chairman, Department of Orthopedic Surgery, Hospital for Joint Diseases, New York, New York.

Reviewers were

Steven A. Abrams, M.D., Professor, Pediatric/Children's Nutrition Research Center, Baylor College of Medicine, Houston, Texas.

Amy Allina, Program and Policy Director, National Women's Health Network, Washington, D.C.

Nell Armstrong, Ph.D., R.N., Program Director, Division of Extramural Activities, National Institute of Nursing Research, National Institutes of Health, Bethesda, Maryland.

David Atkins, M.D., M.P.H., Senior Health Policy Analyst, Center for Practice and Technology Assessment, Agency for Healthcare Research and Quality, U.S. Department of Health and Human Services, Rockville, Maryland.

John Baron, M.D., M.S., M.Sci., Professor of Medicine and of Community and Family Medicine, Biostatistics and Epidemiology, Dartmouth Medical School, Lebanon, New Hampshire.

Douglas Bauer, M.D., Associate Professor of Clinical Medicine, University of California, San Francisco, San Francisco, California.

L. Tony Beck, Ph.D., Program Officer, Division of Clinical Research, National Center for Research Resources, National Institutes of Health, Bethesda, Maryland.

Michele F. Bellantoni, M.D., Associate Professor of Medicine, Division of Geriatric Medicine and Gerontology, Johns Hopkins University School of Medicine (representing American Geriatrics Society), Baltimore, Maryland.

Francis J. Bonner, Jr., M.D., Physiatrist, Department of Physical Medicine, Rehabilitation Hospital of South Jersey, Vineland, New Jersey.

Kathryn Brewer, P.T., G.C.S., M.Ed., Health Educator and Consultant, Arizona Osteoporosis Coalition, Phoenix, Arizona

David Brown, Ph.D., Senior Behavioral Scientist, Division of Nutrition and Physical Activity, Physical Activity and Health Branch, National Center on Chronic Disease Prevention and Health Promotion, Centers for Disease Control and Prevention, Atlanta, Georgia.

Lenore Buckley, M.D., M.P.H., Professor, Division of Rheumatology, Medical College of Virginia, Richmond, Virginia.

Mona S. Calvo, Ph.D., Expert Regulatory Review Scientist, Office of Applied Research and Safety Assessment, Center for Food Safety and Applied Nutrition, Food and Drug Administration, Laurel, Maryland.

Thomas G. Carskadon, Ph.D., Professor of Psychology, Mississippi State University, Mississippi State, Mississippi.

Mary Concannon, M.A., Osteoporosis Prevention Coordinator, Maryland Department of Health and Mental Hygiene, Baltimore, Maryland.

Cyrus Cooper, M.A., D.M., F.R.C.P., Professor, MRC Environmental Epidemiology Unit, Southampton General Hospital, Shirley, Southampton, United Kingdom.

Judith A. Cranford, Executive Director, National Osteoporosis Foundation, Washington, D.C.

Ann Cranney, M.D., M.Sc., Assistant Professor, Division of Rheumatology, Queen's University, Kingston, Ontario, Canada.

William H. Dietz, M.D., Ph.D., Director, Division of Nutrition and Physical Activity, Division of Nutrition and Physical Activity, Centers for Disease Control and Prevention, U.S. Department of Health and Human Services, Atlanta, Georgia.

Marc K. Drezner, M.D., Professor of Medicine, Endocrinology Section, University of Wisconsin, Madison, Wisconsin.

Michael Econs, M.D., Professor of Medicine, School of Medicine, Indiana University Medical Center, Indianapolis, Indiana.

Kristine Ensrud, M.D., M.P.H., Associate Professor, Division of Epidemiology, University of Minnesota, School of Public Health, Minneapolis, Minnesota.

Martin Erlichman, M.S., Senior Health Science Analyst, Center for Practice and Technology Assessment, Agency for Healthcare Research and Quality, U.S. Department of Health and Human Services, Rockville, Maryland.

Bruce Ettinger, M.D., Senior Investigator, Research Division, Kaiser Permanente, San Francisco, California.

Caswell A. Evans, D.M.D., National Institute of Dental and Craniofacial Research, Bethesda, Maryland.

Murray J. Favus, M.D., University of Chicago, Chicago, Illinois.

Nancy Libby Fisher, Coordinator, Disease Prevention and Control, Office of Women's Health, Rhode Island Department of Health, Providence, Rhode Island.

Judith E. Fradkin, M.D., Director, Division of Diabetes Endocrinology and Metabolism, National Institute of Diabetes and Digestive and Kidney Diseases, Bethesda, Maryland.

Harry K. Genant, M.D., Professor Emeritus of Radiology, Orthopaedic Surgery, Medicine, and Epidemiology, University of California San Francisco, San Francisco, California.

Lou Glasse, M.S.W., President Emeritus, Older Women's League, Poughkeepsie, New York.

Joan Goldberg, Executive Director, American Society for Bone and Mineral Research, Washington, D.C.

Frank R. Greer, M.D., Professor, Pediatrics/ Nutritional Sciences, American Academy of Pediatrics, Meriter Hospital, Perinatal Center, Madison, Wisconsin.

Jack Guralnik, M.D., Ph.D., Chief, Epidemiology and Demography Office, National Institute on Aging, National Institutes of Health, Gateway Boulevard, Bethesda, Maryland.

Ralph Hale, M.D., Executive Vice President, American College of Obstetricians and Gynecologists, Washington, D.C.

R. Scott Hanson, M.D., M.P.H., Past President, Rhode Island Public Health Association, Narragansett, Rhode Island.

Olof Johnell, M.D., Professor, Department of Orthopaedics, University General Hospital, Malmo, Sweden.

Clifford Johnson, M.S.P.H., Director, National Health and Nutrition Examination Survey, National Center for Health Statistics, Centers for Disease Control and Prevention, Hyattsville, Maryland.

C. Conrad Johnston, Jr., M.D., Distinguished Professor, School of Medicine, Indiana University, Indianapolis, Indiana.

John Kanis, M.D., Professor, Centre for Metabolic Bone Diseases, University of Sheffield Medical School, Sheffield, S. Yorkshire, United Kingdom.

Theresa Kehoe, M.D., Medical Officer, Food and Drug Administration, Parklawn Building, Rockville, Maryland.

Jennifer Kelsey, Ph.D., Professor, University of Massachusetts Medical School, Clinton, Connecticut.

Jane E. Kerstetter, Ph.D., R.D., Associate Professor, School of Allied Health, University of Connecticut, Stafford Springs, Connecticut.

Patricia A. Kipperman, Omaha, Nebraska.

John H. Klippel, M.D., Medical Director, Arthritis Foundation, Atlanta, Georgia.

Joan M. Lappe, Ph.D., R.N., Associate Professor, Creighton Osteoporosis Research Center, Creighton University, Omaha, Nebraska.

Angelo Licata, M.D., Ph.D., Director of Research, Center for Osteoporosis and Metabolic Bone Disease, Cleveland Clinic Foundation, Cleveland, Ohio.

Robert Lindsay, M.D., Ph.D., Chief of Internal Medicine, Regional Bone Center, Helen Hayes Hospital, West Haverstraw, New York.

Jean L. Lloyd, M.S., R.D., Nutritionist, Office of Community Based Services, U.S. Administration on Aging, U.S. Department of Health and Human Services, Washington, D.C.

Jay Magaziner, Ph.D., M.S., Professor and Director, Division of Gerontology, Epidemiology and Preventive Medicine, University of Maryland, Baltimore, Maryland.

Deborah R. Maiese, Director, Maternal and Child Health Bureau, Office of Women's Health, Health Resources and Services Administration, Rockville, Maryland.

Robert Marcus, M.D., Professor Emeritus, Stanford University, Stanford, California. Medical Advisor, USMD Endocrinology, Eli Lilly, Indianapolis, Indiana.

Ronald Margolis, Ph.D., Senior Advisor for Molecular Endocrinology, Division of Diabetes, Endocrinology and Metabolism, National Institute of Diabetes and Digestive and Kidney Diseases, Bethesda, Maryland.

Joan C. Marini, M.D., Ph.D., Chief, Heritable Disorders Branch, National Institute of Child Health and Human Development, Bethesda, Maryland.

Betsy McClung, R.N., Associate Director, Oregon Osteoporosis Center, Portland, Oregon.

Michael McClung, M.D., F.A.C.E., Director, Oregon Osteoporosis Center, Portland, Oregon.

Daniel McDonald, M.D., Scientific Review Administrator, Center for Scientific Review, National Institutes of Health, Bethesda, Maryland.

Barbara Miller, Ph.D., Category Manager, Professional and Scientific Relations, Procter and Gamble Pharmaceuticals, Mason, Ohio.

Gregory Miller, Ph.D., M.A.C.N., Senior Vice President of Nutrition and Scientific Affairs, National Dairy Council, Rosemont, Illinois.

Ron Nelson, P.A.-C., President/CEO, Health Services Associates, Inc., Fremont, Michigan.

Eric S. Orwoll, M.D., Professor of Medicine, Program Director, General Clinical Research Center, Associate Dean for Clinical Research, Assistant Vice President for Research, Oregon Health and Science University, Portland, Oregon.

Susan Ott, M.D., Associate Professor, Department of Medicine, University of Washington Medical Center, Seattle, Washington.

Susana Perry, M.S., Health Programs Coordinator, Office of Women's Health, Food and Drug Administration, Rockville, Maryland.

Steven Petak, M.D., J.D., F.A.C.E., representing American Association of Clinical Endocrinologists, Houston, Texas.

Sandra C. Raymond, Executive Director, Lupus Foundation of America, Inc., Washington, D.C.

Robert R. Recker, M.D., Director, Osteoporosis Research Center, Creighton University, Omaha, Nebraska.

Trish Reynolds, R.N., M.S., Education Manager/Assistant Project Director, National Institutes of Health Osteoporosis and Related Bone Diseases ~ National Resource Center, Washington, D.C.

Elena Rios, M.D., President, National Hispanic Medical Association, Washington, D.C.

Helena W. Rodbard, M.D., Past President, American Association of Clinical Endocrinologists, Rockville, Maryland.

William Sacks, M.D., Ph.D., Medical Officer, Center for Devices and Radiological Health, Office of Device Evaluation, Food and Drug Administration, Rockville, Maryland.

Paul Scherr, Ph.D., D.Sc., Epidemiologist, Division of Adult and Community Health, Emerging Investigations and Analytic Methods Branch, National Center for Chronic Disease Prevention and Health Promotion, Centers for Disease Control and Prevention, Atlanta, Georgia.

Mary Jean Schumann, Director, Practice and Policy, American Nurses Association, Washington, D.C.

Heller An Shapiro, Executive Director, Osteogenesis Imperfecta Foundation, Gaithersburg, Maryland.

Harriet R. Shapiro, R.N., M.A., Director, Patient and Professional Education, National Osteoporosis Foundation, Washington, D.C.

Frederick R. Singer, M.D., Chairman, Paget Foundation Board of Directors, John Wayne Cancer Institute, Santa Monica, California.

Christine Snow, Ph.D., F.A.C.S.M., Director, Bone Research Laboratory, Professor, Exercise and Sport Science, College of Health and Human Sciences, Oregon State University, Corvallis, Oregon.

Christine Spain, M.A., Director, Research, Planning, and Special Projects, President's Council on Physical Fitness and Sports, Washington, D.C.

Barry Stein, M.D., Surgeon-in-Chief, Urology, Rhode Island Hospital, Providence, Rhode Island.

Susan S. Swift, D.P.A., President, Susan S. Swift, Ltd., New York, New York.

J. Scott Toder, M.D., Physician, Johnston, Rhode Island.

Mehrdad Tondravi, Ph.D., Program Director, Division of Diabetes, Endocrinology and Metabolic Diseases, National Institute of Diabetes and Digestive and Kidney Diseases, Bethesda, Maryland.

Charlene Waldman, Executive Director, The Paget Foundation, New York, New York.

Michael F. White, Principal, Michael F. White and Associates, Women's Health Council, Association of State and Territorial Directors of Chronic Disease Programs, Alexandria, Virginia.

Paul J. Wiesner, M.D., District Health Director, Dekalb County Board of Health, Decatur, Georgia.

T. Franklin Williams, M.D., Professor of Medicine Emeritus, General Medicine and Geriatrics Unit, University of Rochester School of Medicine and Dentistry, Rochester, New York.

Karen Winer, M.D., Fellow, Center for Research for Mothers and Children, Endocrinology, Nutrition, and Growth Branch, National Institute of Child Health and Human Development, Bethesda, Maryland.

Betty H. Wiser, Ed.D., M.S., Director of Older Adult Health Branch, Division of Public Health, North Carolina Department of Health and Human Services, Raleigh, North Carolina.

Susan Wood, Director, Office of Women's Health, Food and Drug Administration, Rockville, Maryland.

Adeline M. Yerkes, R.N., M.P.H., Chief, Chronic Disease, Oklahoma State Department of Health, Oklahoma City, Oklahoma.

Surgeon General Workshop participants were

Amy Allina, Program and Policy Director, National Women's Health Network, Washington, D.C.

Nell Armstrong, Ph.D., R.N., Program Director, Division of Extramural Activities, National Institute of Nursing Research, National Institutes of Health, Bethesda, Maryland.

David Atkins, M.D., M.P.H., Senior Health Policy Analyst, Center for Practice and Technology Assessment, Agency for Healthcare Research and Quality, U.S. Department of Health and Human Services, Rockville, Maryland.

Roberta Biegel, Director of Government Relations, Society for Women's Health Research, Washington, D.C.

Dennis Black, Ph.D., Professor, Department of Epidemiology and Biostatistics, University of California San Francisco, San Francisco, California.

Henry G. Bone, III, M.D., Director, Michigan Bone and Mineral Clinic, Detroit, Michigan.

Joyce M. Briscoe, Cavarocchi Ruscio Dennis Associates, LLC, Washington, D.C.

David Buchner, M.D., M.P.H., Chief, Physical Activity and Health Branch, Division of Nutrition and Physical Activity, Centers for Disease Control and Prevention, Department of Health and Human Services, Atlanta, Georgia.

Mona S. Calvo, Ph.D., Expert Regulatory Review Scientist, Office of Applied Research and Safety Assessment, Center for Food Safety and Applied Nutrition, Food and Drug Administration, Laurel, Maryland.

Thomas G. Carskadon, Ph.D., Professor of Psychology, Mississippi State University, Mississippi State, Mississippi.

Jane Cauley, Dr.P.H., Associate Professor, Department of Epidemiology, University of Pittsburgh, Pittsburgh, Pennsylvania.

Nicholas G. Cavarocchi, Cavorocchi Ruscio Dennis Associates, LLC, Washington, D.C.

David A. Chambers, Ph.D., M.Sc., Program Officer, Dissemination and Implementation Research Program, Services Research and Clinical Epidemiology Branch, National Institute of Mental Health, National Institutes of Health, Bethesda, Maryland.

Katherine Moy Chin, R.D., L.D., Commissioner, State of Maryland Governor's Commission on Asian Pacific American Affairs, Baltimore, Maryland.

Wojtek Chodzko-Zajko, Ph.D., Professor and Department Chair, Department of Kinesiology, University of Illinois, Urbana, Illinois.

Kathleen Cody, Executive Director, Foundation for Osteoporosis Research, and Education, Oakland, California.

Rosaly Correa-de-Araujo, M.D., Health Scientist Administrator, Agency for Healthcare Research and Quality, Rockville, Maryland.

Judith Cranford, Executive Director, National Osteoporosis Foundation, Washington, D.C.

Denise Cyzman, Senior Project Coordinator, Health Promotion and Disease Prevention, Osteoporosis and Other Chronic Conditions, Michigan Public Health Institute, Okemos, Michigan.

Susan Davidson, M.S., R.D., Consultant, Germantown, Maryland.

Bess Dawson-Hughes, M.D., Professor of Medicine, Metabolism Lab, Tufts University, U.S. Department of Agriculture, Human Research Center on Aging, Boston, Massachusetts.

Susan Dentzer, Health Correspondent, NewsHour with Jim Lehrer, Arlington, Virginia.

Barbara DeVinney, Ph.D., AAAS Science Policy Fellow, Office of Behavioral and Social Sciences Research, Office of the Director, National Institutes of Health, Bethesda, Maryland.

Ann L. Elderkin, P.A., Managing Editor and Project Director, Surgeon General's Report, Health Systems Research, Inc., Washington, D.C.

Martin Erlichman, M.S., Senior Health Science Analyst, Center for Practice and Technology Assessment, Agency for Healthcare Research and Quality, U.S. Department of Health and Human Services, Rockville, Maryland.

Christine M. Everett, M.P.H., Special Assistant to the Acting Director, Food and Drug Administration, Rockville, Maryland.

Suzanne Feetham, Ph.D., R.N., F.A.A.N., Senior Advisor, Office of Director, Bureau of Primary Health Care, Health Resources and Services Administration, Bethesda, Maryland.

Lawrence Fields, M.D., Senior Executive Advisor to the Assistant Secretary for Health, Department of Health and Human Services, Washington, D.C.

Michael Fleischman, Intern, President's Council on Physical Fitness and Sports, Washington, D.C.

Susan M. Friedman, Deputy Director, Government Relations, American Osteopathic Association, Washington, D.C.

Deborah A. Galuska, Ph.D., M.P.H., Epidemiologist, Division of Nutrition and Physical Activity, Centers for Disease Control and Prevention, U.S. Department of Health and Human Services, Atlanta, Georgia.

Jean Gearing, Ph.D., M.P.H., Acting Osteoporosis Program Manager, Chronic Disease Prevention and Health Promotion Branch, Georgia Division of Public Health, Atlanta, Georgia.

Deborah T. Gold, Ph.D., Associate Professor, Departments of Psychiatry and Behavioral Sciences, Sociology, and Psychology: Social and Health Sciences, Duke University Medical Center, Durham, North Carolina.

Joan Goldberg, Executive Director, American Society for Bone and Mineral Research, Washington, D.C.

Jean Gonzalez, Lovettsville, Viginia.

Julie Gonzalez, Lovettsville, Viginia.

Christine W. Gould, Director of Health, YWCA of the USA, Washington, D.C.

Amy Greene, Director, Prevention Policy, Adolescent Health, Association of State and Territorial, Health Officials, Washington, D.C.

Susan L. Greenspan, M.D., Professor of Medicine, University of Pittsburgh, Kaufmann Medical Building, Pittsburgh, Pennsylvania.

Betty Lee Hawks, Special Assistant to the Director, Office of Minority Health, Office of Public Health and Science, U.S. Department of Health and Human Services, Rockwall II, Rockville, Maryland.

Leanne Jerome, Writer, Office of the Surgeon General, Department of Health and Human Services, Rockville, Maryland.

Sara Johnson, Ph.D., Director, Health Behavior Change Programs, Pro-Change Behavior Systems, Inc., West Kingston, Rhode Island.

Linda Johnson, Brentwood, Maryland.

Wanda K. Jones, Dr.P.H., Deputy Assistant Secretary and Director of the Office of Women's Health, Office of the Secretary, Office of Public Health and Science, Department of Health and Human Services, Washington, D.C.

Jason Jurkowski, Fellow, Office of the Surgeon General, Department of Health and Human Services, Rockville, Maryland.

Stephen I. Katz, M.D., Ph.D., Director, National Institute of Arthritis and Musculoskeletal and Skin Diseases, National Institutes of Health, Bethesda, Maryland.

Douglas P. Kiel, M.D., M.P.H., Director of Medical Research, Research and Training Institute, Hebrew Rehabilitation Center for the Aged, Boston, Massachusetts.

Raynard S. Kington, M.D., Ph.D., Associate Director, Office of the Director, Office of Behavioral and Social Sciences Research, National Institutes of Health, Department of Health and Human Services, Bethesda, Maryland.

Richard L. Kravitz, M.D., M.S.P.H., Professor of Medicine, Center for Health Services Research in Primary Care, University of California, Davis Medical Center, Sacramento, California.

Peggy Lassanske, President, Elder Floridians Foundation, Tallahassee, Florida.

Marie-Michele Leger, M.P.H., P.A.-C., Director, Professional Education, American Academy of Physician Assistants, Alexandria, Viginia.

Jewel F. Lewis, Retired Chief Judge and Chair, Board of Contract Appeals, Department of Agriculture, Associate General Counsel and General Counsel of Service Corps of Retired Executives, Washington, D.C.

Karen Lim, Acting Executive Director, National Asian Women's Health Organization, San Francisco, California.

Anita M. Linde, Senior Program Analyst, Office of the Director, National Institute of Arthritis and Musculoskeletal and Skin Diseases, Bethesda, Maryland.

Jean Lloyd, M.S., R.D., National Nutritionist, Office of Community Based Services, U.S. Administration on Aging, U.S. Department of Health and Human Services, Washington, D.C.

Anne Looker, Ph.D., Senior Research Epidemiologist, Health Examination Statistics, National Center for Health Statistics, Centers for Disease Control and Prevention, Hyattsville, Maryland.

Robert Lorigan, Orient, Maine.

Annie Lorigan, Orient, Maine.

Kathryn R. Mahaffey, Ph.D., Director, Office of Science Coordination and Policy, Division of Exposure Assessment, Environmental Protection Agency, Washington, D.C.

Edward W. Maibach, M.P.H., Ph.D., Worldwide Director of Social Marketing, Porter Novelli, Washington, D.C.

Deborah Maiese, former Director, Maternal and Child Health Bureau, Office of Women's Health, Health Resources and Services Administration, Rockville, Maryland.

Jean Mandeville, Hopkins, Minnesota.

Ronald Margolis, Ph.D., Senior Advisor for Molecular Endocrinology, Division of Diabetes, Endocrinology and Metabolism, National Institute of Diabetes and Digestive and Kidney Diseases, Bethesda, Maryland.

Joan C. Marini, M.D., Ph.D., Chief, Heritable Disorders Branch, National Institute of Child Health and Human Development, Bethesda, Maryland.

Saralyn Mark, M.D., Senior Medical Advisor, Office on Women's Health, Office of Public Health and Science, National Aeronautics and Space Administration, Department and Health and Human Services, Washington, D.C.

Jeff Martin, Office of the Surgeon General, Department of Health and Human Services, Rockville, Maryland.

Joan A. McGowan, Ph.D., Senior Scientific Editor, Surgeon General's Report, Director, Musculoskeletal Diseases Branch, Extramural Program, National Institute of Arthritis and Musculoskeletal and Skin Diseases, National Institutes of Health, Bethesda, Maryland.

John McGrath, Ph.D., Chief, Public Information and Communications Branch, National Institute of Child Health and Human Development, National Institutes of Health, Bethesda, Maryland.

Taya McMillan, Intern, Office on Women's Health, Office of Public Health and Science, Department of Health and Human Services, Washington, D.C.

L. Joseph Melton, III, M.D., Eisenberg Professor, Department of Health Sciences Research, Mayo Clinic and Foundation, Rochester, Minnesota.

Kenneth P. Moritsugu, M.D., M.P.H., Deputy Surgeon General of the United States, Office of the Surgeon General, Department of Health and Human Services, Rockville, Maryland.

Miriam Nelson, Ph.D., Director, Friedman School of Nutrition Science and Policy, Center for Physical Activity and Nutrition, Tufts University, Boston, Massachusetts.

Debra Nichols, M.D., Public Health Advisor, Office of Disease Prevention and Health Promotion, Office of Public Health and Science, Department of Health and Human Resources, Washington, D.C.

Allan S. Noonan, M.D., M.P.H., CAPT, U.S. Public Health Service, Scientific Editor, Surgeon General's Report, Office of the Surgeon General, Office of the Secretary, Washington, D.C.

Eric S. Orwoll, M.D., Professor of Medicine, Program Director, General Clinical Research Center, Associate Dean for Clinical Research, Assistant Vice President for Research, Oregon Health and Science University, Portland, Oregon.

Lucille Norville Perez, M.D., Past President, National Medical Association, Bethesda, Maryland.

Diana Pethtel, Washington, D.C.

Robert A. Phillips, Ph.D., Chief, Radiological Devices Branch, Center for Devices and Radiological Health, Office of Device Evaluation, Food and Drug Administration, Rockville, Maryland.

Vivian W. Pinn, M.D., Associate Director for Research on Women's Health, Office of the Director, National Institutes of Health, Bethesda, Maryland.

Geraldine B. Pollen, M.A., Research Activities Coordinator, National Institute of Arthritis and Musculoskeletal and Skin Diseases, Extramural Program, National Institutes of Health, One Democracy Plaza, Bethesda, Maryland.

Lawrence G. Raisz, M.D., Scientific Editor, Board of Trustees Distinguished Professor of Medicine, Interim Director, Musculoskeletal Institute, Division of Endocrinology and Metabolism, University of Connecticut Health Center, Farmington, Connecticut.

Claudia Reid Ravin, C.N.M., M.S.N., Associate Director, Women's Health Programs, Association of Women's Health, Obstetric, and Neonatal Nurses, Washington, D.C.

B. Lawrence Riggs, M.D., Distinguished Investigator, Mayo Foundation, Purvis and Roberta Tabor Professor of Medical Research, Mayo Medical School, Division of Endocrinology, Mayo Clinic and Foundation, Rochester, Minnesota.

Edward J. Roccella, Ph.D., M.P.H., Coordinator, National High Blood Pressure Education Program, Office of Prevention, Education and Control, National Heart, Lung and Blood Institute, National Institutes of Health, Bethesda, Maryland.
Clifford Rosen, M.D., Chief of Medicine, Maine Center for Osteoporosis Research, St. Joseph Hospital, Bangor, Maine.

Bruce S. Schneider, M.D., Medical Officer, Division of Metabolic and Endocrine Drug Products, Center for Drug Evaluation and Research, Food and Drug Administration, Rockville, Maryland.

Jean Scott, Dr.P.H., R.N., Senior Epidemiologist, Quality Measurement & Health

Assessment Group, Centers for Medicare and Medicaid Services, Department of Health and Human Services, Baltimore, Maryland.

Jay R. Shapiro, M.D., Director, Osteogenesis Imperfecta Clinic, Kennedy Krieger Institute, Baltimore, Maryland.

Heller An Shapiro, Executive Director, Osteogenesis Imperfecta Foundation, Gaithersburg, Maryland.

Sherry Sherman, Ph.D., Director, Clinical Endocrinology and Osteoporosis Research, National Institute on Aging, National Institutes of Health, Bethesda, Maryland.

Kathy Shipp, P.T., Ph.D., Assistant Research Professor, Physical Therapy, Community and Family Medicine, Duke University Medical Center, Durham, North Carolina.

Ethel S. Siris, M.D., Madeline C. Stabile Professor of Clinical Medicine, Endocrinology Division, Columbia University and Columbia Presbyterian Medical Center, New York, New York.

Eve Slater, M.D., Assistant Secretary for Health, Department of Health and Human Services, Washington, D.C.

Christine Snow, Ph.D., F.A.C.S.M., Director, Bone Research Laboratory, Professor, Exercise and Sport Science, College of Health and Human Sciences, Oregon State University, Corvallis, Oregon.

Christine Spain, M.A., Director, Research, Planning, and Special Projects, President's Council on Physical Fitness and Sports, Washington, D.C.

Larry Stepnick, M.B.A., Consultant, The Severyn Group, Inc., Ashburn, Virginia.

Jeannie Suarez-Reyes, M.P.H., Project Director, Center for Consumers, National Alliance for Hispanic Health, Washington, D.C.

William W. Tipton, Jr., M.D., Executive Vice President, American Academy of Orthopaedic Surgeons, Rosemount, Illinois.

Mehrdad Tondravi, M.D., Program Director, Division of Diabetes, Endocrinology and Metabolic Diseases, National Institute of Diabetes and Digestive and Kidney Diseases, Bethesda, Maryland.

Laura Tosi, M.D., Division Chief, Orthopaedic Surgery and Sports Medicine, Children's National Medical Center, Washington, D.C.

Anna N. Tosteson, Sc.D., Professor, Departments of Medicine and Community and Family Medicine, Dartmouth Medical School, Lebanon, New Hampshire.

Wulf H. Utian, M.D., Ph.D., Executive Director, North American Menopause Society, Mayfield Heights, Ohio.

Charlene Waldman, Executive Director, The Paget Foundation, New York, New York.

Nelson Watts, M.D., Director, Bone Health and Osteoporosis Center, University of Cincinnati, Cincinnati, Ohio.

Connie M. Weaver, Ph.D., Distinguished Professor, Department Head, Foods and Nutrition, Purdue University, West Lafayette, Indiana.

Michael F. White, Consultant, Michael F. White and Associates, Women's Health Council, Association of State and Territorial Directors of Chronic Disease Programs, Alexandria, Virginia.

Susan Whittier, M.H.A., Director, National Institutes for Health Osteoporosis and Related Bone Diseases ~ National Resource Center, Washington, D.C.

Michael P. Whyte, M.D., Professor of Medicine, Pediatrics, and Genetics, Bone and Mineral Diseases, Department of Medicine, Barnes-Jewish Hospital at Washington University School of Medicine, St. Louis, Missouri.

Lynne Wilcox, M.D., M.P.H., CAPT, U.S. Public Health Service, Editor-in-Chief, Preventing Chronic Disease, National Center for Chronic Disease Prevention and Health Promotion, Centers for Disease Control and Prevention, Atlanta, Georgia.

Betty H. Wiser, Ed.D., Director of Older Adult Health Branch, Division of Public Health, North Carolina Department of Health and Human Services, Raleigh, North Carolina.

Susan Wood, Director, Office of Women's Health, Food and Drug Administration, Rockville, Maryland.

Surgeon General's Interagency Work Group on Osteoporosis and Bone Health

Nell Armstrong, Ph.D., R.N., Program Director, Division of Extramural Activities, National Institute of Nursing Research, National Institutes of Health, Bethesda, Maryland.

William H. Dietz, M.D., Ph.D., Director, Division of Nutrition and Physical Activity, Division of Nutrition and Physical Activity, Centers for Disease Control and Prevention, U.S. Department of Health and Human Services, Atlanta, Georgia.

Sherri A. Clark, Aging Services Program Specialist, Administration on Aging, Washington, D.C.

Agnes Donahue, Advisor to Director, Office of Intergovernmental Affairs, Department of Health & Human Services, Washington, D.C.

Ann L. Elderkin, P.A., Managing Editor and Project Director, Surgeon General's Report, Health Systems Research, Inc., Washington, D.C.

Martin N. Erlichman, M.S., Senior Health Science Analyst, Vice-Chair International Network of Agencies for Health Technology Assessment, Center for Practice and Technology Assessment, Agency for Healthcare Research and Quality, Rockville, Maryland.

MAJ Rachel Evans, Ph.D., R.P.T, Director, Bone Health Research Program, U.S. Army Research Institute of Environmental Medicine, Military Performance Division, Natick, Massachusetts.

Christine M. Everett, M.P.H., Special Assistant to the Acting Director, Food and Drug Administration, Rockville, Maryland.

Deborah A. Galuska, Ph.D., M.P.H, Epidemiologist, Division of Nutrition and

Physical Activity Centers for Disease Control and Prevention, Atlanta, Georgia.

Melissa Johnson, M.S., Executive Director, President's Council on Physical Fitness and Sports, Washington, D.C.

Annette Kirshner, PhD, Health Science Administrator, National Institute of Environmental Health Sciences, Division of Extramural Research and Training, Research Triangle Park, North Carolina.

Anita Linde, Senior Program Analyst, Office of the Director, National Institute of Arthritis and Musculoskeletal and Skin Diseases, Bethesda, Maryland.

Jean Lloyd, M.S., R.D., Nutritionist, Center for Community Based Services, U.S. Administration on Aging, Washington, D.C.

Anne Looker, Ph.D., Senior Research Epidemiologist, National Center for Health Statistics, Centers for Disease Control and Prevention, Hyattsville Maryland.

Sabrina Matoff, Acting Director, Office of Women's Health, Maternal and Child Health Bureau, Health Resources and Services Administration, Rockville, Maryland.

Ronald Margolis, Ph.D., Senior Advisor for Molecular Endocrinology, Division of Diabetes, Endocrinology, and Metabolism, National Institute of Diabetes and Digestive and Kidney Diseases, Bethesda, Maryland.

Saralyn Mark, M.D., Senior Medical Advisor, NASA & Office of Women's Health, Department of Health & Human Services, Washington, D.C.

Joan A. McGowan, Ph.D., Senior Scientific Editor, Surgeon General's Report, Director, Musculoskeletal Diseases Branch, Extramural Program, National Institute of Arthritis and Musculoskeletal and Skin Diseases, National Institutes of Health, Bethesda, Maryland.

Debra Nichols, M.D., Office of Disease Prevention and Health Promotion, Department of Health and Human Services, Washington, D.C.

Allan S. Noonan, M.D., M.P.H., CAPT, U.S. Public Health Service, Scientific Editor, Surgeon General's Report, Office of the Surgeon General, Office of the Secretary, Washington, D.C.

Susana Perry, M.S., Health Programs Coordinator, Office of Women's Health, Food and Drug Administration, Rockville, Maryland.

Jean Scott, Dr.P.H., R.N., Senior Epidemiologist, Quality Measurement & Health Assessment Group, Centers for Medicare and Medicaid Services, Department of Health and Human Services, Baltimore, Maryland.

Sherry Sherman, Ph.D., Director, Clinical Endocrinology and Osteoporosis Research, National Institute on Aging, National Institutes of Health, Bethesda, Maryland.

Christine Spain, M.A., Director, Research, Planning, and Special Projects, President's Council on Physical Fitness and Sports, Washington, D.C.

Maxine E. Turnipseed, M.B.A., Insurance Analyst, Partnership Development, Centers for Medicare and Medicaid Services, Baltimore, Maryland.

Valerie A. Welsh, Senior Health Policy Analyst and Evaluation Officer, Office of Minority Health, OS/DHHS, Rockville, Maryland.

Judith Wilson, M.P.H., R.D., Director, Nutrition Services, U.S. Department of Agriculture, Washington, D.C.

Susan Wood, Director, Office of Women's Health, Food and Drug Administration, Rockville, Maryland.

Elizabeth Yetley, Ph.D., Lead Scientist for Nutrition, Food and Drug Administration, College Park, Maryland.

Bone Health and Osteoporosis
A Surgeon General's Report

Part One

WHAT IS BONE HEALTH?

This introductory part of the report explores the answer to this question, defining bone health as a public health issue with an emphasis on prevention and early intervention to promote strong bones and prevent fractures and their consequences. The first chapter describes this public health approach along with the rationale for the report and the charge from Congress and from the Surgeon General.

Chapter 2 provides a brief overview of the fundamentals of bone biology, helping the reader to understand why humans have bones, how bones work, how bones change during life, what keeps bones healthy, what causes bone disease, and what is in store in the future. It begins to outline the role of genetic and environmental factors such as nutrition and physical activity in keeping bones healthy, an issue that is addressed in more detail later in the report.

Chapter 3 offers a summary review of the more common diseases, disorders, and conditions that both directly and indirectly affect bone. While much of Chapter 3 focuses on osteoporosis (including other diseases and medications that can cause it), it also covers other related bone diseases, including rickets and osteomalacia, renal osteodystrophy, Paget's disease of bone, developmental skeletal disorders, and acquired skeletal disorders.

Both Chapters 2 and 3 should be considered as important scientific background for the remainder of the report.

Chapter 1: Key Messages

- Bone health is critically important to the overall health and quality of life of Americans. Healthy bones provide the body with a frame that allows for mobility and for protection against injury. Bones serve as a storehouse for minerals that are vital to the functioning of many other life-sustaining systems in the body. Unhealthy bones, however, perform poorly in executing these functions and can lead to debilitating fractures.

- The bone health status of Americans appears to be in jeopardy, and left unchecked it is only going to get worse as the population ages. Each year an estimated 1.5 million individuals suffer an osteoporotic-related fracture.

- Great improvements in the bone health status of Americans can be made "simply" by applying in a timely manner that which is already known about prevention, assessment, detection, diagnosis, and treatment.

- There is a large gap between what has been learned and what is applied by American consumers and health care providers. The biggest problem is a lack of awareness of bone disease among both the public and health care professionals.

- An area of particular concern relates to serving ethnic and racial minorities and other underserved populations, including the uninsured, underinsured, and those living in rural areas. Closing this gap will not be possible without specific strategies and programs geared toward bringing improvements in bone health to all currently underserved populations.

- The area of bone health is ideally suited to a public health approach to health promotion. This Surgeon General's report is calling for Federal, State, and local governments (including State and local public health departments) to join forces with the private sector and community organizations in a coordinated, collaborative effort to promote bone health. This type of approach can serve as the primary vehicle for improving the bone health status of Americans. Some of the work has already begun, but much more work remains.

Chapter 1

A PUBLIC HEALTH APPROACH TO PROMOTE BONE HEALTH

This first report of the Surgeon General on bone health and osteoporosis, which was requested by Congress, comes at a critical time. Tremendous progress has been made in bone health in the last several decades, particularly in the past 15 years. Research has accelerated markedly, enabling the medical community to develop a much more detailed understanding of the factors that promote bone health and cause bone disease and fractures. This enhanced level of knowledge has led to significant advances in the ability to prevent, assess risk factors for, diagnose, and treat bone disease.

Physical activity and calcium and vitamin D intake are now known to be major contributors to bone health for individuals of all ages. Even though bone disease often strikes late in life, the importance of beginning prevention at a very young age and continuing it throughout life is now well understood. Advances in knowledge about risk factors have allowed work to begin on tools that assess the potential for bone disease in an individual. These risk-factor assessment tools help to identify high-risk individuals in need of further evaluation. With respect to diagnosis, the development of noninvasive tools to measure bone density and bone mass has been one of the most significant advances in the last quarter century. As a result, it is now possible to

detect bone disease early and to identify those at highest risk of fracture. Therapeutic advances in bone disease have equaled if not surpassed advances in the areas of prevention and diagnosis. Within the last 10–15 years, new classes of drugs have been developed that, for the first time, have been shown in large-scale trials to significantly reduce the risk of fractures in individuals with bone disease. Large-scale trials have also confirmed the value of vitamin D and calcium supplementation in reducing bone loss and the risk of fractures in some populations.

Research has also led to a much better understanding of the role of secondary factors in the development of bone disease, including use of certain medications and the presence of certain diseases. For example, glucocorticoids are now known to be a significant contributor to osteoporosis. As a result, interventions are available that help minimize the risk of bone disease in those who need these drugs. Similarly, much more is now understood about a leading cause of fractures in the elderly—falls in those who have weakened bones. Enhanced knowledge about why people fall has led to interventions that target the risk factors for falls, such as avoiding or minimizing use of medications that cause dizziness, making environmental modifications in the home, and training to improve strength and balance.

In short, the last several decades represent an era of great excitement and progress in the field of bone health. Thirty years ago, relatively little was known or could be done about osteoporosis; both the disease and the fractures that go along with it were thought of as an inevitable part of old age. Today, however, advances in scientific knowledge have ushered in a new era in bone health, one in which bone diseases can be prevented in the vast majority of individuals and identified early and treated effectively in those who do get them.

However, the tremendous potential offered by this new era of bone health has yet to become a reality. Bone diseases, including osteoporosis, Paget's disease of the bone, osteogenesis imperfecta, rickets, osteomalacia, renal osteodystrophy, and hyperparathyroidism, remain a major public health problem in this country. They affect more than 10 million individuals today, a figure that will rise significantly in the decades ahead unless action is taken now. They cause approximately 1.5 million fractures each year, fractures that impose tremendous physical and emotional costs on those who suffer them and their family members. They represent a significant financial burden to both individuals and society at large. Many of these costs are avoidable, since much is already known about how to effectively prevent, diagnose, and treat bone disease throughout the life span. However, much of what could be done to reduce this burden is not being done today, largely due to a lack of awareness of the problem and the failure to apply current knowledge. In fact, many in the public and even the medical community believe that osteoporosis is a natural consequence of aging and that nothing can be done about it. This view must be changed. The intent of this first-ever report of the Surgeon General on bone health and osteoporosis is to serve as a catalyst for the development of a public health approach to promoting bone health. The central focus of this effort is to alert individuals and the medical community to the meaning and importance of bone health, including its impact on overall health and well-being, and of the need to take action to ensure the timely prevention, assessment, diagnosis, and treatment of bone disease and fractures throughout life.

This report comes at a very critical time. Like many nations, the United States faces the prospect of an aging population and with it the expectation that the burden of chronic diseases, including osteoporosis, will increase. In fact, without concerted action to address this issue, it is estimated that in 2020 one in two Americans over age of 50 will have, or be at high risk of developing, osteoporosis. If these predictions come true, they will have a devastating impact on the well-being of Americans as they age. In fact, a major theme of this report is that **bone health is critically important to the overall health and quality of life of Americans.** Healthy bones provide the body with a frame that allows for mobility and for protection against injury. Bones also serve as a storehouse for minerals that are vital to the functioning of many other life-sustaining systems in the body. Unhealthy bones, however, perform poorly in executing these functions. They also lead to fractures, which are by far the most important consequence of poor bone health since they can result in disability, diminished function, loss of independence, and premature death.

In recognition of the importance of promoting bone health and preventing fractures, the President has declared 2002–2011 as the *Decade of the Bone and Joint*. With this designation, the United States has joined with other nations throughout the world in committing resources to accelerate progress in a variety of areas related to the musculoskeletal system, including bone disease and arthritis. As a part of its *Healthy People 2010* initiative, the U.S. Department of Health and Human Services (HHS) has developed two overarching goals that are highly relevant to bone health and osteoporosis. The first goal is increased quality and years of healthy life. In other words, the hope is that Americans can *live long and live well.* As life expectancy has increased, attention has turned to living healthfully throughout life. Fractures, the most common and devastating consequence of bone disease, frequently make it difficult, if not impossible, for elderly individuals to continue to live well. The second goal is to eliminate health disparities across different segments of the population. In addition, the President has launched the HealthierUS initiative and, as a part of this effort, HHS has implemented *Steps to a HealthierUS*, both of which emphasize the importance of physical activity and a nutritious diet. This Surgeon General's Report fits into these larger efforts to highlight the importance of the musculoskeletal system to the health status of Americans and to provide individuals, clinicians, public health officials, policymakers, and other stakeholders with the information and tools they need to improve bone health in all Americans.

The Magnitude of the Problem

Realizing the vision of a "bone-healthy" America will be challenging, given the magnitude of the problem. **The bone health status of Americans appears to be in jeopardy**, a fact that represents another key theme of this report. Fractures due to bone disease are common, costly, and often become a chronic burden on individuals and society. An estimated 1.5 million individuals suffer a bone disease-related fracture each year (Riggs and Melton 1995, Chrischilles et al. 1991). However, this figure significantly

understates the true impact of bone disease, because it captures the problem at a point in time. The impact of bone disease is more appropriately evaluated over a lifetime. Four out of every 10 White women age 50 or older in the United States will experience a hip, spine, or wrist fracture sometime during the remainder of their lives; 13 percent of White men in this country will suffer a similar fate (Cummings and Melton 2002). While the lifetime risk for men and non-White women is less across all fracture types, it is nonetheless substantial, and may be rising in certain populations, such as Hispanic women (Zingmond et al. 2004).

Fractures can have devastating consequences for both the individuals who suffer them and their family members. For example, hip fractures are associated with increased risk of mortality. The risk of mortality is 2.8–4 times greater among hip fracture patients during the first 3 months after the fracture, as compared to the comparable risk among individuals of similar age who live in the community and do not suffer a fracture. Those who are in poor health or living in a nursing home at the time of fracture are particularly vulnerable (Leibson et al. 2002, Richmond et al. 2003). For those who do survive, these fractures often precipitate a downward spiral in physical and mental health that dramatically impairs quality of life. Nearly one in five hip fracture patients, for example, ends up in a nursing home, a situation that a majority of participants in one study compared unfavorably to death (Salkeld et al. 2000). Many fracture victims become isolated and depressed, as the fear of falls and additional fractures paralyzes them. Spine fractures, which are not as easily diagnosed and treated as are fractures at other sites, can become a source of chronic pain as well as disfigurement.

Osteoporosis is the most important underlying cause of fractures in the elderly. Although osteoporosis can be defined as low bone mass leading to structural fragility, it is difficult to determine the extent of the condition described in these qualitative terms. Using the World Health Organization's quantitative definition based on bone density measurement, there are roughly 10 million Americans over age 50 with osteoporosis and an additional 34 million with low bone mass or "osteopenia" of the hip, which puts them at risk for osteoporosis, fractures, and their potential complications later in life (NOF 2002).

Left unchecked, the bone health status of Americans is only going to get worse, due primarily to the aging of the population. In fact, the prevalence of osteoporosis and osteoporotic-related fractures will increase significantly unless the underlying bone health status of Americans is significantly improved. By 2010, roughly 12 million individuals over age 50 are expected to have osteoporosis and another 40 million to have low bone mass. By 2020, those figures are expected to jump to 14 million cases of osteoporosis and over 47 million cases of low bone mass (NOF 2002). These demographic changes could cause the number of hip fractures in the United States to double or triple by 2040 (Schneider and Guralnik 1990).

While much less is known about the prevalence and treatment of other bone diseases, they too can have a severe impact on the health and well-being of those who suffer from them, especially if they are not diagnosed and treated in a timely manner. Many of the drugs that are used for osteoporosis are also effective as treatments for other bone diseases. While these diseases cannot be prevented, treatment can reduce levels of deformity and suffering. Further research on osteoporosis is likely to yield additional improvements in the treatment of these diseases, and may even yield insights into how they can be prevented.

Not surprisingly, bone disease takes a significant financial toll on society and individuals who suffer from it. The direct care expenditures for osteoporotic fractures alone range from $12.2–$17.9 billion each year, measured in 2002 dollars (Tosteson and Hammond 2002). Adding in the direct costs of caring for other bone diseases as well as the indirect costs (e.g., lost productivity for patients and family members) would likely add billions of additional dollars to this tab.

The Challenge

Much of this considerable burden can be prevented. There is no question that significant gaps in knowledge (and hence research needs) remain. **However, another important theme of this report is that great improvements in the bone health status of Americans can be made by applying what is already known about early prevention, assessment, diagnosis, and treatment.** In fact, the evidence clearly suggests that individuals can do a great deal to promote their own bone health. Prevention of bone disease begins at birth and is a lifelong challenge. By choosing to engage in regular physical activity, to follow a bone-healthy diet, and to avoid behaviors such as smoking that can damage bone, individuals can improve their bone health throughout life. Health care professionals can play a critical role in supporting individuals in making these choices and in identifying and treating high-risk individuals and those who have bone disease.

As noted earlier, the importance of achieving adequate levels of physical activity and calcium and vitamin D intake is now known, as is the need to begin prevention at a very young age and continue it throughout life. It is never too late for prevention, as even older individuals with poor bone health can improve their bone health status through appropriate exercise and calcium and vitamin D intake. Much is also known about how to ensure timely diagnosis of bone disease. Thanks to the development of bone mineral density (BMD) testing, fractures need not be the first sign of poor bone health. It is now possible to detect osteoporosis early and to intervene before a fracture occurs. Promising new approaches to assessment and screening will likely provide an even better understanding of the early warning signs of bone disease in the future. On the treatment front, a variety of drugs have been developed that improve bone health and reduce the incidence of fractures. New and potentially more effective drugs are currently under development. There are effective treatments not only for osteoporosis, but also for other bone diseases such as Paget's disease, hyperparathyroidism, rickets, and osteomalacia. There are also promising new directions for the treatment of osteogenesis imperfecta.

However, too little of what has been learned thus far about bone health has been applied in practice. As a result, the bone health status of Americans is poorer than it should be. Perhaps the biggest problem is a lack of awareness of bone disease among both the public and health care professionals, many of whom do not understand the magnitude of the problem, let alone the ways in which bone disease can be prevented and treated.

Relatively few individuals follow the recommendations related to the amounts of physical activity, calcium, and vitamin D that are needed to maintain bone health. National surveys suggest that the average calcium intake of individuals is far below the levels recommended for optimal bone health (Wright et al. 2003.). Measurements of vitamin D in nursing home residents, hospitalized patients, and adults with hip fractures suggest a high prevalence of insufficiency (Webb et al.1990, LeBoff et al. 1999, Thomas et al. 1998). Many Americans do not engage regu-

larly in leisure-time physical activity. As shown in Chapter 6, the participation by both adult men and women declines with age, with women being consistently less active than men (Schiller et al. 2004). In addition, only half those 12–21 years old exercise vigorously on a regular basis and 25 percent report no exercise at all (Gordon-Larsen et al. 1999).

Health care professionals can do a better job as well. Studies show that physicians frequently fail to diagnose and treat osteoporosis, even in elderly patients who have suffered a fracture (Solomon et al. 2003, Andrade et al. 2003, Kiebzak et al. 2002, Kamel et al. 2000, Feldstein et al. 2003). For example, in a recent study of four well-established Midwestern health systems, only one-eighth to a quarter of patients who had a hip fracture were tested for their bone density; fewer than a quarter were given calcium and vitamin D supplements; and fewer than one-tenth were treated with effective antiresorptive drugs (Harrington et al. 2002). Other studies have found low usage rates for testing and treatment among the high-risk population, including BMD testing (which ranged from 3–23 percent), calcium and vitamin D supplementation (11–44 percent), and antiresorptive therapy (12–16 percent) (Morris et al. 2004, Smith et al. 2001). In fact, most physicians do not even discuss osteoporosis with their patients, even after a fracture (Pal 1999). Finally, even when physicians do suggest therapy it often does not conform with recommended practice; for example, many patients with low BMD are not treated while others with high BMD are (Solomon et al. 2000).

Managed care organizations and other insurers that provide coverage to individuals under age 65 may not see the full impact of bone disease in their enrollees, since most will have moved on to Medicare by the time they suffer a fracture. Therefore, the commercial providers may not pay sufficient attention to bone health and to the preventive strategies available to and suitable for younger people.

In short, therefore, the gap between clinical knowledge and its application in the community remains large and needs to be closed, a fact that represents another key theme of this report. Of particular concern is the fact that some populations suffer additional barriers in trying to achieve optimal bone health. Overcoming these barriers will not be possible without specific strategies and programs geared towards bringing improvements in bone health to these populations.

Some of the most important barriers relate to men and racial and ethnic minorities. Osteoporosis and fragility fractures are often mistakenly viewed by both the public and health care practitioners as only being a problem for older White women. This commonly held but incorrect view may delay prevention and even treatment in men and minority women who are not seen as being at risk for osteoporosis. While a relatively small percentage of the total number of people affected, these populations still represent millions of Americans who are suffering the debilitating effects of bone disease.

For the poor (especially the low-income elderly population), individuals with disabilities, individuals living in rural areas, and other underserved populations, timely access to care represents an additional important barrier. Poor access to care may be caused by any number of factors, such as limited knowledge about bone health; a lack of available providers; inadequate income or insurance coverage; the high costs of diagnosis and treatment; a lack of transportation; or the inability to take time off from work to attend to personal or family care needs. Whatever the causes, the goal of better bone health for all Americans cannot be reached without greater efforts to educate underserved populations about

bone health and without significant improvements in their access to appropriate preventive services and counseling, screening, diagnosis, and treatment. Today these underserved populations rely on an unorganized patchwork of providers (e.g., emergency rooms) that are ill-equipped to provide or even facilitate the coordinated, ongoing preventive and treatment services that are needed to maintain bone health and overall health and well-being.

Underserved populations not only have difficulty in accessing care, but there are also concerns about the quality of those services they do receive. A recent study by the Institute of Medicine concluded that racial and ethnic minorities tend to receive lower-quality health care than does the majority population, even after accounting for access-related factors (Smedley et al. 2003). These disparities are consistent across a wide range of services, including those critical to bone health. Moreover, in a large study of older adults who had suffered a hip or wrist fracture, certain groups of patients—including men, older persons, non-Whites, and those with comorbid conditions—were less likely than White women to receive treatment for their bone disease after their fractures (Solomon et al. 2003).

The Opportunity

This Surgeon General's Report looks upon the Nation's at-risk bone status as an opportunity to do better rather than as an intractable problem. A variety of factors make bone health an ideal candidate for a public health approach. These factors include: a) the prospects of declining bone health status due to an aging population; b) the significant gap between what we know and what we apply; c) the need for early prevention of an often "silent" disease; d) the fact that most bone disease does not strike until people are on Medicare; and e) the lack of systematic evaluation of the prevalence and impact of bone disease. This Surgeon General's Report is calling for Federal, State, and local governments (including State and local public health departments) to join forces with the private sector and community organizations in a coordinated effort to promote bone health and prevent disease. This type of approach can serve as the primary vehicle for improving the bone health status of Americans. To be successful it must involve all stakeholders—individual citizens; volunteer health organizations; health care professionals; community organizations; private industry; and government—and must emphasize policies and programs that promote the dissemination of best practices for prevention, screening, and treatment for all Americans.

Some of the work on this public health approach has already begun. The aforementioned *Healthy People 2010* initiative lays out 467 specific objectives in 28 different areas of health to be achieved during the first decade of the 21st century. Included in these objectives are targets for reducing the number of individuals with osteoporosis and the number of hip fractures, along with increasing levels of calcium intake and physical activity. (See Table 1-1 for more information on those *Healthy People 2010* goals that relate to osteoporosis and bone health.)

One of the purposes of this Surgeon General's Report is to build support at many levels to include current *Healthy People 2010* objectives in health agendas and activities at the Federal, State, and local levels. Developing data systems to track progress on these objectives will be critical to achieving improvements in bone health status. Going forward, it is anticipated that the number of objectives related to osteoporosis and bone health will increase when *Healthy People 2020* objectives are developed, and that existing measures will be refined as our

understanding of the science and our data collection and measurement systems improve.

The Charge

Recognizing that bone health can have a significant impact on the overall health and well-being of Americans, Congress instructed that this report cover a range of important issues related to improving bone health, including: challenges in the diagnosis and treatment of osteoporosis and related bone diseases; the impact of these diseases on minority populations; promising prevention strategies; how to improve health provider education and promote public awareness; and ways to enhance access to key health services. (See Appendix A for more details.)

To initiate the development of the report, an interagency work group was convened by the Surgeon General with staff representatives from the National Institutes of Health (NIH), the Centers for Disease Control and Prevention (CDC), the Food and Drug Administration (FDA), the Health Resources and Services Administration (HRSA), the Agency for Healthcare Research and Quality (AHRQ), the Administration on Aging, the Centers for Medicare and Medicaid Services (CMS), the Office of Disease Prevention and Health Promotion, the Office on Women's Health, the Office on Minority Health, the President's Council on Physical Fitness and Sports, the Regional Health Administrators, and the U.S. Department of Agriculture.

As a second step, a Surgeon General's Workshop was convened in December 2002 that brought together a wide range of researchers, public health experts, and patient representatives to discuss key areas that should be addressed in the report. Prior to the workshop, public comments on what the priorities for the report should be were solicited through the Surgeon General's

Table 1-1.   Healthy People 2010 Osteoporosis and Bone Health Objectives

Healthy People 2010 Objective Number	Healthy People 2010 Objective	1998 Baseline	2010 Target
Objective 2.9	Reduce cases of osteoporosis	10 percent of adults aged 50 years and older had osteoporosis as measured by low total femur bone mineral density (BMD) in 1988–94 (age adjusted to the year 2000 standard population).	8 percent
Objective 2.10	Reduce hospitalizations for vertebral fracture	17.5 hospitalizations per 10,000 adults aged 65 years and older were for vertebral fractures associated with osteoporosis in 1998 (age adjusted to the year 2000 standard population).	14.0 hospitalizations per 10,000 adults aged 65 years and older
Objective 15.28	Reduce hip fractures		
15-28a	Females aged 65 years and older	1,055.8 per 100,000	416 per 100,000
15-28b	Males aged 65 years and older	592.7 per 100,000	474 per 100,000
Objective 19.11	Increase calcium intake	46 percent of persons aged 2 years and older were at or above approximated mean calcium requirements (based on consideration of calcium from foods, dietary supplements, and antacids) in 1988–94 (age adjusted to the year 2000 standard population).	75 percent
Objectives 22.1–22.15	Increase physical activity (there are 15 objectives for increasing physical activity)	—	—

Data Source 2.9 - National Health and Nutrition Examination Survey (NHANES), CDC, NCHS
Data Source 2.10 - National Hospital Discharge Survey (NHDS), CDC, NCHS
Data Source 15.28 - National Hospital Discharge Survey (NHDS), CDC, NCHS
Data Source 19.11 - National Health and Nutrition Examination Survey (NHANES), CDC, NCHS

Source: USDHHS 2000.

Web site. Following the workshop, a summary of its key findings was released by the Surgeon General (Report 2003).

This report includes contributions from more than 50 authors across the country, while over 100 experts provided valuable guidance and insights in their reviews of initial drafts.

This report is intended to be a catalyst for the advancement of research in bone health, and for accelerating the translation of existing evidence on how to improve bone health status into everyday practice. The net result should be an improvement in the bone health status of Americans.

Evidence Base for the Report

This report is based on a review of the published scientific literature. The scope of the review encompassed studies written in English from throughout the world. The quality of the evidence, based on study design and its rigor, was considered as a part of this review. All studies used in the report are referenced in the text, with full citations at the conclusion of each chapter.

This report does not offer any new standards or guidelines for the prevention, diagnosis, or treatment of bone disease. Rather, it summarizes knowledge that is already known and can be acted upon.

The clinical literature in bone disease includes the full range of studies, from randomized controlled trials to case studies. Comprehensive reviews of the literature have been used for Chapters 2 through 9, and Chapter 11. Chapter 10, which is an attempt to summarize key, actionable findings for busy health care professionals, contains few references, as it largely draws on findings cited elsewhere in the report. Chapter 12 draws on both published studies and case studies of population-based initiatives in bone health,

which were selected in order to highlight particular lessons about such approaches. Additional information on the various kinds of evidence and studies that were used in preparing this report can be found in Appendix B, entitled, "How We Know What We Know: The Evidence Behind the Evidence."

Experts in their respective fields of bone health contributed to this report. Each chapter was prepared under the guidance of a coordinating author for that chapter. Independent, expert peer review was conducted for all chapters. The full manuscript was reviewed by a number of senior reviewers as well as the relevant Federal agencies. All who contributed are listed in the Acknowledgments section of the report.

Organization of the Report

This report attempts to answer five major questions for a wide variety of stakeholders, including policymakers; national, State, and local public health officials; health system leaders; health care professionals; community advocates; and individuals. The report is organized around each of these five questions. The first section strives to define bone health and bone disease in terms that the public can understand. The second section reviews today's less-than-optimal bone health status and documents the magnitude of the problem facing the Nation. The third, fourth, and fifth sections of the report tackle the issue of what can be done to improve bone health—first from the perspective of the individual, then from the perspective of the health care professional, and finally from the perspective of the larger health system. The final section lays out a vision for the future.

Part One: What Is Bone Health?

This introductory part of the report defines bone health as a public health issue with an emphasis on prevention and early intervention to promote strong bones and prevent fractures and their consequences. This first chapter describes this public health approach along with the rationale for the report and the charge from Congress and from the Surgeon General. Chapter 2 provides a brief overview of the fundamentals of bone biology, helping the reader to understand why humans have bones; how bones work; how bones change during life; what keeps bones healthy; what causes bone disease; and what is in store in the future. Chapter 3 offers a summary review of the more common diseases, disorders, and conditions that both directly and indirectly affect bone. While much of Chapter 3 focuses on osteoporosis (including other diseases and medications that can cause it), it also covers other bone diseases, including rickets and osteomalacia, renal osteodystrophy, Paget's disease of bone, developmental skeletal disorders, and acquired skeletal disorders. Both Chapters 2 and 3 should be considered as important scientific background for the remainder of the report.

Part Two: What Is the Status of Bone Health in America?

This part of the report describes the magnitude and scope of the problem from two perspectives. The first is the prevalence of bone disease within the population at large, and the second is the burden that bone diseases impose on society and those who suffer from them. Chapter 4 provides detailed information on the incidence and prevalence of osteoporosis, fractures, and other bone diseases. Where available, it also provides data on bone disease in men and minorities and offers projections for the future. Chapter 5 examines the costs of bone diseases and their effects on well-being and quality of life, both from the point of view of the individual patient and society at large. It includes some real-life vignettes that highlight the impact that os-

teoporosis, Paget's disease, osteogenesis imperfecta, and other related bone diseases can have on those who suffer from them and their family members.

Part Three: What Can Individuals Do To Improve Their Bone Health?

This part of the report examines factors that determine bone health and describes lifestyle approaches that individuals can take to improve their personal bone health. Chapter 6 provides a thorough review of the evidence on how nutrition, physical activity, and other factors influence bone health, including those behaviors that promote it (e.g., physical activity, adequate calcium intake) and those that can impair it (e.g., smoking). Chapter 7 provides practical, real-world guidance on lifestyle approaches that individuals can take to improve their own bone health, including the following: what foods are the best sources of calcium and vitamin D; how to calculate daily calcium intake; when calcium and/or vitamin D supplementation should be considered; and what types of physical activity can contribute to bone health and overall health.

Part Four: What Can Health Care Professionals Do To Promote Bone Health?

This part of the report describes what health care professionals can do with their patients to promote bone health. Chapter 8 examines the potential risk factors for bone disease; highlights red flags that signal the need for further assessment; reviews the use of formal assessment tools to determine who should get a bone density test; and provides detailed information on how to use BMD for both assessment and monitoring purposes. The chapter also provides a glimpse into the future of bone disease assessment and diagnosis. It includes real-life vignettes that highlight the need for the medical profession to become aware of the potential for severe osteoporosis to develop in younger men and women. Chapter 9 focuses on preventive and therapeutic measures for those who have or are at risk for bone disease. It reviews a "pyramid approach" to treating bone diseases and to preventing falls and fractures, with maintenance of bone health through calcium, vitamin D, physical activity, and fall prevention representing the base of the pyramid for all individuals, including those with bone disease. The second level of the pyramid relates to addressing and treating secondary causes of osteoporosis. The third level of the pyramid is pharmacotherapy. The chapter describes currently available anti-resorptive, anabolic therapies and hormone therapies and offers a glimpse into future directions for pharmacologic treatment of osteoporosis. The chapter also reviews the treatment and rehabilitation of osteoporotic fractures and highlights treatment options for other bone diseases. Chapter 10 "puts it all together" for health care professionals by translating the research into practical advice for preventing, diagnosing, and treating bone disease in patients of all ages. Key symptoms of major metabolic bone diseases are identified, as are red flags that signal a need for further intervention.

Part Five: What Can Health Systems and Population-Based Approaches Do To Promote Bone Health?

This part of the report examines how health systems and population-based approaches can promote bone health. Chapter 11 looks at the key systems-level issues and decisions that affect bone health care, including evidence-based medicine; clinical practice guidelines; training and education of health care professionals; quality assurance; coverage policies; and disparities in prevention and treatment. It also evaluates the key roles of various stakeholders in promoting a more systems-based approach to bone health care, including individual clinicians; medical groups; health plans and other insurers; public health departments; and other stakeholders. Chapter 12 describes the various potential components of population-based approaches at the local, State, and Federal levels to promote bone health and reviews the evidence supporting their use. This chapter also includes several detailed profiles of innovative and/or effective population-based programs, each of which was selected to illustrate an important concept in population-based health. Chapter 12 also draws lessons for bone health from population-based approaches that have been used in other areas of health, such as the National Cholesterol Education Program, to reduce cholesterol levels in Americans.

Part Six: Challenges and Opportunities: A Vision for the Future

The final part summarizes the key themes of the report, highlights those opportunities that have been identified for promoting bone health, and lays out a vision for how these opportunities can be realized so that bone health can be improved today and far into the future. The key to success will be for public and private stakeholders—including individual consumers; voluntary health organizations and professional associations; health care professionals; health systems; academic medical centers; researchers; health plans and insurers; public health departments; and all levels of government—to join forces in developing a collaborative approach to promoting timely prevention, assessment, diagnosis, and treatment of bone disease throughout life.

References

Andrade SE, Majumdar SR, Chan KA, Buist DS, Go AS, Goodman M, Smith DH, Platt R, Gurwitz JH. Low frequency of treatment of osteoporosis among postmenopausal women following a fracture. Arch Intern Med. 2003 Sep 22;163(17):2052-7.

Chrischilles EA, Butler CD, Davis CS, Wallace RB. A model of lifetime osteoporosis impact. Arch Intern Med. 1991 Oct;151(10):2026-32.

Cummings SR, Melton LJ 3rd. Epidemiology and outcomes of osteoporotic fractures. Lancet 2002 May 18;359(9319):1761-7.

Feldstein AC, Nichols GA, Elmer PJ, Smith DH, Aickin M, Herson M. Older women with fractures: Patients falling through the cracks of guideline-recommended osteoporosis screening and treatment. J Bone Joint Surg Am 2003 Dec;85-A(12):2294-302.

Gordon-Larsen P, McMurray RG, Popkin BM. Adolescent physical activity and inactivity vary by ethnicity: The National Longitudinal Study of Adolescent Health. J Pediatr 1999 Sep;135(3):301-6.Harrington JT, Broy SB, Derosa AM, Licata AA, Shewmon DA. Hip fracture patients are not treated for osteoporosis: a call to action. Arthritis Rheum 2002 Dec 15;47(6):651-4.

Kamel HK, Hussain MS, Tariq S, Perry HM, Morley JE. Failure to diagnose and treat osteoporosis in elderly patients hospitalized with hip fracture. Am J Med 2000 Sep;109(4):326-8.

Kiebzak GM, Beinart GA, Perser K, Ambrose CG, Siff SJ, Heggeness MH. Undertreatment of osteoporosis in men with hip fracture. Arch Intern Med. 2002 Oct 28;162(19):2217-22.

LeBoff MS, Kohlmeier L, Hurwitz S, Franklin J, Wright J, Glowacki J. Occult vitamin D deficiency in postmenopausal US women with acute hip fracture. JAMA 1999 Apr 28;281(16):1505-11.

Leibson CL, Tosteson AN, Gabriel SE, Ransom JE, Melton LJ. Mortality, disability, and nursing home use for persons with and without hip fracture: A population-based study. J Am Geriatr Soc. 2002 Oct; 50(10): 1644-50.

Morris CA, Cheng H, Cabral D, Solomon DH. Predictors of screening and treatment of osteoporosis: A structured review of the literature. Endocrinologist. 2004 Mar/Apr;14(2):70-75.

National Osteoporosis Foundation. America's Bone Health: The State of Osteoporosis and Low Bone Mass in Our Nation. Washington, DC: National Osteoporosis Foundation; 2002.

Pal B. Questionnaire survey of advice given to patients with fractures. BMJ 1999 Feb 20;318(7182):500-1.

Report of the Surgeon General's Workshop on Osteoporosis and Bone Health; 2002 Dec 12-13;Washington (DC) [report on the Internet]: U.S. Department of Health and Human Services; c2003 [cited 2004 June 28]. Available from: http://www.surgeongeneral.gov/topics/bonehealth/.

Richmond J, Aharonoff GB, Zuckerman JD, Koval KJ. Mortality Risk After Hip Fracture. J Orthop Trauma. 2003 Sep;17(8 Suppl):S2-5.

Riggs BL, Melton LJ 3rd. The worldwide problem of osteoporosis: insights afforded by epidemiology. Bone 1995 Nov;17(5 Suppl):505S-11S.

Salkeld G, Cameron ID, Cumming RG, Easter S, Seymour J, Kurrle SE, Quine S. Quality of life related to fear of falling and hip fracture in older women: A time trade off study. BMJ 2000 Feb 5;320(7231):341-6.

Schiller JS, Coriaty-Nelson Z, Barnes P. Early release of selected estimates based on data from the 2003 National Health Interview Survey. National Center for Health Statistics. c2004 [cited 2004 July 9]. Available from: http://www.cdc.gov/nchs/about/major/nhis/released200406.htm.

Schneider EL, Guralnik JM. The aging of America: Impact on health care costs. JAMA 1990 May 2;263(17):2335-40.

Smedley, Brian D; Stith, Adrienne Y; Nelson, Alan R. editors. Unequal treatment: confronting racial and ethnic disparities in health care. Committee on Understanding and Eliminating Racial and Ethnic Disparities in Health Care, Board on Health Sciences Policy. Institute of Medicine. Washington, DC: National Academies Press; 2003. 764 p.

Smith MD, Ross W, Ahern MJ. Missing a therapeutic window of opportunity: An audit of patients attending a tertiary teaching hospital with potentially osteoporotic hip and wrist fractures. J Rheum 2001 Nov;28(11):2504-8.

Solomon DH, Levin E, Helfgott SM. Patterns of medication use before and after bone densitometry: Factors associated with appropriate treatment. J Rheumatol 2000 Jun;27(6):1496-500.

Solomon DH, Finkelstein JS, Katz JN, Mogun H, Avorn J. Underuse of osteoporosis medications in elderly patients with fractures. Amer J Med 2003 Oct 1;115(5):398-400.

Thomas MK, Lloyd-Jones DM, Thadhani R, Shaw AC, Deraska DJ, Kitch BT, Vamvakas E, Dick IM, Prince RL, Finkelstein JS. Hypovitaminosis D in medical inpatients. N Engl J Med 1998 Mar 19;338(12):777-83.

Tosteson AN, Hammond CS. Quality-of-life assessment in osteoporosis: health-status and preference-based measures. Pharmaco-economics 2002;20(5):289-303.

U.S. Department of Health and Human Services. Healthy People 2010. Washington, DC: January 2000.

Webb AR, Pilbeam C, Hanafin N, Holick MF. An evaluation of the relative contributions of exposure to sunlight and of diet to the circulating concentrations of 25-hydroxyvitamin D in an elderly nursing home population in Boston. Am J Clin Nutr 1990;51(6):1075-81.

Wright JD, Wang CY, Kennedy-Stevenson J, Ervin RB. Dietary intakes of ten key nutrients for public health, United States: 1999-2000. Adv Data 2003 Apr 17;(334):104. Hyattsville, Maryland: National Center on Health Statistics. 2003.

Zingmond DS, Melton LJ 3rd, Silverman SL. Increasing hip fracture incidence in California Hispanics, 1983 to 2000. Osteoporos Int. 2004 Mar 4 [Epub ahead of print].

Chapter 2: Key Messages

- The bony skeleton is a remarkable organ that serves both a structural function, providing mobility, support, and protection for the body, and a reservoir function, as the storehouse for essential minerals.

- During childhood and adolescence bones are sculpted by a process called *modeling*, which allows for the formation of new bone at one site and the removal of old bone from another site within the same bone. This process allows individual bones to grow in size and to shift in space.

- Much of the cellular activity in a bone consists of removal and replacement at the same site, a process called *remodeling*. The remodeling process occurs throughout life and becomes dominant by the time that bone reaches its peak mass (typically by the early 20s). Remodeling continues throughout life so that most of the adult skeleton is replaced about every 10 years.

- Both genes and the environment contribute to bone health. Some elements of bone health are determined largely by genes, and errors in signaling by these genes can result in birth defects. External factors, such as diet and physical activity, are critically important to bone health throughout life, and these factors can be modified.

- The growth of the skeleton, its response to mechanical forces, and its role as a mineral storehouse are all dependent on the proper functioning of a number of systemic or circulating hormones that respond to changes in blood calcium and phosphorus. If calcium or phosphorus are in short supply, the regulating hormones take them out of the bone to serve vital functions in other systems of the body. Too many withdrawals can weaken the bone.

- Many things can interfere with the development of a strong and healthy skeleton. *Genetic abnormalities* can produce weak, thin bones, or bones that are too dense. *Nutritional deficiencies* can result in the formation of weak, poorly mineralized bone. Many *hormonal disorders* can also affect the skeleton. Lack of exercise, immobilization, and smoking can also have negative effects on bone mass and strength.

- Osteoporosis, the most common bone disease, typically does not manifest until late in life, when bone loss begins due to bone breakdown and decreased levels of bone formation. Loss of bone mass leads to the development of structural abnormalities that make the skeleton more fragile.

Chapter 2

THE BASICS OF BONE IN HEALTH AND DISEASE

The purpose of this chapter is to provide an overview of bone biology that will help the reader to understand:

- why humans have bones;
- how bones work;
- how bones change during life;
- what keeps bones healthy;
- what causes bone disease, including the most common form, osteoporosis; and
- the future of bone biology and what it means for preventing and treating bone disease.

While dealing with a subject that is highly technical in nature, this chapter attempts to explain bone biology in terms that a lay person can generally understand. It is intended to provide the reader with the background needed to understand the basis for some of the preventive, diagnostic, and treatment approaches related to bone disease that are discussed in detail later in this report. Those interested in a more detailed review of bone biology and bone disease can consult any of a number of recent texts (Bilezikian et al. 2001, Marcus et al. 2001, Favus 2003).

Why Do We Have Bones?

The bony skeleton is a remarkable organ that serves both a structural function—providing mobility, support, and protection for the body—and a reservoir function, as the storehouse for essential minerals. It is not a static organ, but is constantly changing to better carry out its functions. The development of the bony skeleton likely began many eons ago, when animals left the calcium-rich ocean, first to live in fresh water where calcium was in short supply, and then on dry land where weight bearing put much greater stress on the skeleton. The architecture of the skeleton is remarkably adapted to provide adequate strength and mobility so that bones do not break when subjected to substantial impact, even the loads placed on bone during vigorous physical activity. The shape or structure of bone is at least as important as its mass in providing this strength.

The skeleton is also a storehouse for two minerals, calcium and phosphorus, that are essential for the functioning of other body systems, and this storehouse must be called upon in times of need. The maintenance of a constant level of calcium in the blood as well as an adequate supply of calcium and phosphorus in cells is critical for the function of all body organs, but particularly for the nerves and muscle. Therefore, a complex system of regulatory hormones has developed that helps to maintain adequate supplies of these minerals in a variety of situations. These hormones act not only on bone but on other tissues, such as the intestine and the kidney, to regulate the supply of these elements. Thus one reason that bone health is difficult to maintain is that the skeleton is simultaneously serving two different functions that are in competition with each other. First, bone must be responsive to changes in mechanical loading or weight bearing, both of which require strong bones that have ample supplies of calcium and phosphorus. When these elements are in short supply the regulating hormones take them out of the bone to serve vital functions in other systems of the body. Thus the skeleton can be likened to a bank where we can deposit calcium or phosphorus and then withdraw them later in times of need. However, too many withdrawals weaken the bone and can lead to the most common bone disorder, fractures.

Both the amount of bone and its architecture or shape are determined by the mechanical forces that act on the skeleton. Much of this is determined genetically so that each species, including humans, has a skeleton that is adapted to its functions. However, there can be great variation within a species, so that some individuals will have strong bones and others will have weak bones, largely because of differences in their genes (Huang et al. 2003). Moreover, bone mass and architecture are further modified throughout life as these functions and the mechanical forces required to fulfill them change. In other words, bones will weaken if they are not subjected to adequate amounts of loading and weight bearing for sufficient periods of time. If they are not (such as in the weightless condition of space travel), rapid bone loss can occur. In other words, as with muscle, it is "use it or lose it" with bone as well. Conversely, the amount and architecture of the bones can be improved by mechanical loading. However, as described in Chapter 6, some types of exercise may be better than others in strengthening the skeleton.

To respond to its dual roles of support and regulation of calcium and phosphorus, as well as to repair any damage to the skeleton, bone is constantly changing. Old bone breaks down and new bone is formed on a continuous basis. In fact, the tissue of the skeleton is replaced many times during life. This requires an exquisitely controlled regulatory system that involves specialized cells that communicate with each other. These cells must respond to many different signals, both internal and external, mechanical and hormonal, and systemic (affecting the whole skeleton) and local (affecting only a small region of the skeleton). It is not surprising that with so many different tasks to perform and so many different factors regulating how the skeleton grows, adapts, and responds to changing demands, there are many ways that these processes can go astray.

How Bones Work

Bone is a composite material, consisting of crystals of mineral bound to protein. This provides both strength and resilience so that the skeleton can absorb impact without breaking. A structure made only of mineral would be more brittle and break more easily, while a structure made only of protein would be soft and bend too easily. The mineral phase of bone consists of small crystals containing calcium and phosphate, called hydroxyapatite. This mineral is bound in an orderly manner to a matrix that is made up largely of a single protein, collagen. Collagen is made by bone cells and assembled as long thin rods containing three intertwined protein chains, which are then assembled into larger fibers that are strengthened by chemical connections between them. Other proteins in bone can help to strengthen the collagen matrix even further and to regulate its ability to bind mineral. Very small changes in the shape of the bone can act on the cells inside bone (the osteocytes), which produce chemical signals that allow the skeleton to respond to changes in mechanical loading. Abnormalities in the collagen scaffold can occur as a result of a genetic disorder called osteogenesis imperfecta, while the failure of mineral deposition can be the result of rickets and osteomalacia, conditions that result in marked weakening of the skeleton (see below and Chapter 3).

To provide the body with a frame that is both light and strong, bones are hollow. The outer dense shell is called cortical bone, which makes up roughly three-quarters of the total skeletal mass. Inside the cortical shell is a fine network of connecting plates and rods called trabecular bone that makes up the remaining 25 percent (Figure 2-1). Most bones are hollow structures in which the outer cortical bone shell defines the shape of the bone. This cortical shell is essential because it provides strength, sites for firm attachment of the tendons, and muscles and protection without excessive weight. The inner trabecular network has two important functions. It provides a large bone surface for mineral exchange. In addition, trabecular bone helps to maintain skeletal strength and integrity, as it is particularly abundant in the spine and at the ends of the long bones, sites that are under continuous stress from motion and weight-bearing. Fractures are common at these sites when the bone is weakened (Kontulainen, Sievanen et al. 2003). The rods and plates of trabecular bone are aligned in a pattern that provides maximal strength without too much bulk, much in the way that architects and engineers design buildings and bridges. The shape and size of both cortical and trabecular bone can respond to different kinds of stress produced by physical activity. For example, in most people the cortex of their dominant arm is larger than that of their non-dominant arm. The difference in cortex size is even larger for tennis players and other athletes who routinely use a dominant arm in their sporting activities. Bones do not work in isolation, but rather are part of the musculoskeletal system, providing the "lever" that allows muscles to move (by pulling on the lever). Thus muscle activity is important for the normal function of the bone. When the mechanical force produced by muscle is lost—for example, in patients with muscular dystrophy or paralysis—bone mass and strength are also rapidly lost. Many bones in the skeleton also have connecting joints that provide greater flexibility of movement. These joints are sites of great mechanical stress and are subject to injury and to degeneration with aging. The most common type of joint degeneration is osteoarthritis, a painful, degenerative condition that affects the hip, knees, neck, lower back, and/or small joints of the hand. These joint diseases result from very different causes and require very different management than do bone diseases, and consequently they are not covered in this report. However it is important to recognize that the bones, joints, and muscles are the key parts of an integrated "musculoskeletal system." Problems with any one component of this system can affect the other components. Thus, weakness of the muscles can lead to loss of bone and joint damage, while degeneration of the joints leads to changes in the underlying bone, such as the bony spurs or protuberances that occur in osteoarthritis.

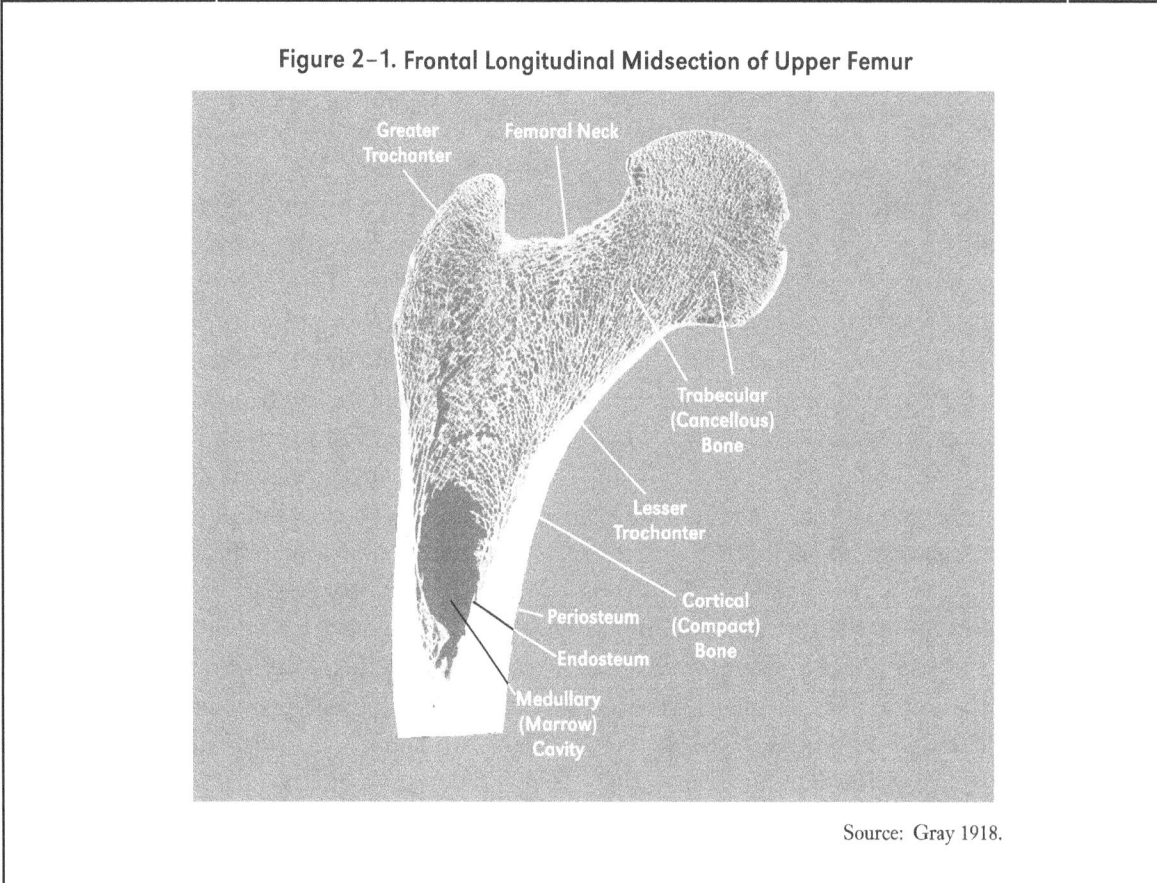

Figure 2–1. Frontal Longitudinal Midsection of Upper Femur

Source: Gray 1918.

How Bones Change Throughout Life

Throughout life, bones change in size, shape, and position. Two processes guide these changes—modeling and remodeling. When a bone is formed at one site and broken down in a different site its shape and position is changed. This is called modeling (Figure 2-2). However, much of the cellular activity in a bone consists of removal and replacement at the same site, a process called remodeling. The remainder of this section explains why and how these processes occur.

Why We Need Modeling and Remodeling

During childhood and adolescence bones are sculpted by modeling, which allows for the formation of new bone at one site and the removal of old bone from another site within the same bone (Seeman 2003) (Figure 2-2). This process allows individual bones to grow in size and to shift in space. During childhood bones grow because resorption occurs inside the bone while formation of new bone occurs on its outer (periosteal) surface. At puberty the bones get thicker because formation can occur on both the outer and inner (endosteal) surfaces. As people get older, resorption occurs on inner surfaces while formation occurs on outer surfaces, which can partially compensate for the loss of strength due to the thinning of the cortex. The size and shape of the skeleton follows a genetic program, but can be greatly affected by the loading or impact that occurs with physical activity. Ultimately bones achieve a shape and size that fits best to their function. In other words, "form follows function."

The remodeling process occurs throughout life and becomes the dominant process by the time that bone reaches its peak mass (typically by the early 20s). In remodeling, a small amount of bone on the surface of trabeculae or in the interior of the cortex is removed and then replaced at the same site (Figure 2-2). The remodeling process does not change the shape of the bone, but it is nevertheless vital for bone health, for a variety of reasons. First, remodeling repairs the damage to the skeleton that can result from repeated stresses by replacing small cracks or deformities in areas of cell damage. Remodeling also prevents the accumulation of too much old bone, which can lose its resilience and become brittle. Remodeling is also important for the function of the skeleton as the bank for calcium and phosphorus. Resorption (the process of breaking down bone), particularly on the surface of trabecular bone, can supply needed calcium and phosphorus when there is a deficiency in the diet or for the needs of the fetus during pregnancy or an infant during lactation. When calcium and phosphorus supplies are ample the formation phase of remodeling can take up these minerals and replenish the bank.

Modeling and remodeling continue throughout life so that most of the adult skeleton is replaced about every 10 years. While remodeling predominates by early adulthood, modeling can still occur particularly in response to weakening of the bone. Thus with aging, if excessive amounts of bone are removed from the inside, some new bone can be laid down on the outside, thus preserving the mechanical strength of the bone despite the loss of bone mass.

How Modeling and Remodeling Occur

The process of building the skeleton and continuously reshaping it to respond to internal and external signals is carried out by specialized cells that can be activated to form or break down bone. Both modeling and remodeling involve the cells that form bone called osteoblasts and the cells that break down bone, called osteoclasts (Figure 2-3). In remodeling there is an important local interaction between osteoblasts or their precursors (the cells that will develop into osteoblasts by acquiring more specialized functions—a process called differentiation) and osteoclasts or their precursors. Since remodeling is the main way that bone changes in adults and abnormalities in remodeling are the primary cause of bone disease, it is critically important to understand this process. In addition, recent research has provided exciting information about these cell interactions.

Osteoblasts are derived from precursor cells that can also be stimulated to become muscle, fat or cartilage; however, under the right conditions these cells change (or differentiate) to form new bone, producing the collagen that forms the scaffolding or bone matrix. This calcium- and phosphate-rich mineral is added to the matrix to form the hard, yet resilient, tissue that is healthy bone. Osteoblasts lay down bone in orderly layers that add strength to the matrix. Some of the osteoblasts are buried in the matrix as it is being produced and these are now called osteocytes. Others remain as thin cells that cover the surface and are called lining cells. Osteocytes are the most numerous cells in bone and are extensively connected to each other and to the surface of osteoblasts by a network of small thin extensions. This network is critical for the

Figure 2–2. Modeling and Remodeling

Modeling

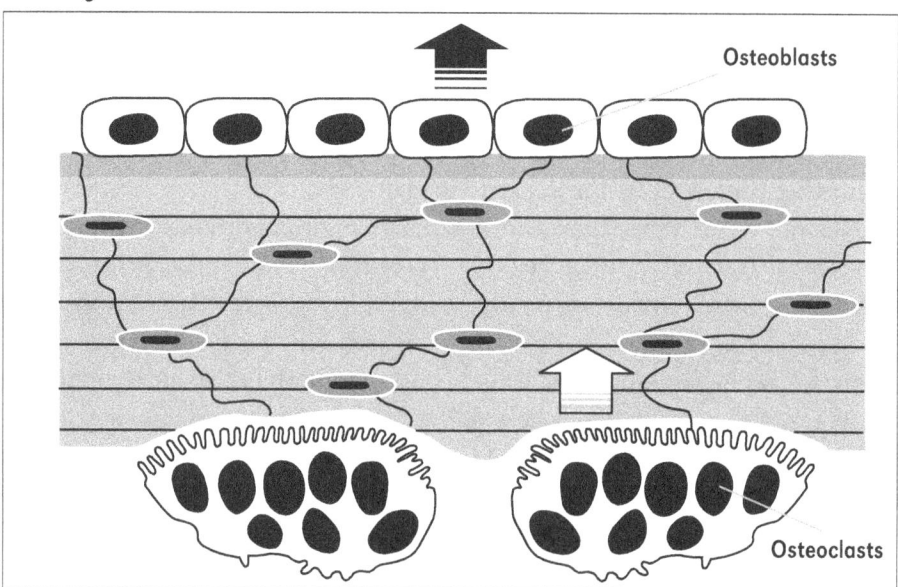

Remodeling

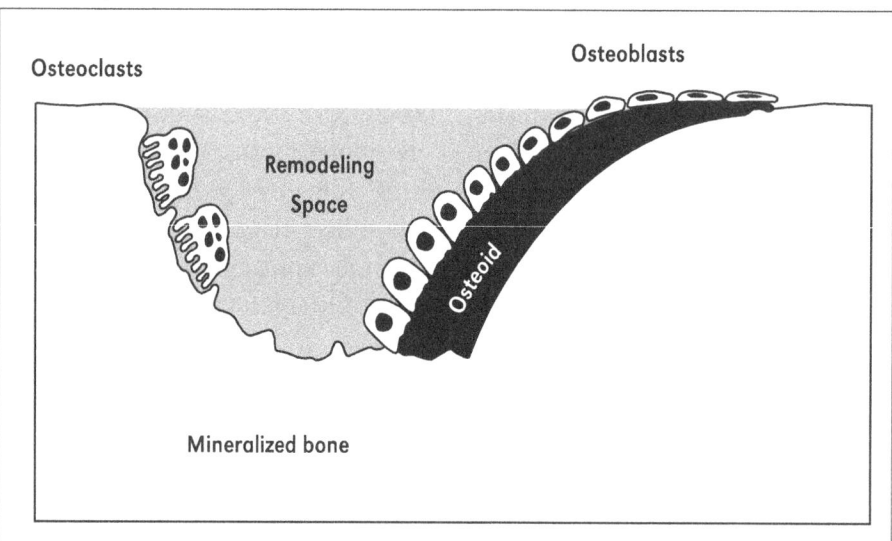

Note: In modeling, osteoblast and osteoclast action are not linked and rapid changes can occur in the amount, shape, and position of bone. In remodeling, osteoblast action is coupled to prior osteoclast action. Net changes in the amount and shape of bone are minimal unless there is a remodeling imbalance.

Source: Rauch 2004.

ability of bone to respond to mechanical forces and injury. When the skeleton is subjected to impact there is fluid movement around the osteocytes and the long-cell extensions that provides signals to the bone cells on the surface to alter their activity, either in terms of changes in bone resorption or formation. Failure of the osteoblasts to make a normal matrix occurs in a congenital disorder of the collagen molecule called osteogenesis imperfecta. Inadequate bone matrix formation also occurs in osteoporosis, particularly in the form of osteoporosis produced

Figure 2–3. Bone Remodeling

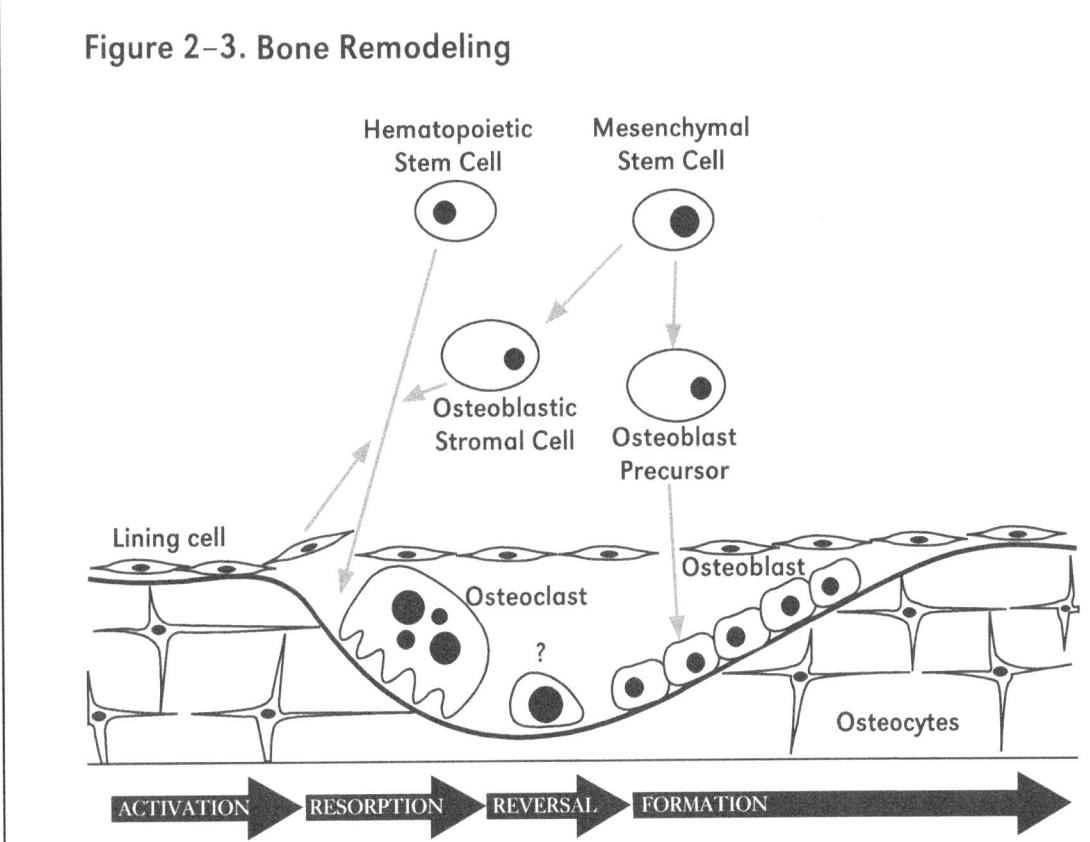

Note: The sequence of *activation, resorption, reversal,* and *formation* is illustrated here. The activation step depends on cells of the osteoblast lineage, either on the surface of the bone or in the marrow, acting on blood cell precursors *(hematopoietic cells)* to form bone-resorbing osteoclasts. The resorption process may take place under a layer of lining cells as shown here. After a brief reversal phase, the osteoblasts begin to lay down new bone. Some of the osteoblasts remain inside the bone and are converted to osteocytes, which are connected to each other and to the surface osteoblasts. The resorption phases last only a few weeks but the formation phase is much slower, taking several months to complete, as multiple layers of new bone are formed by successive waves of osteoblasts.

by an excess of the adrenal hormones called glucocorticoid-induced osteoporosis. This form of osteoporosis differs from primary osteoporosis and most other forms of secondary osteoporosis because with glucocorticoid-induced osteoporosis inhibition of bone formation is the dominant mechanism for weakening of the skeleton.

The osteoclasts remove bone by dissolving the mineral and breaking down the matrix in a process that is called bone resorption. The osteoclasts come from the same precursor cells in the bone marrow that produce white blood cells. These precursor cells can also circulate in the blood and be available at different sites in need of bone breakdown. Osteoclasts are formed by fusion of small precursor cells into large, highly active cells with many nuclei. These large cells can fasten onto the bone, seal off an area on the surface, and develop a region of intense activity in which the cell surface is highly irregular, called a ruffled border. This ruffled border contains transport molecules that transfer hydrogen ions from the cells to the bone surface where they can dissolve the mineral. In addition, packets of enzymes are secreted from the ruffled border that can break down the matrix. Excessive bone breakdown by osteoclasts is an important cause of bone fragility not only in osteoporosis, but also in other bone diseases such as hyperparathyroidism, Paget's disease, and fibrous dysplasia (see Chapter 3). Inhibitors of osteoclastic bone breakdown have been developed to treat these disorders (see Chapter 9).

Removal and replacement of bone in the remodeling cycle occurs in a carefully orchestrated sequence that involves communication between cells of the osteoblast and osteoclast lineages (Hauge, Qvesel et al. 2001; Parfitt 2001). It is controlled by local and systemic factors that regulate bone remodeling to fulfill both its structural and metabolic functions. The activation of this process involves an interaction between cells of the osteoblastic lineage and the precursors that will become osteoclasts. What stops this process is not known, but the osteoclasts machinery clearly slows down and the osteoclasts die by a process that is called programmed cell death. Thus the amount of bone removed can be controlled by altering the rate of production of new osteoclasts, blocking their activity, or altering their life span. Most current treatments for osteoporosis work by slowing down osteoclastic bone breakdown through use of antiresorptive agents.

The activation and resorption phases are followed by a brief reversal phase (Everts, Delaisse et al. 2002). During the reversal phase the resorbed surface is prepared for the subsequent formation phase, in part by producing a thin layer of protein, rich in sugars, which is called the cement line and helps form a strong bond between the old bone and the newly formed bone.

These three phases are relatively rapid, probably lasting only 2 to 3 weeks in humans. The final phase of bone formation takes much longer, lasting up to 3 or 4 months. Thus active remodeling at many sites can weaken the bone for a considerable period of time (even if formation catches up eventually), as many defects form in the bony structure that have not yet been filled. Formation is carried out by large active osteoblasts that lay down successive layers of matrix in an orderly manner that provides added strength. The addition of minerals to the collagenous matrix completes the process of making strong bone. Any error in this complex process can lead to bone disease.

Since remodeling serves both the structural and metabolic functions of the skeleton, it can be stimulated both by the hormones that regulate mineral metabolism and by mechanical loads and local damage acting through local factors.

Repair of local damage is an important function of remodeling. Over time repeated small stresses on the skeleton can produce areas of defective bone, termed micro-damage. Replacement of that damaged bone by remodeling restores bone strength. Signals for these responses are probably developed by the network of osteocytes and osteoblasts, which, through their multiple connections, can detect changes in the stress placed upon bone and in the health of the small areas of micro-damage. Factors that affect the formation, activity, and life span of osteoclasts and osteoblasts as they develop from precursor cells can affect the remodeling cycle. Drugs have been developed that act in these ways, with the goal of reducing bone loss or increasing bone formation and maintaining skeletal health.

What Keeps Bones Healthy?

Both genes and the environment contribute to bone health. Some elements of bone health (e.g., the size and shape of the skeleton) are determined largely by genes, and errors in signaling by these genes can result in birth defects. External factors, such as diet and physical activity, are critically important to bone health throughout life and can be modified. As noted above, the mechanical loading of the skeleton is essential for maintenance of normal bone mass and architecture. In addition, the skeleton needs certain nutritional elements to build tissue. Not only does the skeleton require the same nutritional elements as the rest of the body, but it also has a special requirement for large amounts of calcium and phosphorus. While adequate levels of these minerals can be obtained from the mother during pregnancy and nursing, they must come from the diet thereafter.

The growth of the skeleton, its response to mechanical forces, and its role as a mineral storehouse are all dependent on the proper functioning of a number of systemic or circulating hormones produced outside the skeleton that work in concert with local regulatory factors. The systemic hormones that affect the supply of calcium and phosphorus and the formation and breakdown of bone are listed in Table 2-1. This complex system of regulatory hormones responds to changes in blood calcium and phosphorus, acting not only on bone but also on other tissues such as the intestine and the kidney. The system is illustrated for calcium regulation in Figure 2-4. Under normal conditions only part of the dietary calcium is absorbed and some calcium is secreted into the intestinal tract so that the net amount of calcium entering the body normally is only a small proportion of dietary calcium. In healthy young adults there is calcium balance, where the amount taken in is equal to the amount excreted. The bones are constantly remodeling, but breakdown and formation are equal. The kidney filters the blood, including a large amount of calcium, but most of this is taken back into the body by the kidney cells. When calcium and/or phosphorus are in short supply, the regulating hormones take them out of the bone to serve vital functions in other systems of the body. Too many withdrawals can weaken the bone. The regulatory hormones also play critical roles in determining how much bone is formed at different phases of skeletal growth and how well bone strength and mass is maintained throughout life. For example, sex hormones and the growth hormone system described below are increased during puberty, a time of rapidly increased skeletal growth. Finally, it is important to remember that the effects of hormones and mechanical forces on the skeleton are closely linked. For example, the ability of bone to respond to mechanical loading is impaired in animals lacking the receptor for estrogen (Lee et al. 2003).

Genes, hormones, local factors, and lifestyle all play a role in determining one's peak bone mass, a level that is typically achieved by the time an individual reaches his or her late teens or early 20s. The stronger the bones are at this time, the better able they are to deal with any withdrawals of calcium and phosphorus that are needed and with any other changes to bone that occur with aging.

What follows is a brief description of the most important regulating hormones with respect to bone health.

Calcium-Regulating Hormones

Three calcium-regulating hormones play an important role in producing healthy bone: 1) parathyroid hormone or PTH, which maintains the level of calcium and stimulates both resorption and formation of bone; 2) calcitriol, the hormone derived from vitamin D, which stimulates the intestines to absorb enough calcium and phosphorus and also affects bone directly; and 3) calcitonin, which inhibits bone breakdown and may protect against excessively high levels of calcium in the blood.

Parathyroid hormone or PTH

PTH is produced by four small glands adjacent to the thyroid gland. These glands precisely control the level of calcium in the blood. They are sensitive to small changes in calcium concentration so that when calcium concentration decreases even slightly the secretion of PTH increases. PTH acts on the kidney to conserve calcium and to stimulate calcitriol production, which increases intestinal absorption of calcium. PTH also acts on the bone to increase movement of calcium from bone to blood. Excessive production of PTH, usually due to a small tumor of the parathyroid glands, is called hyperparathyroidism and can lead to bone loss. PTH stimulates bone formation as well as resorption. When small amounts are injected intermittently,

Table 2–1. Most Critical Systemic Hormones Regulating Bone

Calcium Regulating Hormones
Parathyroid Hormone
Calcitriol (Active Vitamin D)
Calcitonin
Sex Hormones
Estrogen
Testosterone
Other Systemic Hormones
Growth Hormone/Insulin-Like Growth Factor
Thyroid Hormone
Cortisol

bone formation predominates and the bones get stronger (Rubin, Cosman et al. 2002). This is the basis for a new treatment for osteoporosis (see Chapter 9).

In recent years a second hormone related to PTH was identified called parathyroid hormone-related protein (PTHrP). This hormone normally regulates cartilage and bone development in the fetus, but it can be over-produced by individuals who have certain types of cancer. PTHrP then acts like PTH, causing excessive bone breakdown and abnormally high blood calcium levels, called hypercalcemia of malignancy (Stewart 2002).

Figure 2–4. Regulation of the Calcium Levels in the Body Fluids

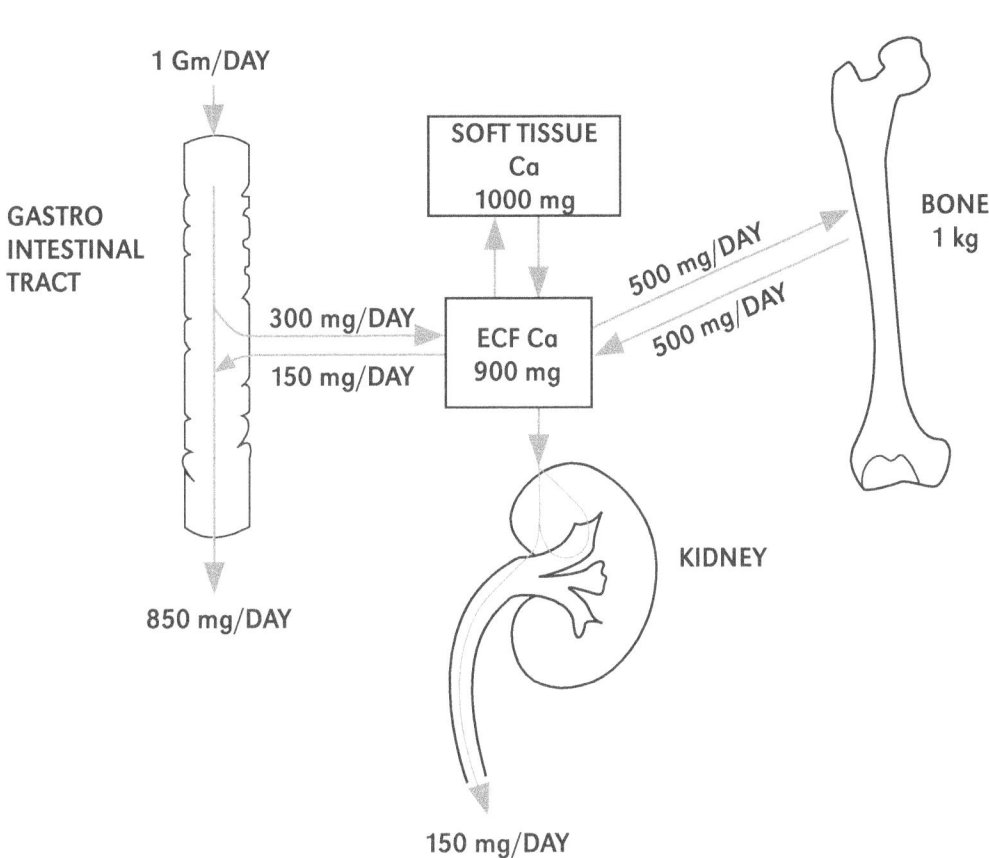

Note: The extracellular fluid (ECF) calcium level is regulated not only by bone, but also by the intestine and kidney as shown in this figure. In addition to the limited absorption of calcium from the intestine, there is secretion of calcium into the intestine as part of the intestinal juices so that the net absorption in an average normal individual may be only 150 mg/day. The movement of calcium in and out of bone in a normal young adult is in balance, that is, bone resorption and bone formation are equal. A large amount of calcium is filtered through the kidney but brought back into the circulation by reabsorption. All of these movements are controlled by hormones, particularly parathyroid hormone, and 1,25 dihydroxy vitamin D (calcitriol). The constant level in the ECF is essential for normal cell function and also for maintaining the right amount of calcium inside the cell.

Source: Mundy and Guise 1999.

Calcitriol

Calcitriol is the hormone produced from vitamin D (Norman, Okamura et al. 2002). Calcitriol, also called 1,25 dihydroxy vitamin D, is formed from vitamin D by enzymes in the liver and kidney. Calcitriol acts on many different tissues, but its most important action is to increase intestinal absorption of calcium and phosphorus, thus supplying minerals for the skeleton. Vitamin D should not technically be called a vitamin, since it is not an essential food element and can be made in the skin through the action of ultra violet light from the sun on cholesterol. Many people need vitamin D in their diet because they do not derive adequate levels from exposure to the sun. This need occurred as people began to live indoors, wear clothes, and move further north. In northern latitudes the sun's rays are filtered in the winter and thus are not strong enough to make sufficient vitamin D in the skin. Vitamin D deficiency leads to a disease of defective mineralization, called rickets in children and osteomalacia in adults. These conditions can result in bone pain, bowing and deformities of the legs, and fractures. Treatment with vitamin D can restore calcium supplies and reduce bone loss.

Calcitonin

Calcitonin is a third calcium-regulating hormone produced by cells of the thyroid gland, although by different cells than those that produce thyroid hormones (Sexton, Findlay et al. 1999). Calcitonin can block bone breakdown by inactivating osteoclasts, but this effect may be relatively transient in adult humans. Calcitonin may be more important for maintaining bone development and normal blood calcium levels in early life. Excesses or deficiencies of calcitonin in adults do not cause problems in maintaining blood calcium concentration or the strength of the bone. However, calcitonin can be used as a drug for treating bone disease.

Sex Hormones

Along with calcium-regulating hormones, sex hormones are also extremely important in regulating the growth of the skeleton and maintaining the mass and strength of bone. The female hormone estrogen and the male hormone testosterone both have effects on bone in men and women (Falahati-Nini, Riggs et al. 2000). The estrogen produced in children and early in puberty can increase bone growth. The high concentration that occurs at the end of puberty has a special effect—that is, to stop further growth in height by closing the cartilage plates at the ends of long bone that previously had allowed the bones to grow in length.

Estrogen acts on both osteoclasts and osteoblasts to inhibit bone breakdown at all stages in life. Estrogen may also stimulate bone formation. The marked decrease in estrogen at menopause is associated with rapid bone loss. Hormone therapy was widely used to prevent this, but this practice is now controversial because of the risks of increased breast cancer, strokes, blood clots, and cardiovascular disease with hormone therapy (see Chapter 9).

Testosterone is important for skeletal growth both because of its direct effects on bone and its ability to stimulate muscle growth, which puts greater stress on the bone and thus increases bone formation. Testosterone is also a source of estrogen in the body; it is converted into estrogen in fat cells. This estrogen is important for the bones of men as well as women. In fact, older men have higher levels of circulating estrogen than do postmenopausal women.

Other Important Hormones

Growth hormone from the pituitary gland is also an important regulator of skeletal growth. It acts by stimulating the production of another hormone called insulin-like growth factor-1 (IGF-1), which is produced in large amounts in the liver and released into circulation. IGF-1 is also produced locally in other tissues, particularly in bone, also under the control of growth hormone. The growth hormone may also directly affect the bone—that is, not through IGF-1 (Wang et al. 2004). Growth hormone is essential for growth and it accelerates skeletal growth at puberty. Decreased production of growth hormone and IGF-1 with age may be responsible for the inability of older individuals to form bone rapidly or to replace bone lost by resorption (Yakar and Rosen 2003). The growth hormone/IGF-1 system stimulates both the bone-resorbing and bone-forming cells, but the dominant effect is on bone formation, thus resulting in an increase in bone mass.

Thyroid hormones increase the energy production of all body cells, including bone cells. They increase the rates of both bone formation and resorption. Deficiency of thyroid hormone can impair growth in children, while excessive amounts of thyroid hormone can cause too much bone breakdown and weaken the skeleton (Vestergaard and Mosekilde 2002). The pituitary hormone that controls the thyroid gland, thyrotropin or TSH, may also have direct effects on bone (Abe et al. 2003).

Cortisol, the major hormone of the adrenal gland, is a critical regulator of metabolism and is important to the body's ability to respond to stress and injury. It has complex effects on the skeleton (Canalis and Delany 2002). Small amounts are necessary for normal bone development, but large amounts block bone growth. Synthetic forms of cortisol, called glucocorticoids, are used to treat many diseases such as asthma and arthritis. They can cause bone loss due both to decreased bone formation and to increased bone breakdown, both of which lead to a high risk of fracture (Kanis et al. 2004).

There are other circulating hormones that affect the skeleton as well. Insulin is important for bone growth, and the response to other factors that stimulate bone growth is impaired in individuals with insulin deficiency (Lu et al. 2003, Suzuki et al. 2003). A recently discovered hormone from fat cells, leptin, has also been shown to have effects on bone (Elefteriou et al. 2004, Cornish et al. 2002).

What Causes Diseases of Bone?

Maintaining a strong and healthy skeleton is a complicated process that requires having the right amount of bone with the right structure and composition in the right place. There are many things that can go wrong along the way.

Genetic abnormalities can produce weak, thin bones, or bones that are too dense. The disease osteogenesis imperfecta is caused by abnormalities in the collagen molecule that make the matrix weak and can lead to multiple fractures. In another congenital disorder, osteopetrosis, the bones are too dense because of failure of osteoclast formation or function. This failure of the remodeling process results in persistence of trabecular bone in the marrow space so that the marrow cavity may not be large enough to form red and white blood cells normally. These dense bones cannot remodel well in response to mechanical forces or micro damage and hence may be weaker and subject to fracture even though bone mass is increased. There are also other abnormalities of the genes that affect the size and shape of the skeleton and can cause deformities or abnormal growth.

Nutritional deficiencies, particularly of vitamin D, calcium, and phosphorus, can result in the formation of weak, poorly mineralized bone. In children, vitamin D deficiency produces rickets in which there is not only a marked weakness of bone and fractures but also bowing of the long bones and a characteristic deformity due to overgrowth of cartilage at the ends of the bones. In adults, vitamin D deficiency leads to a softening of the bone (a condition known as osteomalacia) that can also lead to fractures and deformities.

Many hormonal disorders can also affect the skeleton. Overactive parathyroid glands or hyperparathyroidism can cause excessive bone breakdown and increase the risk of fractures. In severe cases, large holes or cystic lesions appear in the bone, which makes them particularly fragile. A deficiency of the growth hormone/IGF-1 system can inhibit growth, leading to short stature. Loss of gonadal function or hypogonadism in children and young adults can cause severe osteoporosis due to loss of the effects of testosterone and estrogen. In addition, too much cortisol production by the adrenal gland can occur in Cushing's syndrome.

Use of glucocorticoids as medication is a common cause of bone disease. Excess glucocorticoids will stop bone growth in children and cause marked thinning of the bone in adults, often leading to fracture.

Many bone disorders are local, affecting only a small region of the skeleton. Inflammation can lead to bone loss, probably through the production of local resorbing factors by the inflammatory white cells. This process can occur around the affected joints in patients with arthritis. Bacterial infections, such as severe gum inflammation or periodontal disease, can produce loss of the bones around the teeth, and osteomyelitis can produce a loss of bone at the site of infection. This type of bone loss is due to the direct damaging effect of bacterial

products as well as the production of resorbing factors by white cells. Paget's disease is a multifaceted condition in which the first change is the formation of large, highly active, and unregulated osteoclasts that produce abnormal bone resorption. The precise cause of Paget's disease is not known, but it appears to be the consequence of both genetic factors and environmental factors, possibly a viral infection. The osteoblasts try to repair this damage by increasing bone formation. However, the normal bone architecture has been disrupted, leading to weak bones and the potential for fractures and deformities (even though the bones may appear dense on an x-ray). One reason for this is that the new bone formed is disorderly, "woven" bone, which does not have the proper alignment of mineral crystals and collagen matrix. In addition, the new bone may not be in the right place to provide strength.

What Is Osteoporosis?

Osteoporosis is by far the most common bone disease. Osteoporosis is "a skeletal disorder characterized by compromised bone strength, predisposing to an increased risk of fracture" (Osteoporosis 2000). The composition of the mineral and matrix, the fine structure of the trabecular bone, the porosity of the cortical bone, and the presence of micro-fractures and other forms of damage in bone are all important in determining bone strength. Changes in the fine structure or micro-architecture of trabecular bone are particularly important since the most common fractures in osteoporosis occur at the spine, wrist, and hip, sites where trabecular bone predominates. As shown in Figure 2-5, the structure of normal trabecular bone consists of well-connected plates or broad bands that provide great strength. In individuals with osteoporosis these bands are disrupted and often become thin, weakened rods.

Figure 2–5. Normal vs. Osteoporotic Bone

Normal Bone	Osteoporotic Bone
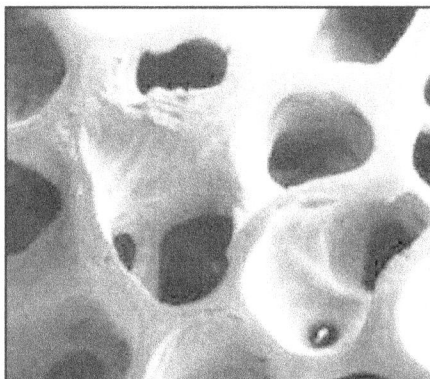	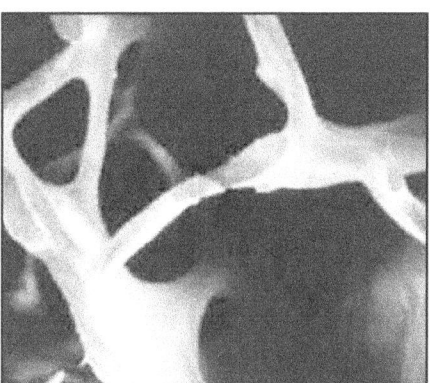

Note: These pictures, called scanning electron micrographs, are from biopsies of a normal and an osteoporotic patient. The normal bone shows a pattern of strong interconnected plates of bone. Much of this bone is lost in osteoporosis and the remaining bone has a weaker rod-like structure. Moreover some of the rods are completely disconnected. These bits of disconnected bone may be measured as bone mass, but contribute nothing to bone strength.

Source: Reproduced from J Bone Miner Res 1986: 1:16-21 with permission from American Society for Bone and Mineral Research.

Some of these rods are no longer connected to another piece of bone, meaning that they no longer contribute to bone strength.

Unfortunately, however, it is not possible to measure bone strength directly, or to detect changes in the micro-architecture of bone in living patients. The mass of bone, its density, and its general shape can be determined by radiographs and absorptiometry (see Chapter 8). These measures are used as "proxies" for bone strength in assessing the risk of osteoporosis today.

There are a number of different ways in which osteoporosis can develop, with the skeleton becoming more fragile and the risk of fracture increasing (Raisz and Rodan 2003). Some of the most important mechanisms that lead to skeletal fragility and fractures are listed in Table 2-2. Many people have relatively weak bones even as young adults because of their genes or because of suboptimal nutrition and lifestyle. However, fractures due to bone fragility rather than severe injury are uncommon in young adults. It is typically not until later in life that bone loss begins due to bone breakdown, a process that accelerates around the time of menopause in women. At the same time, bone formation tends

Table 2–2. Causes of Bone Loss and Fractures in Osteoporosis

Failure to develop a strong skeleton
Genetics–limited growth or abnormal bone composition
Nutrition–Calcium, phosphorous and vitamin D deficiency, poor general nutrition
Lifestyle–lack of weight-bearing exercise, smoking

Loss of bone due to excessive breakdown (resorption)
Decreased sex hormone production
Calcium and vitamin D deficiency, increased parathyroid hormone
Excess production of local resorbing factors

Failure to replace lost bone due to impaired formation
Loss of ability to replenish bone cells with age
Decreased production of systemic growth factors
Loss of local growth factors

Increased tendency to fall
Loss of muscle strength
Slow reflexes and poor vision
Drugs that impair balance

to decrease with age in both men and women, typically failing to keep up with the rate of bone resorption. An imbalance between bone resorption and bone formation results in loss of bone mass, leading to the development of structural abnormalities that make the skeleton more fragile. There are a number of different combinations of increased resorption and decreased formation that can result in a weakened skeletal structure (see Figure 2-5). Each of these pathways can be involved in producing skeletal fragility at different times or sites within an individual patient. Since bone breakdown is the first step in this process, blocking bone resorption is one way to decrease bone loss and prevent fractures. It is currently the most widely used therapeutic approach in osteoporosis. Stimulation of bone formation can also reverse skeletal fragility; new therapies based on this approach have recently been developed (Chapter 9).

The Future: Where a Better Understanding of Bone Biology Can Take Us

This brief overview of the basics of bone health and disease provides a framework for the discussion of what is known about the causes, prevention, and treatment of skeletal disorders today. Many knowledge gaps remain, and it is still unclear precisely why so many people suffer fractures. Fortunately there have recently been a number of exciting new discoveries about skeletal regulation, and there are undoubtedly many more to come. These discoveries will further increase our understanding of bone health and disease.

For example, recent discoveries have shown how osteoblastic and osteoclastic cells communicate and provide signals to begin the process of resorption (Figure 2-6). The osteoblastic cells produce macrophage colony stimulating factor

(M-CSF) and receptor activator of nuclear factor kappa B ligand (RANKL) (Khosla 2001), proteins that bind to receptors on the osteoclast precursors, stimulate their proliferation and differentiation, and increase osteoclast activity. Osteoblastic cells also produce a protein called osteoprotegerin that can bind RANKL and prevent it from interacting with osteoclastic cells. The hormones and local factors that stimulate bone resorption act on this system. The balance between RANKL and osteoprotegerin (OPG) production is probably critical in determining how fast bone breaks down. RANKL in bone is increased in individuals with estrogen deficiency (Eghbali-Fatourechi et al. 2003). While RANKL excess or osteoprotegerin deficiency would be expected to cause bone loss, measurements of the amounts of these proteins in circulating blood do not support this theory. OPG levels are higher and RANKL levels are lower in patients with fractures or low bone mass (Schett et al. 2004, Jorgensen et al. 2004). On the other hand, OPG or drugs that act like it by interfering with the binding of RANKL could be useful in the treatment of osteoporosis.

Recently another signaling system was discovered in bone involving a receptor called lipoprotein receptor-related protein 5. Patients with over-activity in this receptor have strong bones that typically do not fracture (Boyden, Mao et al. 2002; Little, Carulli et al. 2002). Patients in whom this receptor does not function form severe osteoporosis (Gong, Slee et al. 2001). Smaller variations in the gene for this receptor may have an important influence on bone size and strength (Ferrari et al. 2004). Many other genes have also recently been identified as influencing bone mass and strength. A gene for an enzyme called lipoxygenase was recently found to affect bone mass in mice (Klein et al. 2004). Genetics studies in Iceland have shown that variants in one of the genes for bone morphogenetic proteins are associated with osteoporosis (Styrkarsdottir et al. 2003). There are also unidentified genes on specific sites on chromosomes that appear to control bone mass and architecture.

All of these new findings could ultimately lead to much better ways of determining whether or not an individual will develop a disorder of the skeleton. Enough information exists today about the causes, prevention, diagnosis, and treatment of bone diseases to increase the bone health and decrease the risk of fracture among Americans today. The goal of this report is to describe how this can be accomplished and how both personal and public health measures can promote bone health in our population.

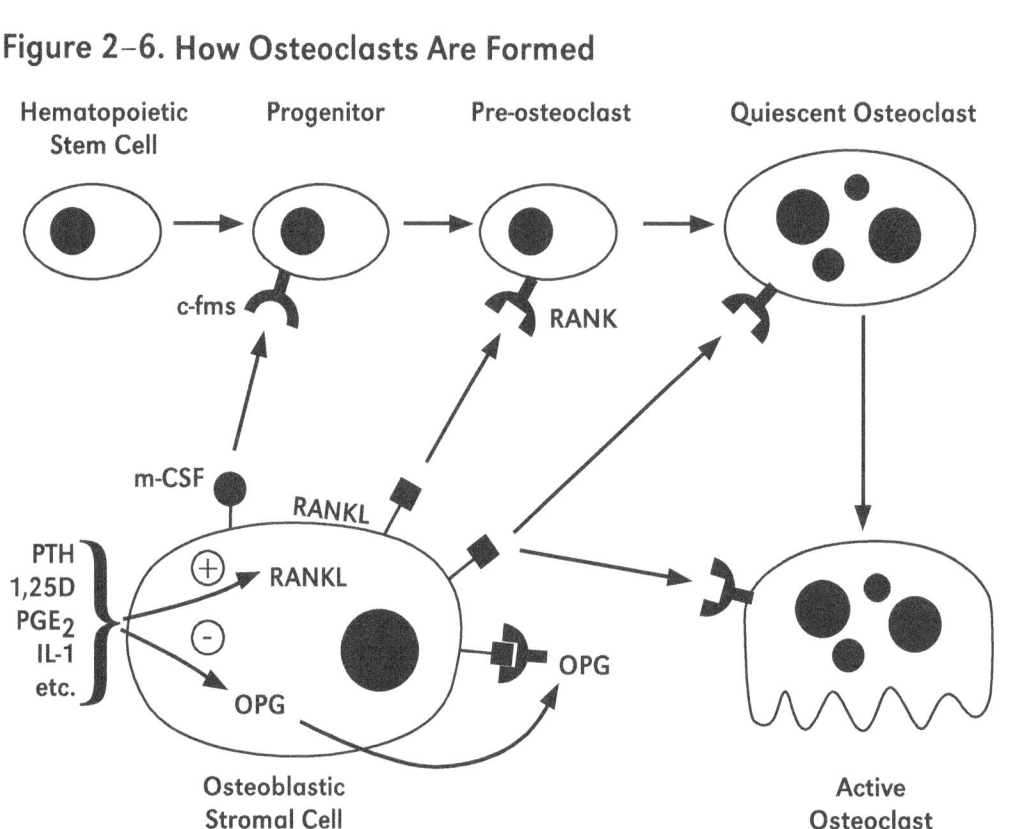

Figure 2–6. How Osteoclasts Are Formed

Note: The interaction between cells of the osteoblastic lineage and the osteoclast lineage is illustrated here. The osteoblastic cells produce several proteins that regulate osteoblast formation and activity. One is *macrophage colony stimulating factor* (M-CSF) that acts on its receptor to increase the number of precursors available to form osteoclasts. The osteoclasts also produce a protein called *receptor activator of nuclear factor kappa B ligand.* (RANKL) that can bind to a receptor on the osteoclast precursors (RANK) and stimulate them to develop into fully differentiated osteoclasts. The RANKL/RANK interaction also increases osteoclast activity. Finally the osteoblastic cells can produce *osteoprotegerin* (OPG), a protein that can be secreted outside the cell and then bind RANKL and prevent it from interacting with RANK, thus blocking the formation and activation of osteoclasts. Hormones and local factors such as parathyroid hormone (PTH), calcitriol or 1,25 dihydroxy D (1,25 D), prostaglandin E2 (PGE$_2$) and Interleukin-1 (IL-1) are shown in this figure as acting on the osteoblastic cells to increase production of RANKL and decrease production of OPG. The balance between RANKL and OPG production determines how fast bone breaks down.

Key Questions for Future Research

Remarkable progress in furthering our understanding of the cellular, molecular biology, and genetics of skeletal tissues in the last quarter century has provided answers to many key questions. As expected, these answers have given rise to additional research questions, as outlined below. The answers to these new questions should, in turn, lead to new approaches to diagnosis, prevention, and treatment. Thus it is important to maintain strong support for basic research, even as existing research findings are applied to the everyday practice of medicine.

- How does the normal skeleton respond to mechanical forces and maintain the best structure?
- How is this response lost in those individuals who develop bone disease?

Local factors that contribute to this process have been identified but their specific roles are not known. In addition, there is a general understanding of bone remodeling, but there are many specific steps—in particular the reversal phase—about which little is known.

- How precisely does estrogen maintain bone mass and strength?
- What is the relative importance of other circulating hormones in maintaining bone health? These include not only the calcium and growth-regulating hormones, but also recently identified hormones such as leptin.
- How do newly identified genes and proteins (e.g., the Wnt signaling pathway) that affect bone cells work?

References

Abe E, Marians RC, Yu W, Wu XB, Ando T, Li Y, Iqbal J, Eldeiry L, Rajendren G, Blair HC, et al. TSH is a negative regulator of skeletal remodeling. Cell. 2003 Oct17;115(2):151-62.

Bilezikian JP, Marcus R, Levine MA, editors. The parathyroids, 2nd ed. San Diego (CA): Academic Press; 2001.

Boyden LM, Mao J, Belsky J, Mitzner L, Farhi A, Mitnick MA, Wu D, Insogna K, Lifton RP. High bone density due to a mutation in LDL-receptor-related protein 5. N Engl J Med. 2002 May 16;346(20):1513-21.

Canalis E, and Delany AM. Mechanisms of glucocorticoid action in bone. Ann N Y Acad Sci. 2002 Jun;966:73-81.

Cornish J, Callon KE, Bava U, Lin C, Naot D, Hill BL, Grey AB, Broom N, Myers DE, Nicholson GC, et al. Leptin directly regulates bone cell function in vitro and reduces bone fragility in vivo. J Endocrinol. 2002 Nov;175(2):405-15.

Eghbali-Fatourechi G, Khosla S, Sanyal A, Boyle WJ, Lacey DL, Riggs BL. Role of RANK ligand in mediating increased bone resorption in early postmenopausal women. J Clin Invest. 2003 Apr;111(8):1221-30.

Elefteriou F, Takeda S, Ebihara K, Magre J, Patano N, Kim CA, Ogawa Y, Liu X, Ware SM, Craigen WJ, et al. Serum leptin level is a regulator of bone mass. Proc Natl Acad Sci U S A. 2004 Mar 2;101(9):3258-63.

Everts V, Delaisse JM, Korper W, Jansen DC, Tigchelaar-Gutter W, Saftig P, Beertsen W. The bone lining cell: Its role in cleaning Howship's lacunae and initiating bone formation. J Bone Miner Res. 2002 Jan;17(1):77-90.

Falahati-Nini A, Riggs BL, Atkinson EJ, O'Fallon WM, Eastell R, Khosla S. Relative contributions of testosterone and estrogen in regulating bone resorption and formation in normal elderly men. J Clin Invest. 2000 Dec;106(12):1553-60.

Favus, MJ, editor. Primer on the metabolic bone diseases and disorders of mineral metabolism. 5th Edition. Washington (DC): American Society for Bone and Mineral Research; 2003.

Ferrari SL, Deutsch S, Choudhury U, Chevalley T, Bonjour JP, Dermitzakis ET, Rizzoli R, Antonarakis SE. Polymorphisms in the low-density lipoprotein receptor-related protein 5 (LRP5) gene are associated with variation in vertebral bone mass, vertebral bone size, and stature in whites. Am J Hum Genet 2004 May;74(5):866-75.

Gong Y, Slee RB, Fukai N, Rawadi G, Roman-Roman S, Reginato AM, Wang H, Cundy T, Glorieux FH, Lev D, et al. LDL receptor-related protein 5 (LRP5) affects bone accrual and eye development. Cell. 2001 Nov 16;107(4): 513-23.

Gray H. Anatomy of the Human Body. Philadelphia: Lea & Febiger, 1918; New York: Bartleby.com, 2000 [cited 2004 Jun 9]. Available from www.bartleby.com/107/illus247.html.

Hauge EM, Qvesel D, Eriksen EF, Mosekilde L, Melsen F. Cancellous bone remodeling occurs in specialized compartments lined by cells expressing osteoblastic markers. J Bone Miner Res. 2001 Sep;16(9): 1575-82.

Huang QY, Recker RR, Deng HW. Searching for osteoporosis genes in the post-genome era: Progress and challenges. Osteoporos Int. 2003 Sep;14(9): 701-15.

Jorgensen HL, Kusk P, Madsen B, Fenger M, Lauritzen JB. Serum osteoprotegerin (OPG) and the A163G polymorphism in the OPG promoter region are related to peripheral measures of bone mass and fracture odds ratios. J Bone Miner Metab. 2004;22(2):132-8.

Kanis JA, Johansson H, Oden A, Johnell O, De Laet C, Melton III LJ, Tenenhouse A, Reeve J, Silman AJ, Pols HA, Eisman JA, McCloskey EV, Mellstrom D. A meta-analysis of prior corticosteroid use and fracture risk. J Bone Miner Res 2004 Jun;19(6):893-99.

Khosla, S. Minireview: the OPG/RANKL/RANK system. Endocrinology. 2001 Dec;142(12):5050-5.

Klein RF, Allard J, Avnur Z, Nikolcheva T, Rotstein D, Carlos AS, Shea M, Waters RV, Belknap JK, et al. Regulation of bone mass in mice by the lipoxygenase gene Alox15. Science. 2004 Jan 9;303(5655): 229-32.

Kontulainen S, Sievanen H, Kannus P, Pasanen M, Vuori I. Effect of long-term impact-loading on mass, size, and estimated strength of humerus and radius of female racquet-sports players: A peripheral quantitative computed tomography study between young and old starters and controls. J Bone Miner Res. 2003 Feb;18(2): 352-9.

Lee K, Jessop H, Suswillo R, Zaman G, Lanyon L. Endocrinology: Bone adaptation requires oestrogen receptor. Nature. 2003;424:389.

Little RD, Carulli JP, Del Mastro RG, Dupuis J, Osborne M, Folz C, Manning SP, Swain PM, Zhao SC, Eustace B, et al. A mutation in the LDL receptor-related protein 5 gene results in the autosomal dominant high-bone-mass trait. Am J Hum Genet. 2002 Jan;70(1): 11-9. Epub 2001 Dec 03.

Lu H, Kraut D, Gerstenfeld LC, Graves DT. Diabetes interferes with the bone formation by affecting the expression of transcription factors that regulate osteoblast differentiation. Endocrinology. 2003 Jan;144(1):346-52.

Marcus R, Feldman D, Kelsey J, editors. Osteoporosis, Second Edition. Volume 2. San Diego (CA): Academic Press; 2001:207-27.

Mundy GR, Guise TA. Hormonal control of calcium homeostasis. Clin Chem 1999 Aug;45(8 Pt 2):1347-52.

Norman AW, Okamura WH, Bishop JE, Henry HL. Update on biological actions of 1alpha,25(OH)(2)-vitamin D(3) (rapid effects) and 24R,25(OH)(2)-vitamin D(3). Mol Cell Endocrinol. 2002 Nov 29;197(1-2): 1-13.

Osteoporosis Prevention, Diagnosis, and Therapy. NIH Consensus Statement Online 2000 March 27-29; [cited 2004 Mar 26]; 17(1): 1-36.

Parfitt AM. The bone remodeling compartment: A circulatory function for bone lining cells. J Bone Miner Res. 2001 Sep;16(9):1583-5.

Raisz LG, Rodan GA. Pathogenesis of osteoporosis. Endocrinol Metab Clin North Am. 2003 Mar;32(1):15-24.

Rauch F and Glorieux FH. Osteogenesis imperfecta. Lancet. 2004 Apr 24;363(9418):1377-85.

Rubin MR, Cosman F, Lindsay R, Bilezikian JP. The anabolic effects of parathyroid hormone. Osteoporos Int. 2002;13(4):267-77.

Schett G, Kiechl S, Redlich K, Oberhollenzer F, Weger S, Egger G, Mayr A, Jocher J, Xu Q, Pietschmann P, et al. Soluble RANKL and risk of nontraumatic fracture. JAMA 2004 Mar 3;291(9):1108-13.

Seeman E. Periosteal bone formation—a neglected determinant of bone strength. N Engl J Med. 2003 Jul 24;349(4):320-3.

Sexton PM, Findlay DM, Martin TJ. Calcitonin. Curr Med Chem. 1999 Nov;6(11):1067-93.

Stewart A F. Hyperparathyroidism, humoral hypercalcemia of malignancy, and the anabolic actions of parathyroid hormone and parathyroid hormone-related protein on the skeleton. J Bone Miner Res. 2002 May;17(5):758-62.

Styrkarsdottir U, Cazier JB, Kong A, Rolfsson O, Larsen H, Bjarnadottir E, Johannsdottir VD, Sigurdardottir MS, Bagger Y, Christiansen C,et al. Linkage of Osteoporosis to Chromosome 20p12 and Association to BMP2. PLoS Biol. 2003 Dec;1(3):E69.

Suzuki K, Miyakoshi N, Tsuchida T, Kasukawa Y, Sato K, Itoi E. Effects of combined treatment of insulin and human parathyroid hormone (1-34) on cancellous bone mass and structure in streptozotocin-induced diabetic rats. Bone. 2003 Jul;33(1):108-14.

Vestergaard P, Mosekilde L. Fractures in patients with hyperthyroidism and hypothyroidism: A nationwide follow-up study in 16,249 patients. Thyroid. 2002 May;12(5):411-9.

Yakar S, Rosen CJ. From mouse to man: Redefining the role of insulin-like growth factor-I in the acquisition of bone mass. Exp Biol Med (Maywood). 2003 Mar;228(3):245-52.

Wang J, Zhou J, Cheng CM, Kopchick JJ, Bondy CA. Evidence supporting dual, IGF-I-independent and IGF-I-dependent, roles for GH in promoting longitudinal bone growth. J Endocrinol. 2004 Feb;180(2):247-55.

Chapter 3: Key Messages

- Osteoporosis affects millions of Americans. Individuals with osteoporosis are at high risk of suffering one or more fractures, which are often physically debilitating and can potentially lead to a downward spiral in physical and mental health.

- The most common form of osteoporosis is known as "primary osteoporosis." It is the result of the cumulative impact of bone loss and deterioration of bone structure as people age. This bone loss can be minimized and osteoporosis prevented through adequate nutrition, physical activity, and, if necessary, appropriate treatment.

- There are a wide variety of diseases and certain medications and toxic agents that can cause or contribute to the development of osteoporosis. If recognized as a potential threat, this form of the disease—known as secondary osteoporosis—can often be prevented through proper nutrition and physical activity, along with appropriate therapy if needed.

- A number of childhood diseases cause rickets, a condition that results from a delay in depositing calcium phosphate mineral in growing bones. This delay leads to skeletal deformities, especially bowed legs. In adults, the equivalent disease is called osteomalacia. Both diseases can generally be prevented by ensuring adequate levels of vitamin D, but they can have devastating consequences for affected individuals.

- Patients with chronic renal disease are at risk for developing a complex bone disease known as renal osteodystrophy. While dialysis and transplantation have extended the life-expectancy of these patients, it may not prevent further progression of bone disease.

- Paget's disease of bone is a progressive, often crippling disorder of bone remodeling that commonly involves the spine, pelvis, legs, or skull (although any bone can be affected). If diagnosed early, its impact can be minimized.

- A large number of genetic and developmental disorders affect the skeleton. Among the more common of these is osteogenesis imperfecta (OI). Patients with this condition have bones that break easily.

- Some skeletal disorders tend to develop later in life. One of the most common of these acquired skeletal disorders is a malignancy of the bone. These malignancies can originate in the bone (primary tumors) or, much more commonly, result from the seeding of bone by tumors outside of the skeleton (metastatic tumors). Primary bone cancer also occurs in children. Both types of tumors can destroy bone.

Chapter 3

DISEASES OF BONE

The body systems that control the growth and maintenance of the skeleton, which are described in Chapter 2, can be disrupted in different ways that result in a variety of bone diseases and disorders. These include problems that can occur at or before birth, such as genetic abnormalities and developmental defects, as well as diseases such as osteoporosis and Paget's disease of bone that damage the skeleton later in life. In addition to conditions that affect bone directly, there are many other disorders that indirectly affect bone by interfering with mineral metabolism. This chapter reviews some of the more common diseases, disorders, and conditions that both directly and indirectly affect bone.

Osteoporosis

As pointed out in Chapter 2, osteoporosis is a disease characterized by low bone mass and deterioration of bone structure that causes bone fragility and increases the risk of fracture. For practical purposes, the World Health Organization has defined osteoporosis as a bone mineral density (BMD) value more than 2.5 standard deviations below the mean for normal young White women. Osteoporosis is a common disease affecting millions of Americans. As described in Chapters 4 and 5, it can have devastating consequences. Individuals with osteoporosis are at high risk of suffering one or more fractures, injuries that can often be

Classical Case

"A classical case of osteoporosis may start in a woman about 55 years of age with a wrist fracture. Ten years later she may present with back pain, with or without minor trauma, and thoracolumbar spine x-rays may show a vertebral fracture. She might have one of several risk factors: low body weight, premature menopause, a family history of fractures, smoking, heavy alcohol consumption, inactivity, calcium or vitamin D deficiency, or corticosteroid use. The back pain may remit and relapse with subsequent vertebral fractures. Approximately 10–15 years later, at the age of 75–80 years, the patient may fall and sustain a hip fracture, resulting in hospitalization, a 20 percent excess risk of death, considerable functional impairment and possibly a loss of independence if she survives. Although this scenario is instantly recognizable, osteoporosis may present with any of a wide range of fractures and at a variety of ages; it is also increasingly recognized among men" (WHO 2003). Recognition that the first fracture was a sentinel event may have triggered a detailed assessment that could potentially have prevented additional fractures. See Chapter 8 for more information on such assessments.

physically debilitating and potentially lead to a downward spiral in physical and mental health (Figure 3-1). Generalized osteoporosis is the most common form of the disease, affecting most of the skeleton. Osteoporosis can also occur in localized parts of the skeleton as a result of injury or conditions that reduce muscle forces on the bone, such as limb paralysis. There are a variety of different types of osteoporosis. The most common form of osteoporosis is known as "primary osteoporosis"—that is, osteoporosis that is not caused by some other specific disorder. Bone loss caused by specific diseases or medications (see below) is referred to as "secondary osteoporosis." Each of these major categories of osteoporosis is discussed in more detail on the following pages.

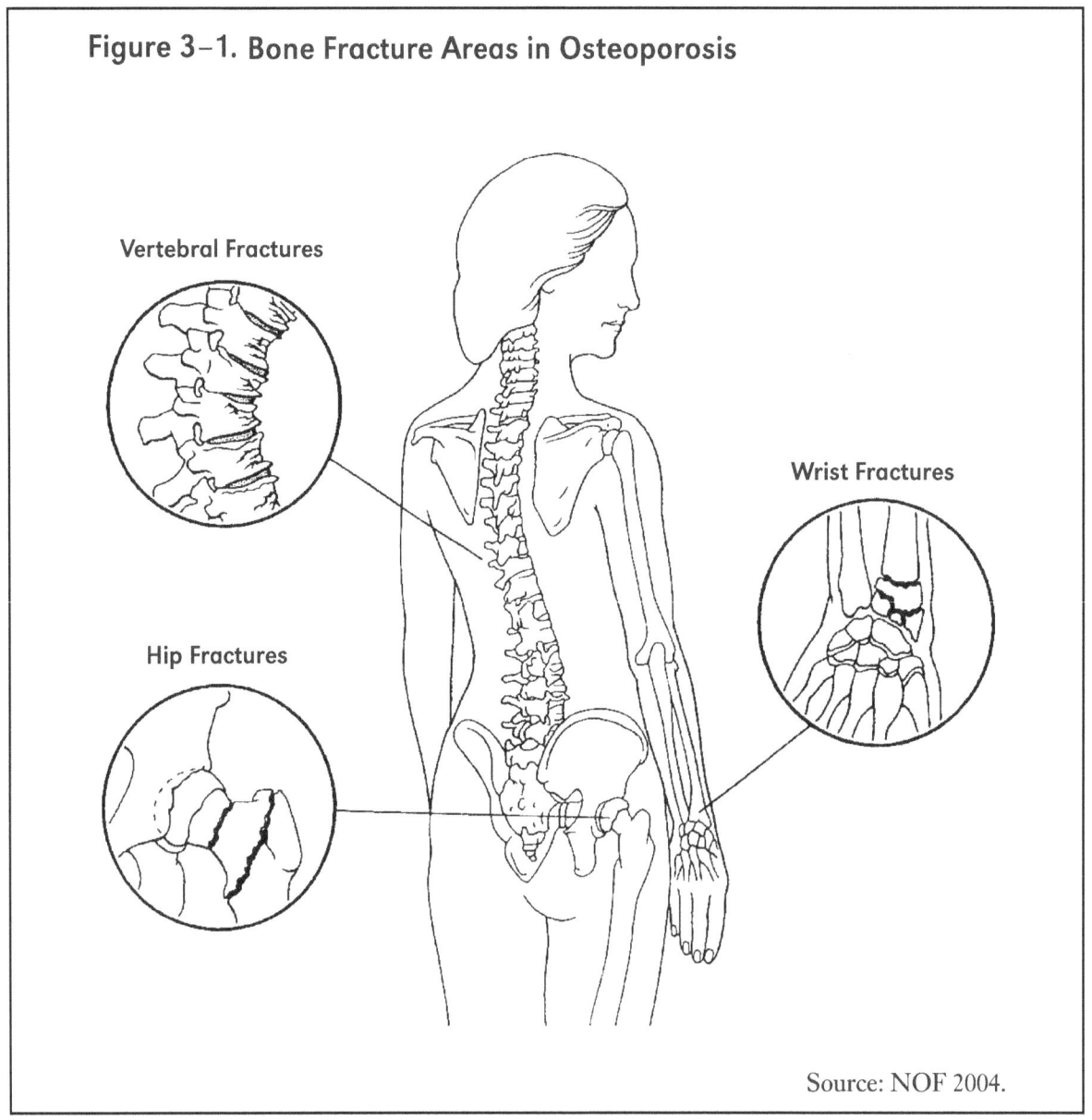

Figure 3–1. Bone Fracture Areas in Osteoporosis

Vertebral Fractures

Wrist Fractures

Hip Fractures

Source: NOF 2004.

Primary Osteoporosis

Primary osteoporosis is mainly a disease of the elderly, the result of the cumulative impact of bone loss and deterioration of bone structure that occurs as people age (Seeman 2003). This form of osteoporosis is sometimes referred to as age-related osteoporosis. Since postmenopausal women are at greater risk, the term "postmenopausal" osteoporosis is also used. Younger individuals (including children and young adults) rarely get primary osteoporosis, although it can occur on occasion. This rare form of the disease is sometimes referred to as "idiopathic" osteoporosis, since in many cases the exact causes of the disease are not known, or idiopathic. Since the exact mechanisms by which aging produces bone loss are not all understood (that is, it is not always clear why some postmenopausal women develop osteoporosis while others do not), age-related osteoporosis is also partially idiopathic. A brief review of "idiopathic" primary osteoporosis and a more detailed review of the more common condition of age-related osteoporosis follows.

Idiopathic Primary Osteoporosis

There are several different forms of idiopathic osteoporosis that can affect both children and adolescents, although these conditions are quite rare (Norman 2003). Juvenile osteoporosis affects previously healthy children between the ages of 8 and 14. Over a period of several years, bone growth is impaired. The condition may be relatively mild, causing only one or two collapsed bones in the spine (vertebrae), or it may be severe, affecting virtually the entire spine. The disease almost always goes into remission (spontaneously) around the time of puberty with a resumption of normal bone growth at that time. Patients with mild or moderate forms of the disease may be left with a curvature of the spine (kyphosis) and short stature, but those with a more severe form of the disease may be incapacitated for life.

Primary osteoporosis is quite rare in young adults. In this age-group, the disease is usually caused by some other condition or factor, such as anorexia nervosa or glucocorticoid use (Khosla et al. 1994). When idiopathic forms of primary osteoporosis do occur in young adults, they appear in men as often as they do in women (this is in contrast to age-related primary osteoporosis, which occurs more often in women). The characteristics of the disease can vary broadly and may involve more than one disorder. Some young adults with idiopathic primary osteoporosis may have a primary defect in the regulation of bone cell function, resulting in depressed bone formation, increased bone resorption, or both (see Chapter 2). Others with a mild form of the disease may simply have failed to achieve an adequate amount of skeletal mass during growth. In some patients, the disease runs a mild course, even without treatment, and the clinical manifestations are limited to asymptomatic spinal compression fractures. More typically, however, multiple spine fractures occur over a 5–10 year period leading to a height loss of up to 6 inches.

Age-Related Osteoporosis

Age-related osteoporosis is by far the most common form of the disease (Figure 3-2). There are many different causes of the ailment, but the bone loss that leads to the disease typically begins relatively early in life, at a time when corrective action (such as changes in diet and physical activity) could potentially slow down its course. While it occurs in both sexes, the disease is two to three times more common in women (see Chapter 4). This is partly due to the fact that women have two phases of age-related bone loss—a rapid phase that begins at menopause and lasts 4–8 years, followed by a slower continuous phase that lasts throughout the rest of life (Riggs et al. 2002). By contrast, men go through only the slow, continuous phase. As a result, women typically lose more bone than do men. The rapid phase of bone loss alone in women results in losses of 5–10 percent of cortical bone (which makes up the hard outer shell of the skeleton) and 20–30 percent of trabecular bone (which fills the ends of the limb bones and the vertebral bodies in the spine, the sites of most osteoporotic fractures). The slow phase of bone loss results in losses of 20–25 percent of cortical and trabecular bone in both men and women, but over a longer period of time (Riggs et al. 2002).

Although other factors such as genetics and nutrition contribute, both the rapid phase of bone loss in postmenopausal women and the slow phase of bone loss in aging women and men appear to be largely the result of estrogen deficiency. (This is demonstrated by the fact that correction of estrogen deficiency can prevent these changes.) For women, the rapid phase of bone loss is initiated by a dramatic decline in estrogen production by the ovaries at menopause. The loss of estrogen action on estrogen receptors in bone results in large increases in bone resorption (see Chapter 2), combined with reduced bone formation. The end result is thinning of the cortical outer shell of bone and damage to the trabecular bone structure (see Figure 2-5, Chapter 2). There may be some countervailing forces on this process, as the outside diameter of the bone can increase with age, thus helping to maintain bone strength (Ahlborg et al. 2003).

By contrast, the slower phase of bone loss is thought to be caused by a combination of factors including age-related impairment of bone formation, decreased calcium and vitamin D intake, decreased physical activity, and the loss of estrogen's positive effects on calcium balance

in the intestine and kidney as well as its effects on bone (Riggs et al. 2002). This leads to further impairment of absorption of calcium by the intestine and reduced ability of the kidney to conserve calcium. If the amount of calcium absorbed from the diet is insufficient to make up for the obligatory calcium losses in the stool and urine, serum calcium begins to fall. Parathyroid hormone levels will then increase, removing calcium from bone to make up for the loss, as illustrated in Figure 3-3. The net result of this process is an increase in bone resorption. It is important to realize that these mineral losses need not be great to result in osteoporosis. A negative balance of only 50–100 mg of calcium per day (far less than the 300 mg of calcium in a single glass of milk) over a long period of time is sufficient to produce the disease.

For aging men, sex steroid deficiency also appears to be a major factor in age-related osteoporosis. Although testosterone is the major sex steroid in men, some of it is converted by the aromatase enzyme into estrogen. In men, however, the deficiency is mainly due to an increase in sex hormone binding globulin, a substance that holds both testosterone and estrogen in a form that is not available for use by the body. Between 30–50 percent of elderly men are deficient in biologically active sex steroids (Khosla et al. 1998). In fact, except for the lack of the early postmenopausal phase, the process of bone loss in older men is similar to that for older women. As with women, the loss of sex steroid activity in men has an effect on calcium absorption and conservation, leading to progressive secondary increases in parathyroid hormone levels. As in older women, the resulting imbalance between bone resorption and formation results in slow bone loss that continues over life. Since testosterone may stimulate bone formation more than estrogen does, however, decreased bone

Figure 3–2. Progressive Spinal Deformity in Osteoporosis

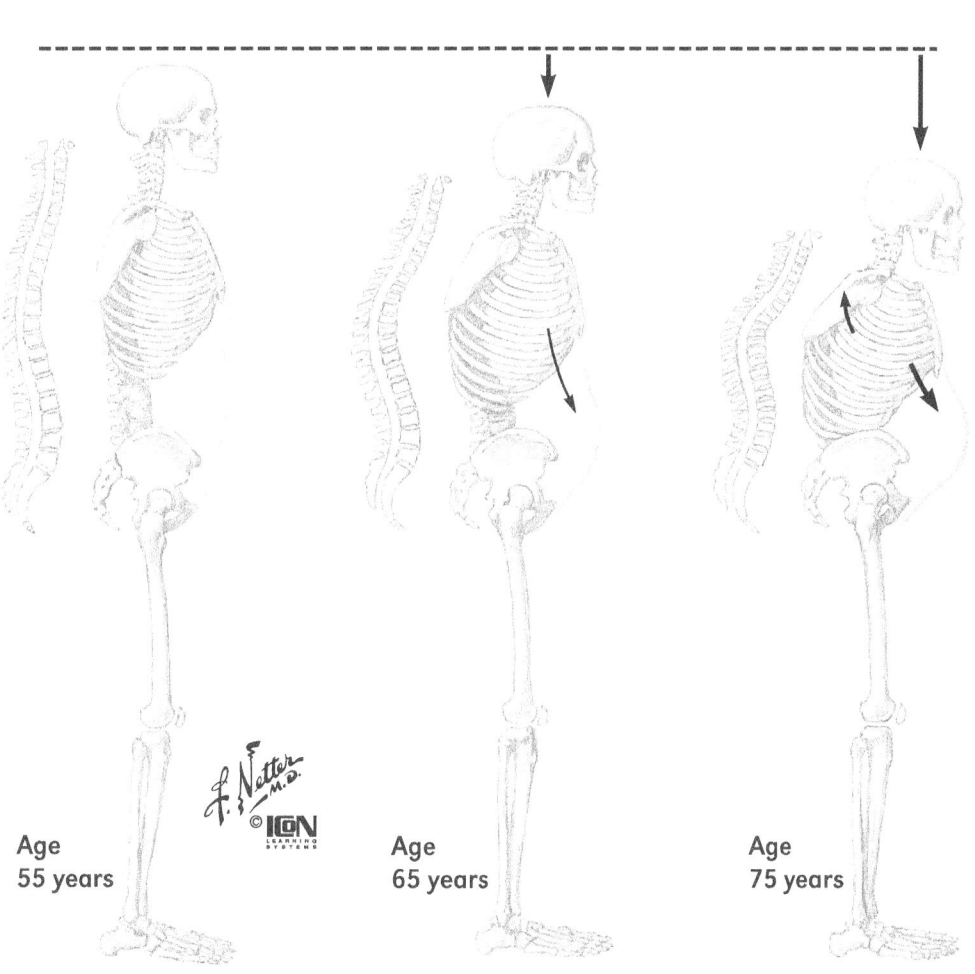

Age
55 years

Age
65 years

Age
75 years

Note: Compression fractures of thoracic vertebrae lead to loss of height and progressive thoracic kyphosis (dowager's hump). Lower ribs eventually rest on ileac crests, and downward pressure on viscera causes abdominal distention.

Source: Netter 1987. Netter Illustrations used with permission from Icon Learning Systems, a division of MediMedia, USA, Inc. All rights reserved.

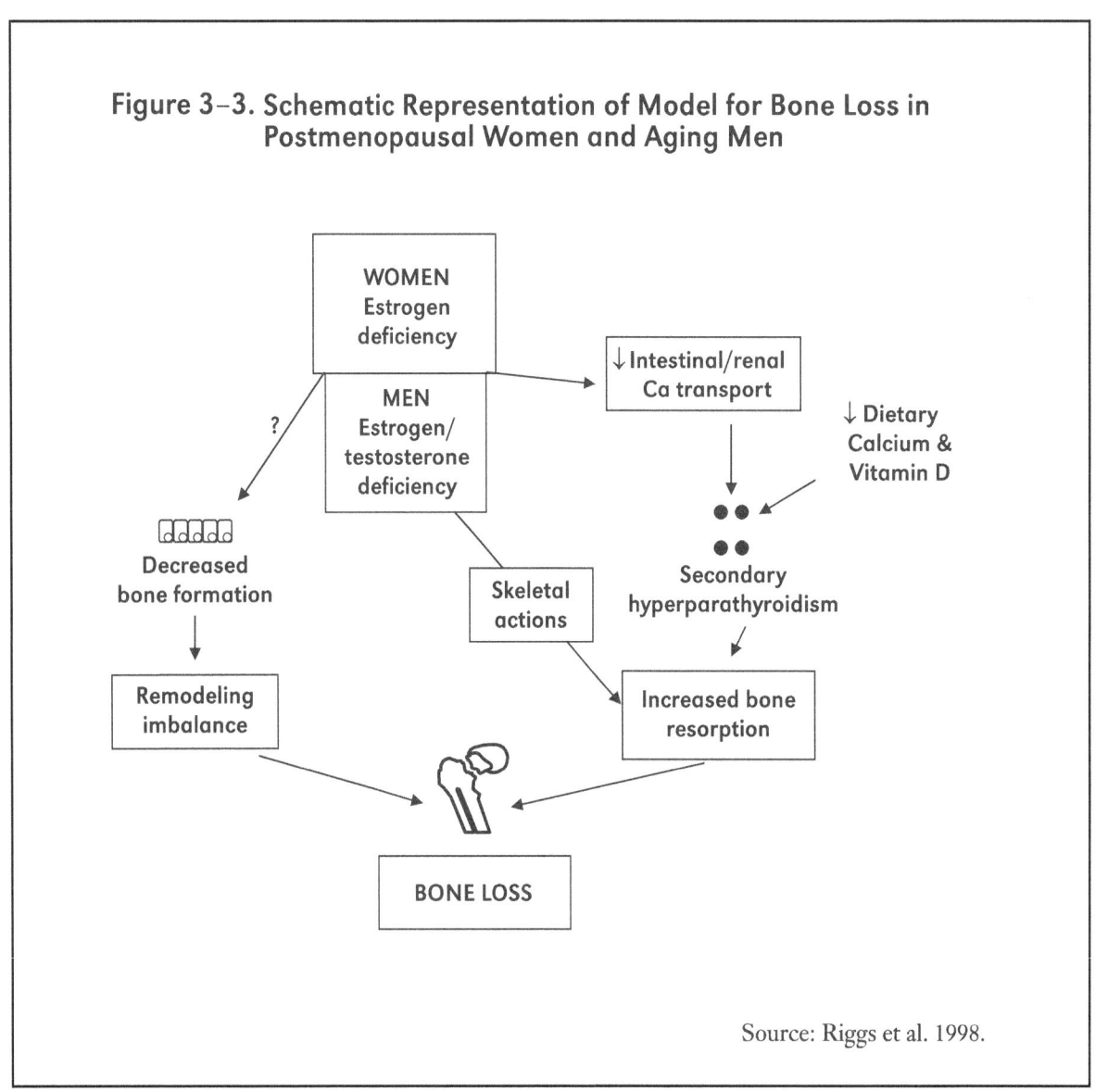

Figure 3–3. Schematic Representation of Model for Bone Loss in Postmenopausal Women and Aging Men

Source: Riggs et al. 1998.

formation plays a relatively greater role in the bone loss experienced by elderly men.

Secondary Osteoporosis

Young adults and even older individuals who get osteoporosis often do so as a byproduct of another condition or medication use. In fact, there are a wide variety of diseases (Table 3-1) along with certain medications and toxic agents (Table 3-2) that can cause or contribute to the development of osteoporosis (Stein and Shane 2003). Individuals who get the disease due to these "outside" causes are said to have "secondary" osteoporosis. They typically experience greater levels of bone loss than would be expected for a normal individual of the same age, gender, and race. Secondary causes of the disease are common in many premenopausal women and men with osteoporosis (Khosla et al. 1994); in fact, by some estimates the majority of men with osteoporosis exhibit secondary

Table 3–1. Diseases That Cause or Contribute to Secondary Osteoporosis

Genetic Disorders

Cystic Fibrosis	Homocystinuria	Osteogenesis Imperfecta
Ehlers-Danlos	Hypophosphatasia	Porphyria
Glycogen Storage Diseases	Idiopathic Hypercalciuria	Riley-Day Syndrome
Gaucher's Disease	Marfan Syndrome	
Hemochromatosis	Menkes Steely Hair Syndrome	

Hypogonadal States

Androgen Insensitivity	Hyperprolactinemia	Turner's and Klinefelter's
Anorexia Nervosa	Panhypopituitarism	Syndrome
Athletic Amenorrhea	Premature ovarian failure	

Endocrine Disorders

Acromegaly	Cushing's Syndrome	Hyperparathyroidism
Adrenal Insufficiency	Diabetes Mellitus (Type I)	Thyrotoxicosis

Gastrointestinal Diseases

Gastrectomy	Malabsorption	Primary Biliary Cirrhosis
Inflammatory Bowel Disease	Celiac Disease	

Hematologic Disorders

Hemophilia	Multiple Myeloma	Systemic Mastocytosis
Leukemias and Lymphomas	Sickle Cell Disease	Thalassemia

Rheumatic and Auto-Immune Diseases

Ankylosing Spondylitis	Lupus	Rheumatoid Arthritis

Miscellaneous

Alcoholism	Emphysema	Multiple Sclerosis
Amyloidosis	End Stage Renal Disease	Muscular Dystrophy
Chronic Metabolic Acidosis	Epilepsy	Post-transplant Bone
Congestive Heart Failure	Idiopathic Scoliosis	Disease
Depression	Immobilization	Sarcoidosis

causes of the disease (Orwoll 1998). In addition, up to a third of postmenopausal women with osteoporosis also have other conditions that may contribute to their bone loss (Tannenbaum et al. 2002). This section briefly describes some of the more common diseases, disorders, and medications that can cause or contribute to the development of osteoporosis.

Diseases and Disorders That Can Cause Osteoporosis

Several genetic diseases have been linked to secondary osteoporosis. Idiopathic hyper-calciuria and cystic fibrosis are the most common. Patients with cystic fibrosis have markedly decreased bone density and increased fracture rates (Ott and Aitken 1998) due to a variety of factors, including calcium and vitamin D malabsorption, reduced sex steroid production and delayed puberty, and increased inflammatory cytokines (see Chapter 2). Some patients with idiopathic hypercalciuria have a renal defect in the ability of the kidney to conserve calcium. This condition may be aggravated if they are advised to lower their dietary calcium intake to prevent kidney stones. Several studies have documented low bone density in these individuals, and they may respond to drugs that decrease calcium excretion in the urine. Other genetic disorders (listed in Table 3-1), although rare, should be considered in patients with osteoporosis after more common causes have been excluded.

Estrogen or testosterone deficiency during adolescence (due to Turner's, Kallman's, or Klinefelter's syndrome, anorexia nervosa, athletic amenorrhea, cancer, or any chronic illness that interferes with the onset of puberty) leads to low peak bone mass (Riggs et al. 2002). Estrogen deficiency that develops after peak bone mass is achieved but before normal menopause (due to premature ovarian failure for

example) is associated with rapid bone loss. Low sex steroid levels may also be responsible for reduced bone density in patients with androgen insensitivity or acromegaly. By contrast, excess thyroid hormone (thyrotoxicosis), whether spontaneous or caused by overtreatment with thyroid hormone, may be associated with substantial bone loss (Ross 1994); while bone turnover is increased in these patients, bone resorption is increased more than bone formation. Likewise, excess production of glucocorticoids caused by tumors of the pituitary or adrenal glands (Cushing's syndrome) can lead to rapidly progressive and severe osteoporosis, as can treatment with glucocorticoids (see below). The relationship between diabetes and osteoporosis is more controversial (Stein and Shane 2003). For example, hip fractures are increased in some studies of diabetic patients, but not in others. In general, patients with type 1 (insulin-dependent) diabetes, particularly those with poor control of their blood sugar (Heap et al. 2004), are at greater risk of osteoporosis than are those with type 2 (non-insulin dependent) diabetes (Piepkorn et al. 1997).

Primary hyperparathyroidism is a relatively common condition in older individuals, especially postmenopausal women, that is caused by excessive secretion of parathyroid hormone. Most often, the cause is a benign tumor (adenoma) in one or more parathyroid glands; very rarely (less than 0.5 percent of the time) the cause is parathyroid cancer (Wynne et al. 1992). Since most patients now come to clinical attention when they are unexpectedly found on routine examination to have an abnormally high calcium level in the blood (Wermers et al. 1997), the clinical presentation has changed over the past 30 years from an uncommon but highly symptomatic disorder involving renal stones and bone disease (osteitis fibrosa cystica) to a common but relatively asymptomatic condition (Silverberg and Bilezikian 2001). Typically, cortical bone (for example, in the distal forearm) is affected to a greater extent than trabecular bone (for example, in the spine) in primary hyperparathyroidism (Silverberg et al. 1989). It is presumed that the reduction in bone mass is associated with the increased risk of fracture seen in these patients (Khosla and Melton 2002).

Diseases that reduce intestinal absorption of calcium and phosphorus, or impair the availability of vitamin D, can also cause bone disease. Moderate malabsorption results in osteoporosis, but severe malabsorption may cause osteomalacia (see below). Celiac disease, due to inflammation of the small intestine by ingestion of gluten, is an important and commonly overlooked cause of secondary osteoporosis (Bianchi and Bianchi 2002). Likewise, osteoporosis and fractures have been found in patients following surgery to remove part of the stomach (gastrectomy), especially in women. Bone loss is seen after gastric bypass surgery even in morbidly obese women who do not have low bone mass initially (Coates et al. 2004). Increased osteoporosis and fractures are also seen in patients with Crohn's disease and ulcerative colitis (Bernstein et al. 2000). Glucocorticoids, commonly used to treat both disorders, probably contribute to the bone loss. Similarly, diseases that impair liver function (primary biliary cirrhosis, chronic active hepatitis, cirrhosis due to hepatitis B and C, and alcoholic cirrhosis) may result in disturbances in vitamin D metabolism and may also cause bone loss by other mechanisms. Primary biliary cirrhosis is associated with particularly severe osteoporosis. Fractures are more frequent in patients with alcoholic cirrhosis than any other types of liver disease, although this may be related to the increased risk of falling among heavy drinkers (Crawford et al. 2003). Human immunodeficiency virus (HIV) infected patients also have a higher prevalence of osteopenia or osteoporosis (Brown et al. 2004). This may involve multiple endocrine, nutritional, and metabolic factors and may also be affected by the antiviral therapy that HIV patients receive (Thomas and Doherty 2003).

Autoimmune and allergic disorders are associated with bone loss and increased fracture risk. This is due not only to the effect of immobilization and the damage to bone by the products of inflammation from the disorders themselves, but also from the glucocorticoids that are used to treat these conditions (Lien et al. 2003, Orstavik et al. 2004). Rheumatic diseases like lupus and rheumatoid arthritis have both been associated with lower bone mass and an increased risk of fractures. A study found that 12 percent of women with systemic lupus erythematosus reported at least one fracture since the onset of disease, a 4.7-fold higher risk of fracture than for the typical woman. Fractures in these women were found to be associated with the following: older age at diagnosis, longer disease duration, longer duration of steroid use, and post-menopausal status (Ramsey-Goldman et al. 1999, Haugeberg et al. 2003).

Many neurologic disorders are associated with impaired bone health and an increased risk of fracture (Whooley, Kip et al. 1999; Lloyd, Spector et al. 2000). This may be due in part to the effects of these disorders on mobility and balance or to the effects of drugs used in treating these disorders on bone and mineral metabolism. Unfortunately, however, health care providers often fail to assess the bone health of patients who have these disorders or to provide appropriate preventive and therapeutic measures. For example, patients with stroke, spinal cord injury, or neurologic disorders show rapid bone loss in the affected areas (Dauty, Perrouin Verbe et al. 2000; Poole, Reeve et al. 2002; Tuzun, Altintas et al. 2003). There are many disabling conditions that can lead to bone loss, and thus it is important to pay attention to bone health in patients with developmental disabilities, such as cerebral palsy, as well as diseases affecting nerve and muscle, such as poliomyelitis and multiple sclerosis. Children and adolescents with these disorders are unlikely to achieve optimal peak bone mass, due both to an increase in bone resorption and a decrease in bone formation. In some cases very rapid bone loss can produce a large enough increase in blood calcium levels to produce symptoms (Carey and Raisz 1985; Go 2001). Fractures are common in these individuals not only because of bone loss, but also because of muscular weakness and neurologic impairment that increases the likelihood of falls. Bone loss can be slowed—but not completely prevented—by antiresorptive therapy (Sato, Asoh et al. 2000). Epilepsy is another neurologic disorder that increases the risk of bone disease, primarily because of the adverse effects of anti-epileptic drugs. Many of the drugs used in epilepsy can impair vitamin D metabolism, probably by acting on the liver enzyme which converts vitamin D to 25 hydroxy vitamin D (Farhat, Yamout et al. 2000, Sheth 2002). In addition, there may be a direct effect of these agents on bone cells. Due to the negative bone-health effects of drugs, most epilepsy patients are at risk of developing osteoporosis. In those who have low vitamin D intakes, intestinal malabsorption, or low sun exposure, the additional effect of anti-epileptic drugs can lead to osteomalacia. Supplemental vitamin D may be effective in slowing bone loss, although patients who develop osteoporosis may require additional therapy such as bisphosphonates.

Psychiatric disorders can also have a negative impact on bone health. While anorexia nervosa is the psychiatric disorder that is most regularly associated with osteoporosis, major depression, a much more common disorder, is also associated with low bone mass and an increased risk of fracture (Coelho, Silva et al. 1999; Cizza, Ravn et al. 2001; Robbins, Hirsch et al. 2001). Many studies show lower BMD in depressed patients (Michelson et al. 1996). In addition, one large study found an increased incidence of falls and fractures among depressed women, even though there was no difference between their BMD and that of non-depressed women included in the study (Whooley, Kip et al. 1999). Higher scores for depressive symptoms have also been reported in women with osteoporosis. Yet what these studies do not make clear is whether major depression causes low BMD and increased fracture risk, or whether the depression is a consequence of the diminished quality of life and disability that occurs in many osteoporotic patients. One factor that may cause bone loss in severely depressed individuals is increased production of cortisol, the adrenal stress hormone. Whatever the cause of low BMD and increased fracture risk, measurement of BMD is appropriate in both men and women with major depression. While the response of individuals with major depression to calcium, vitamin D, or antiresorptive therapy has not been specifically documented, it would seem reasonable to provide these preventive measures to patients at high risk.

Finally, several diseases that are associated with osteoporosis are not easily categorized. Aseptic necrosis (also called osteonecrosis or avascular necrosis) is a well-known skeletal disorder that may be a complication of injury, treatment with glucocorticoids, or alcohol abuse (Pavelka 2000). This condition commonly affects the ends of the femur and the humerus. The precise cause is unknown, but at least two theories have been suggested. One is that blood supply to the bone is blocked by collapsing bone. The other is that microscopic fat particles block blood flow and result in bone cell death. Chronic obstructive pulmonary disease (emphysema and chronic bronchitis) is also now recognized as being associated with osteoporosis and fractures even in the absence of glucocorticoid therapy. Immobilization is clearly associated with rapid bone loss; patients with spinal cord lesions are at particularly high risk for fragility fractures (Kiratli 2001). However, even modest reductions in physical activity can lead to bone loss (see Chapter 6). Hematological disorders, particularly malignancies, are commonly associated with osteoporosis and fractures as well. These are discussed in more detail later in the chapter.

Medications and Therapies That Can Cause Osteoporosis

Osteoporosis can also be a side effect of particular medical therapies (Table 3-2).

Table 3-2. Medications Associated With Secondary Osteoporosis

Anticoagulants (heparin)
Anticonvulsants
Cyclosporine A and Tacrolimus
Cancer Chemotherapeutic Drugs
Glucocorticoids (and ACTH)
Gonadotropin-releasing Hormone Agonists
Lithium
Methotrexate
Parenteral Nutrition
Thyroxine

Glucocorticoid-Induced Osteoporosis (GIO). GIO is by far the most common form of osteoporosis produced by drug treatment. While it has been known for many years that excessive production of the adrenal hormone cortisol can cause thinning of the bone and fractures, this condition, a form of Cushing's syndrome, remains uncommon. With the increased use of prednisone and other drugs that act like cortisol for the treatment of many inflammatory and autoimmune diseases, this form of bone loss has become a major clinical concern. The concern is greatest for those diseases in which the inflammation itself and/or the immobilization caused by the illness also caused increased bone loss and fracture risk. Glucocorticoids, which are used to treat a wide variety of inflammatory conditions (e.g., rheumatoid arthritis, asthma, emphysema, chronic lung disease), can cause profound reductions in bone formation and may, to a lesser extent, increase bone resorption (Saag 2002), leading to loss of trabecular bone at the spine and hip, especially in postmenopausal women and older men. The most rapid bone loss occurs early in the course of treatment, and even small doses (equivalent to 2.5–7.5 mg prednisone per day) are associated with an increase in fractures (van Staa et al. 2002). As shown in Figure 3-4, the risk of fractures increases rapidly in patients treated with glucocortocoids, even before much bone has been lost. This rapid increase in fracture risk is attributed to damage to the bone cells, which results in less healthy bone tissue. To avoid this problem, health care providers are urged to use the lowest possible dose of glucocorticoids for as short a time as possible. For some diseases, providers should also consider giving glucocorticoids locally (e.g., asthma patients can inhale them), which results in much less damage to the bone.

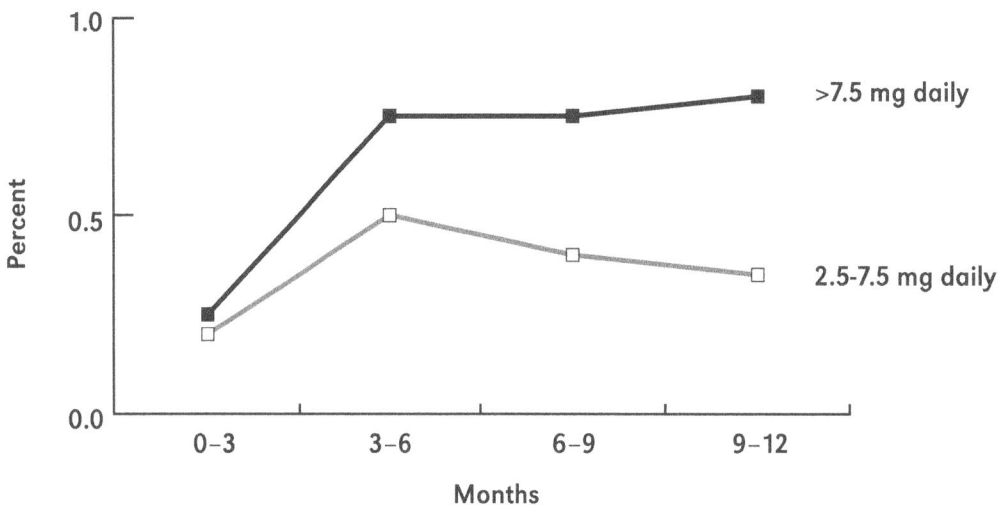

Figure 3–4. Rapid Increase in Vertebral Fracture Rates in Patients Treated With Glucocorticoids

Note: Before glucocorticoid treatment was started, the rate of fractures was less than 0.2% per year. On the higher doses (more than 7.5 mg of prednisone or equivalent per day) the rate increased at least four fold by 6 months, and there was a significant increase even on doses of 2.5 to 5 mg/day. Non-vertebral fractures also showed an increase which began in the first 3 months of treatment.

Source: van Staa et al. 2002.

Other Medications That Can Cause Osteoporosis. Cyclosporine A and tacrolimus are widely used in conjunction with glucocorticoids to prevent rejection after organ transplantation, and high doses of these drugs are associated with a particularly severe form of osteoporosis (Cohen and Shane 2003). Bone disease has also been reported with several frequently prescribed anticonvulsants, including diphenylhydantoin, phenobarbital, sodium valproate, and carbamazepine (Stein and Shane 2003). Patients who are most at risk of developing this type of bone disease include those on long-term therapy, high medication doses, multiple anticonvulsants, and/or simultaneous therapy with medications that raise liver enzyme levels. Low vitamin D intake, restricted sun exposure, and the presence of other chronic illnesses increase the risk, particularly among elderly and institutionalized individuals. In contrast, high intakes of vitamin A (retinal) may increase fracture risk (Michaelsson et al 2003). Methotrexate, a folate antagonist used to treat malignancies and (in lower doses) inflammatory diseases such as rheumatoid arthritis, may also cause bone loss, although research findings are not consistent. In addition, gonadotropin-releasing hormone (GnRH) agonists, which are used to treat endometriosis in women and prostate cancer in men, reduce both estrogen and testosterone levels, which may cause significant bone loss and fragility fractures (Smith 2003).

Rickets and Osteomalacia

Rickets (which affects children) and osteomalacia (which affects adults) are relatively uncommon diseases in the United States, since they can generally be prevented by ensuring adequate levels of vitamin D. These diseases can have devastating consequences to those who get them (Chesney 2001, Pettifor 2002 and 2003).

A number of childhood diseases cause rickets, a condition that results from a delay in depositing calcium phosphate mineral in growing bones, thus leading to skeletal deformities, especially bowed legs. In adults, the equivalent disease is called osteomalacia. Since longitudinal growth has stopped in adults, deficient bone mineralization does not cause skeletal deformity but can lead to fractures, particularly of weight-bearing bones such as the pelvis, hip, and feet. Even when there is no fracture, many patients with rickets and osteomalacia suffer from bone pain and can experience severe muscle weakness.

Rickets and osteomalacia are typically caused by any of a variety of environmental abnormalities. While rare, the disorder can also be inherited (Drezner 2003) as a result of mutations in the gene producing the enzyme that converts 25-hydroxy vitamin D to the active form, 1,25-dihydroxy vitamin D, or in the gene responsible for the vitamin D receptor. Osteomalacia can also be caused by disorders

that cause marked loss of phosphorus from the body. This can concur as a congenital disorder or can be acquired in patients who have tumors that produce a protein that affects phosphorus transport in the kidney.

Since vitamin D is formed in the skin by sunlight, the most common cause is reduced sun exposure. This is particularly important in northern latitudes where the winter sun does not have the power to form vitamin D in the skin. Thus the disease is often seen in individuals living at northern latitudes, particularly immigrants who have pigmented skin that decreases the formation of vitamin D or who habitually cover themselves. This problem can also occur in children who are confined indoors and in individuals who are house-bound (e.g., due to chronic ill health or frailty). Patients with diseases of the gastrointestinal tract, such as gastrectomy, malabsorption syndromes, and small bowel resection, are also at higher risk, since these conditions reduce vitamin D absorption from the diet.

There is also a second form of rickets and osteomalacia that is caused by phosphate deficiency. This condition can be inherited (this is known as X-linked hypophosphatemic rickets), but it is more commonly the result of other factors. Individuals with diseases affecting the kidney's ability to retain phosphate rapidly are at risk of this condition, as are those with diseases of the renal tubule that affect the site of phosphate reabsorption. While most foods are rich in phosphate, phosphate deficiency may also result from consumption of very large amounts of antacids containing aluminum hydroxide, which prevents the absorption of dietary phosphate. Finally, rickets due to phosphate deficiency may occur in individuals with acquired or inherited defects in acid secretion by the kidney tubule and those who take certain drugs (Table 3-3) that interfere with phosphate absorption or the bone mineralization process.

There are also patients who develop tumors that secrete a factor that causes loss of phosphate from the body. This condition is called tumor-induced or oncogenic osteomalacia.

Table 3-3. Causes of Drug-Induced Rickets/Osteomalacia

Drugs resulting in hypocalcemia
Inhibitors of vitamin D formation or intestinal absorption
Sunscreens Cholestyramine
Increased catabolism of vitamin D or its metabolites
Anticonvulsants
Drugs resulting in hypophosphatemia
Inhibitors of intestinal phosphate absorption • Aluminum-containing antacids Impaired renal phosphate reabsorption • Cadmium • Ifosfamide • Saccharated ferric oxide
Direct impairment of mineralization
Parenteral aluminum Fluoride Etidronate

Source: Pettifor 2003. Reproduced from J Bone Miner Res 1998: May; 13(5): 763-73 with permission of the American Society for Bone and Mineral Research.

Renal Osteodystrophy

Patients with chronic renal disease are not only at risk of developing rickets and osteomalacia (Elder 2002), but they are also at risk of a complex bone disease known as renal osteodystrophy (Cunningham et al. 2004). This condition is characterized by a stimulation of bone metabolism caused by an increase in parathyroid hormone and by a delay in bone mineralization that is caused by decreased kidney production of 1,25-dihydroxyvitamin D. In addition, some patients show a failure of bone formation, called adynamic bone disease. As a result of this complexity, bone biopsies are often needed to make a correct diagnosis (Martin et al. 2004). By the time the patient progresses to end-stage renal failure, clinical manifestations of the disease appear, including bone cysts that result from stimulation of osteoclasts by the excess parathyroid hormone. While dialysis can significantly extend the life-expectancy of patients with chronic renal failure, it does nothing to prevent further progression of the osteodystrophy. In fact, the managing of the patient through dialysis may lead to further bone abnormalities that become superimposed on the underlying osteodystrophy, thus increasing the risk of fractures (Alem et al. 2000). While a renal transplant (offered to a growing number of patients on dialysis) may reverse many features of renal osteodystrophy, the use of antirejection medication in transplant patients may cause bone loss and fractures.

Paget's Disease of Bone

Paget's disease of bone (Siris and Roodman 2003) is a progressive, often crippling disorder of bone remodeling (see Chapter 2) that commonly involves the spine, pelvis, legs, or skull (although any bone can be affected). If diagnosed early, its impact can be minimized.

Individuals with this condition experience an increase in bone loss at the affected site due to excess numbers of overactive osteoclasts. While bone formation increases to compensate for the loss, the rapid production of new bone leads to a disorganized structure. The resulting bone is expanded in size and associated with increased formation of blood vessels and connective tissue in the bone marrow. Such bone becomes more susceptible to deformity or fracture (Figure 3-5). Depending on the location, the condition may produce no clinical signs or symptoms, or it may be associated with bone pain, deformity, fracture, or osteoarthritis of the joints adjacent to the abnormal bone. Paget's disease of bone can also cause a variety of neurological complications as a result of compression of nerve tissue by pagetic bone. In very rare cases (probably less than 1 percent of the time) the disease is complicated by the development of an osteosarcoma.

Although Paget's disease is the second most common bone disease after osteoporosis (see Chapter 4), many questions remain regarding its pathogenesis. There is a strong familial predisposition for Paget's disease, but no single genetic abnormality has been identified that can explain all cases. Paget's disease can be transmitted (or inherited) across generations in an affected family; 15–40 percent of patients have a relative with the disorder (Morales-Piga et al. 1995). Studies in the United States (Siris et al. 1991) suggest that a close relative of a pagetic patient is seven times more likely to develop Paget's disease than is someone who does not have an affected relative. However, environmental factors are likely play a role in the majority of cases. For example, some studies have suggested that Paget's disease may result from a "slow virus" infection with measles (Friedrichs et al. 2002).

Paget's Disease of Bone

Paget's disease may present in many different ways since it can affect bones throughout the body. A typical case might be a man in his 60s who complains to his doctor of pain in the hip. The doctor might tell him he has arthritis and suggest that he take ibuprofen or acetaminophen (Tylenol). Then, several years later, a routine screening may show a high alkaline phosphatase level. This test would then prompt use of a bone scan and radiographs, which would finally show Paget's disease of his femur and pelvic bone. Unfortunately, by this time the man likely has developed some bowing of the leg and suffered damage to the joints, neither of which can be reversed by treatment. However, treatment with a bisphosphonate can stop the progression of the disease. As a result, the man lives the rest of his life with some pain and he walks with a limp. Not surprisingly, the man, his family, and his doctor all wish that the diagnosis had been made earlier. Since Paget's disease runs in families, they decide to test the man's relatives. These tests show that the man's younger brother has a similar problem. He is treated immediately and no deformities ever develop.

Developmental Skeletal Disorders

A large number of genetic and developmental disorders affect the skeleton. Among the more common and more important of these is a group of inherited disorders referred to as osteogenesis imperfecta or OI (Whyte 2003, Rauch and Glorieux 2004). Patients with this condition have bones that break easily (therefore, the condition is also known as brittle bone disease). There are

Figure 3–5. Paget's Disease of Bone

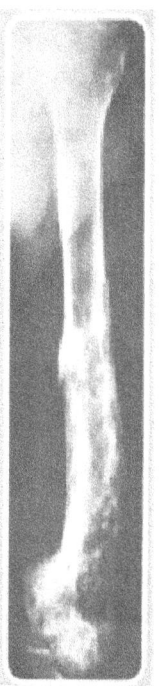
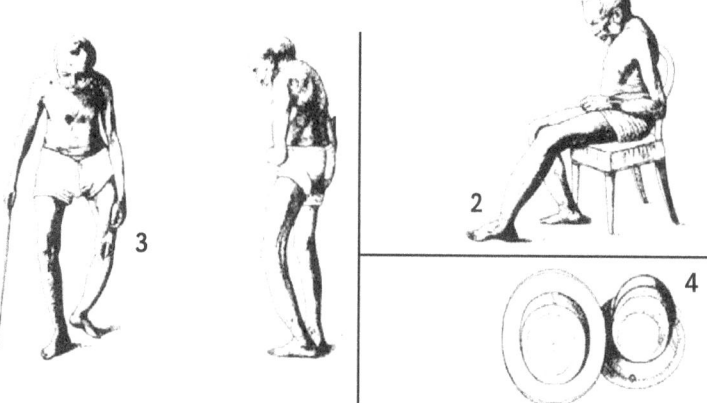

Note: On left, radiograph of humerus showing pagetic change in the distal half, with cortical thickening, expansion, and mixed areas of lucency and sclerosis, contrasted with normal bone in the proximal half. On right, drawing of Sir James Paget's first patient, published in his original paper, demonstrating the characteristic appearance that occurs with severe disease: 1) kyphosis (curvature) of the spine, 2) tibial thickening and bowing, 3) bowing of the femur and tibia in the leg, 4) increase in hat size indicative of skull enlargement.

Sources: Favus 2003, Reproduced from Primer on the metabolic bone diseases and disorders of mineral metabolism, 5th ed., Washington, D.C.: 2003, with permission of the American Society for Bone and Mineral Research. Paget 1877.

a number of forms of OI (see Table 3-4) that result from different types of genetic defects or mutations. These defects interfere with the body's production of type I collagen, the underlying protein structure of bone. As illustrated in Table 3-4, most, but not all, forms of OI are inherited. The disease manifests through a variety of clinical signs and symptoms, ranging from severe manifestations that are incompatible with life (that is, causing a stillbirth) to a relatively asymptomatic disease. However, most OI patients have low bone mass

(osteopenia) and as a result suffer from recurrent fractures and resulting skeletal deformities. There are four main types of OI, which vary according to the severity and duration of the symptoms. The most common form (Type I) is also the mildest version; and patients may have relatively few fractures. The second mildest form of the disease (which is called Type IV, because it was the fourth type of OI to be discovered) results in mild to moderate bone deformity, and sometimes in dental problems and hearing loss. These patients also sometimes have a blue, purple, or gray discoloration in the whites of their eyes, a condition known as blue sclera. A more severe form of the disease (Type III) results in relatively frequent fractures, and often in short stature, hearing loss, and dental problems. Finally, patients with the most severe form of the disease (Type II) typically suffer numerous fractures and severe bone deformity, generally leading to early death.

OI is not the only group of developmental skeletal disorders. An even larger group of rare diseases (sclerosing bone disorders) causes an increase in bone mass (Whyte 2003). One of these, osteopetrosis (marble bone disease), is more or less the opposite of osteoporosis. Instead of overactive osteoclasts, osteopetrosis results from a variety of genetic defects that impair the ability of osteoclasts to resorb bone. This interferes with the normal development of the skeleton and leads to excessive bone accumulation. Although such bone is very dense, it is also brittle and thus fractures often result. In addition, by compressing various nerves, the excess bone in patients with osteopetrosis may cause neurological symptoms, such as deafness or blindness. These patients may also suffer anemia, as blood-forming cells in the bone marrow are "crowded out" by the excess bone. Similar symptoms can result from over-activity of these bone cells, as in fibrous dysplasia where bone-forming cells produce too much connective tissue.

Malignancy and the Skeleton

Some other skeletal disorders are not inherited but rather develop only later in life. One of the most common of these acquired skeletal disorders is a tumor of the bone. Bone tumors can originate in the bone (these are known as primary tumors) or, much more commonly, result from the seeding of bone by tumors outside of the skeleton (these are known as metastatic tu-

Osteogenesis Imperfecta (OI)

There is an enormous range of severity in OI cases, from children who are stillborn due to multiple fractures in the womb and the inability to breathe, to children who suffer a few fractures, to mild cases where fractures do not occur until later in life, much like in patients with osteoporosis.

One scenario that causes tremendous hardship for the patient and the family is the occurrence of multiple fractures in the first few years of life in a child without the telltale sign of OI—a blue color in the "whites" of their eyes. Often the parents of these children are accused of child abuse. While it may be possible to make a diagnosis by analyzing the child's tissues, this expensive, difficult-to-perform test is not widely available. Typically, the frequency of fractures decreases over time and may even stop entirely at puberty. As an adult, an OI patient may be left with considerable deformity and short stature, but he or she can generally function well with the right environment and support. When females with OI reach menopause they sometimes start to fracture again. Since treatment is now available, it is important to identify OI patients at all stages of life, and to alert family members of the possibility that they may also be affected. Pediatricians, orthopedists, emergency room physicians, and others who see children with fractures need to consider OI as a possible cause, particularly in cases involving multiple fractures or a family history of fractures. These points are covered in detail in a recent book (Chiasson et al. 2004).

Table 3–4. Clinical Heterogeneity and Biochemical Defects in Osteogenesis Imperfecta (OI)

OI type	Clinical features	Inheritance	Biochemical defects
I	Normal stature, little or no deformity, blue sclerae, hearing loss in about 50% of individuals. Dentinogenesis imperfecta is rare and may distinguish a subset	AD	Decreased production of type I procollagen. Substitution for residue other than glycine in triple-helix of $\alpha_1(I)$
II	Lethal in the perinatal period, minimal calvarial mineralization, beaded ribs, compressed femurs, marked long bone deformity, platyspondyly	AD (new mutation) AR (rare)	Rearrangements in the COLA1 and COLA2 genes. Substitutions for glycyl residues in the triple-helical domain of the $\alpha_1(I)$ $\alpha_2(I)$ chain. Small deletion in $\alpha_2(I)$ on the background of a null allele
III	Progressively deforming bones, usually with moderate deformity at birth. Sclerae variable in hue, often lighten with age. Dentinogenesis imperfecta is common, hearing loss is common. Stature very short	AD AR	Point mutations in the $\alpha_1(I)$ or $\alpha_2(I)$ chain Frameshift mutation that prevents incorporation of pro $\alpha_2(I)$ into molecules (noncollagenous defects)
IV	Normal sclerae, mild to moderate bone deformity, and variable short stature. Dentinogenesis imperfecta is common, and hearing loss occurs in some	AD	Point mutations in the $\alpha_1(I)$ chain. Rarely point mutations in the $\alpha_1(I)$ chain. Small deletions in the $\alpha_1(I)$ chain

AD, autosomal dominant; AR, autosomal recessive.

Source: Byers 2001.

mors, since they have spread from elsewhere). Both types of tumors can destroy bone, although some metastatic tumors can actually increase bone formation. Primary bone tumors can be either benign (noncancerous) or malignant (cancerous). The most common benign bone tumor is osteochondroma, while the most common malignant ones are osteosarcoma and Ewing's sarcoma. Metastatic tumors are often the result of breast or prostate cancer that has spread to the bone (Coleman 2001). These may destroy bone (osteolytic lesion) or cause new bone formation (osteoblastic lesion). Breast cancer metastases are usually osteolytic, while most prostate cancer metastases are osteoblastic, though they still destroy bone structure (Berruti et al. 2001). Many tumor cells produce parathyroid hormone related peptide, which increases bone resorption (Bryden et al. 2002). This process of tumor-induced bone resorption leads to the release of growth factors stored in bone, which in turn increases tumor growth still further.

Bone destruction also occurs in the vast majority (over 80 percent) of patients with another type of cancer, multiple myeloma, which is a malignancy of the plasma cells that produce antibodies (Berenson 2002). The myeloma cells secrete cytokines (see Chapter 2), substances that may stimulate osteoclasts and inhibit osteoblasts (Roodman 2001, Tian et al. 2003). The bone destruction can cause severe bone pain, pathologic fractures, spinal cord compression, and life-threatening increases in blood calcium levels (Callander and Roodman 2001). A benign form of overproduction of antibodies, called monoclonal gammopathy, may also be associated with increased fracture risk (Melton et al. 2004).

Bone-resorbing cytokines are also produced in acute and chronic leukemia, Burkitt's lymphoma, and non-Hodgkins's lymphoma; patients with these chronic lymphoproliferative disorders often have associated osteoporosis. Both osteoporosis and osteosclerosis (thickening of trabecular bone) have been reported in association with systemic mastocytosis, a condition of abnormal mast cell proliferation (Schneider and Shane 2001). In addition, there are other infiltrative processes that affect bone, including infections and marrow fibrosis (myelofibrosis).

Oral Health and Bone Disease

Oral bone, like the rest of the skeleton, comprises both trabecular and cortical bone and undergoes formation and resorption throughout the life span. When oral bone loss exceeds gain, it can cause a loss of tooth-anchoring support or it can diminish the remaining ridge in those areas where partial or complete tooth loss has occurred.

The prevalence of oral bone loss is significant among adult populations worldwide, and it increases with age for both sexes. Oral bone loss and attendant tooth loss are associated with estrogen deficiency and osteoporosis. As a consequence, osteoporosis or osteopenia in postmenopausal women may have an impact on the need for, and the outcomes from, a variety of periodontal and prosthetic procedures, including guided tissue regeneration and tooth implantation. Furthermore, it is possible that oral examination and radiographic findings may be useful signs of extra-oral bone loss (Jeffcoat et al. 2000, Geurs et al. 2000).

Key Questions for Future Research

The major diseases of bone have been broadly characterized, but many questions remain unanswered, as outlined below:

- Within the spectrum of clinical disorders that represent "primary osteoporosis," are there differences in the mechanisms that lead to bone loss and bone fragility? What implications do these differences have for diagnosis and treatment?

- How do the environmental and genetic determinants of bone mass and strength interact in individuals with certain diseases? For example, are there genetic differences in the response to estrogen or calcium deficiency that affect their relative importance in the pathogenesis of osteoporosis?

- Are the animal studies on the role of cytokines relevant to human disease?

- What are the implications of research on the pathogenetic mechanisms for diseases other than osteoporosis? For example, further research on Paget's disease could uncover more about the ways in which excessive osteoclastic bone resorption can occur.

- What is the role of phosphate in bone mineralization?

- How is bone affected in patients who have cancer? What implications do these changes have with respect to both the spread of the cancer and to other skeletal disorders?

References

Ahlborg HG, Johnell O, Turner CH, Rannevik G, Karlsson MK. Bone loss and bone size after menopause. N Engl J Med. 2003 Jul 24;349(4):327-34.

Alem MA, Sherrard DJ, Gillen DL, Weiss NS, Beresford SA, Heckbert SR, Wong C, Stehman-Breen C . Increased risk of hip fracture among patients with end-stage renal disease. Kidney Int 2000;58(1):396-9.

Berenson JR. Advances in the biology and treatment of myeloma bone disease. Semin Oncol. 2002 Dec;29(6 Suppl 17):11-6.

Bernstein CN, Blanchard JF, Leslie W, Wajda A, Yu BN. The incidence of fracture among patients with inflammatory bowel disease. A population-based cohort study. Ann Intern Med 2000 Nov 21;133(10):795-9.

Berruti A, Dogliotti L, Tucci M, Tarabuzzi R, Fontana D, Angeli A. Metabolic bone disease induced by prostate cancer: Rationale for the use of bisphosphonates. J Urol. 2001 Dec;166(6):2023-31.

Bianchi ML, Bardella MT. Bone and celiac disease. Calcif Tissue Int. 2002 Dec; 71(6):465-71.

Bilezikian JP. Primary hyperparathyroidism. In: Primer on the metabolic bone diseases and disorders of mineral metabolism. 5th Edition. Favus MJ, editor. Washington (DC): American Society for Bone and Mineral Research; 2003:230-5.

Brown TT, Ruppe MD, Kassner R, Kumar P, Kehoe T, Dobs AS, Timpone J. Reduced bone mineral density in human immunodeficiency virus-infected patients and its association with increased central adiposity and postload hyperglycemia. J Clin Endocrinol Metab. 2004 Mar;89(3):1200-6.

Bryden AA, Hoyland JA, Freemont AJ, Clarke NW, George NJ. Parathyroid hormone related peptide and receptor expression in paired primary prostate cancer and bone metastases. Br J Cancer. 2002 Feb 1;86(3):322-5.

Byers PH. Disorders of collagen biosynthesis and structure. In: Scriver CR, Beaudet AL, Sly WA, Valle D, Childs B, Vogelstein B, eds. The Metabolic and Molecular Bases of Inherited Disease. 8th ed. New York: The McGraw Hill Companies; 2001. 5241-85.

Callander NS, Roodman GD. Myeloma bone disease. Semin Hematol. 2001 Jul;38(3):276-85.

Carey DE, Raisz LG. Calcitonin therapy in prolonged immobilization hypercalcemia. Arch Phys Med Rehabil. 1985 Sep;66(9):640-4.

Chesney RW. Vitamin D deficiency and rickets. Rev Endocr Metab Disord. 2001 Apr;2(2):145-51.

Chiasson RM, Munns C, Zeitlin L, Interdisciplinary treatment approach for children with osteogenesis imperfecta. Montreal, Canada: Shriner's Hospitals for Children; 2004.

Cizza G, Ravn P, Chrousos GP, Gold PW. Depression: A major, unrecognized risk factor for osteoporosis? Trends Endocrinol Metab. 2001 Jul; 12(5): 198-203.

Coates PS, Fernstrom JD, Fernstrom MH, Schauer PR, Greenspan SL. Gastric bypass surgery for morbid obesity leads to an increase in bone turnover and a decrease in bone mass. J Clin Endocrinol Metab. 2004 Mar;89(3): 1061-5.

Coelho R, Silva C, Maia A, Prata J, Barros H. Bone mineral density and depression: A community study in women. J Psychosom Res. 1999 Jan; 46(1):29-35.

Cohen A, Shane E. Osteoporosis after solid organ and bone marrow transplantation. Osteoporos Int. 2003 Aug;14(8):617-30.

Epub 2003 Aug 08.

Coleman RE. Metastatic bone disease: Clinical Features, pathophysiology and treatment strategies. Cancer Treat Rev. 2001 Jun;27(3):165-76.

Crawford BA, Kam C, Donaghy AJ, McCaughan GW. The heterogeneity of bone disease in cirrhosis: A multivariate analysis. Osteoporos Int. 2003 Dec:14(12):987-94.

Cunningham J, Sprague SM, Cannata-Andia J, Coco M, Cohen-Solal M, Fitzpatrick L, Goltzmann D, Lafage-Proust MH, Leonard M, Ott S, Rodriguez M, et al. Osteoporosis in chronic kidney disease. Am J Kidney Dis. 2004 Mar;43(3): 566-71.

Dauty M, Perrouin Verbe B, Maugars Y, Dubois C, Mathe JF. Supralesional and sublesional bone mineral density in spinal cord-injured patients. Bone. 2000 Aug; 27(2): 305-9.

Drezner MK. Hypophosphatemic rickets. Endocr Dev. 2003;6:126-55.

Elder G. Pathophysiology and recent advances in the management of renal osteodystrophy. J Bone Miner Res. 2002 Dec;17(12):2094-105.

Farhat G, Yamout B, Mikati MA, Demirjian S, Sawaya R, El-Hajj Fuleihan G. Effect of antiepileptic drugs on bone density in ambulatory patients. Neurology. 2000 May 14; 58(9): 1348-53.

Favus MJ, Ed. Primer on the metabolic bone diseases and disorders of mineral metabolism. 5th ed. Washington (DC): American Society for Bone and Mineral Research; 2003: cover.

Friedrichs WE, Reddy SV, Bruder JM, Cundy T, Cornish IJ, Singer FR, Roodman GD. Sequence analysis of measles virus nucleocapsid transcripts in patients with Paget's disease. J Bone Miner Res. 2002 Jan;17(1):145-51.

Geurs NC, Lewis CE, Jeffcoat MK. Osteoporosis and periodontal disease progression. Periodontol 2000. 2003;32:105-10.

Go T. Low-dose oral etidronate therapy for immobilization hypercalcaemia associated with Guillain-Barre syndrome. Acta Paediatr. 2001 Oct; 90(10):1202-4.

Haugeberg G, Orstavik RE, Kvien TK. Effects of rheumatoid arthritis on bone. Curr Opin Rheumatol 2003 Jul;15(4):469-75.

Heap J, Murray MA, Miller SC, Jalili T, Moyer-Mileur LJ. Alterations in bone characteristics associated with glycemic control in adolescents with type 1 diabetes mellitus. J Pediatr. 2004 Jan;144(1):56-62.

Jeffcoat MK, Lewis CE, Reddy MS, Wang CY, Redford M. Post-menopausal bone loss and its relationship to oral bone loss. Periodontol 2000. 2000 Jun;23:94-102.

Khosla S, Lufkin EG, Hodgson SF, Fitzpatrick LA, Melton LJ 3rd. Epidemiology and clinical features of osteoporosis in young individuals. Bone. 1994 Sep-Oct;15(5):551-5.

Khosla S, Melton LJ 3rd, Atkinson EJ, O'Fallon WM, Klee GG, Riggs BL. Relationship of serum sex steroid levels and bone turnover markers with bone mineral density in men and women: A key role for bioavailable estrogen. J Clin Endocrinol Metab. 1998 Jul;83(7):2266-74.

Khosla S, Melton J 3rd. Fracture risk in primary hyperparathyroidism. J Bone Miner Res. 2002 Nov;17Suppl 2:N103-7.

Kiratli BJ. Immobilization osteopenia. In: Osteoporosis, Second Edition. Volume 2. Marcus R, Feldman D, Kelsey J, editors. San Diego (CA): Academic Press; 2001:207-27.

Lien G, Flato B, Haugen M, Vinje O, Sorskaar D, Dale K, Johnston V, Egeland T, Forre O. Frequency of osteopenia in adolescents with early-onset juvenile idiopathic arthritis: A long-term outcome study of one hundred five patients. Arthritis Rheum. 2003 Aug;48(8):2214-23.

Lloyd ME, Spector TD, Howard R. Osteoporosis in neurological disorders. J Neurol Neurosurg Psychiatry. 2000 May; 68(5):543-7.

Martin KJ, Olgaard K, Coburn JW, Coen GM, Fukagawa M, Langman C, Malluche HH, McCarthy JT, Massry SG, Mehls O, et al. Diagnosis, assessment, and treatment of bone turnover abnormalities in renal osteo-dystrophy. Am J Kidney Dis. 2004 Mar;43(3):558-65.

Melton LJ 3rd, Rajkumar SV, Khosla S, Achenbach SJ, Oberg AL, Kyle RA. Fracture risk in monoclonal gammopathy of undetermined significance. J Bone Miner Res. 2004 Jan;19(1):25-30.

Michaelsson K, Lithell H, Vessby B, Melhus H. Serum retinol levels and the risk of fracture. N Engl J Med. 2003 Jan 23;348(4): 287-94.

Michelson D, Stratakis C, Hill L, Reynolds J, Galliven E, Chrousos G, Gold P. Bone mineral density in women with depression. N Engl J Med. 1996 Oct 17;335(16):1176-81.

Morales-Piga AA, Rey-Rey JS, Corres-Gonzalez J, Garcia-Sagredo IM, Lopez-Abente G. Frequency and characteristics of familial aggregation of Paget's disease of bone. J Bone Miner Res. 1995 Apr;10(4):663-70.

National Osteoporosis Foundation: Osteoporosis: What is it? [homepage on the Internet]. Washington, DC: National Osteoporosis Foundation. [Cited 2004 Mar 1]. Available from: http://www.nof.org/osteoporosis/index.htm

Netter, Frank H., The Ciba collection of medical illustrations. In: Woodburne, Russell T.; Crelin, Edmund S.; Kaplan, Frederick, S., editors. Vol. 8, Part 1, Musculoskeletal system: Anatomy, Physiology, and Metabolic Disorders. West Cauldwell, NJ: Ciba-Geigy Pharmaceutical Products; 1987. p.260.

Norman, ME. Juvenile osteoporosis. In: Favus, MJ, editor. Primer on the metabolic bone diseases and disorders of mineral metabolism. 5th ed. Washington, DC: American Society for Bone and Mineral Research; 2003. p. 382-6.

Orstavik RE, Haugeberg G, Uhlig T, Mowinckel P, Falch JA, Halse JI, Kvien TK. Self reported non-vertebral fractures in rheumatoid arthritis and population based controls: Incidence and relationship with bone mineral density and clinical variables. Ann Rheum Dis. 2004 Feb;63(2): 177-82.

Orwoll E. Osteoporosis in men. Endocrinol Metab Clin North Am. 1998 Jun;27(2)349-67.

Ott S, Aitken ML. Osteoporosis in patients with cystic fibrosis. Clin Chest Med. 1998 Sep;19(3):555-67.

Paget J. On a form of chronic inflammation of bones (osteitis deformans). Medico-chirurgical transactions 1877;60:37-63.

Pavelka K. Osteonecrosis. Baillieres Best Pract Res Clin Rheumatol. 2000 Jun;14(2):399-414.

Pettifor JM. Rickets. Calcif Tissue Int. 2002 May; 70(5):398-9.

Pettifor JM. Nutritional and drug-induced rickets and osteomalacia. In: Favus MJ, editor. Primer on the metabolic bone diseases and disorders of mineral metabolism. 5th ed. Washington, DC: American Society for Bone and Mineral Research; 2003. p. 399-407.

Piepkorn B, Kann P, Forst T, Andreas J, Pfützner A, Beyer J. Bone mineral density and bone metabolism in diabetes mellitus. Horm Metab Res. 1997 Nov;29(11):584-91.

Poole KE, Reeve J, Warburton EA. Falls, fractures, and osteoporosis after stroke: Time to think about protection? Stroke. 2002 May; 33(5):1432-6.

Ramsey-Goldman R, Dunn JE, Huang CF, Dunlop D, Rairie JE, Fitzgerald S, Manzi S. Frequency of fractures in women with systemic lupus erythematosus: Comparison with United States population data. Arthritis Rheum 1999 May;42(5):882-90.

Rauch F, Glorieux FH. Osteogenesis imperfecta. Lancet 2004 Apr 24;363(9418):1377-85.

Riggs BL, Khosla S, Melton LJ 3rd. A unitary model for involutional osteoporosis: estrogen deficiency causes both type I and type II osteoporosis in postmenopausal women and contributes to bone loss in aging men. J Bone Miner Res. 1998 May;13(5):763-73.

Riggs BL, Khosla S, Melton LJ 3rd. Sex steroids and the construction and conservation of the adult skeleton. Endocr Rev. 2002 Jun;23(3):279-302.

Robbins J, Hirsch C, Whitmer R, Cauley J, Harris T. The association of bone mineral density and depression in an older population. J Am Geriatr Soc. 2001 Jun; 49(6): 732-6.

Roodman GD. Biology of osteoclast activation in cancer. J Clin Oncol. 2001 Aug 1;19(15):3562-71.

Ross DS. Hyperthyroidism, thyroid hormone therapy, and bone. Thyroid. 1994 Fall;4(3):319-26.

Saag K. Glucocorticoid-induced osteoporosis. Endocrinol Metab Clin North Am. 2003 Mar;32(1):135-57, vii.

Sato Y, Asoh T, Kaji M, Oizumi K. Beneficial effect of intermittent cyclical etidronate therapy in hemiplegic patients following an acute stroke. J Bone Miner Res. 2000 Dec; 15(12): 2487-94.

Schneider A, Shane E. Osteoporosis secondary to illness and medications. In: Marcus R, Feldman D, Kelsey J, editors. Osteoporosis. 2nd ed. San Diego: Academic Press; 2001. p. 303-27.

Seeman E. Invited Review: Pathogenesis of osteoporosis. J Appl Physiol. 2003 Nov; 95(5):2142-51.

Sheth RD. Bone health in epilepsy. Epilepsia. 2002 Dec; 43(12):1453-4.

Silverberg SJ, Shane E, de la Cruz L, Dempster DW, Feldman F, Seldin D, Jacobs TP, Siris ES, Cafferty M, Parisien MV, et al. Skeletal disease in primary hyperparathyroidism. J Bone Miner Res. 1989 Jun;4(3):283-91.

Silverberg SJ, Bilezikian JP. Clinical presentation of primary hyperparathyroidism in the United States. In: Bilezikian JP, Marcus R, Levine MA, editors. The parathyroids, 2nd ed. San Diego (CA): Academic Press; 2001:349-60.

Siris ES, Ottman R, Flaster E, Kelsey JL. Familial aggregation of Paget's disease of bone. J Bone Miner Res. 1991 May;6(5):495-500.

Siris, ES; Roodman, GD. Paget's disease of bone. In: Favus, MJ, editor. Primer on the metabolic bone diseases and disorders of mineral metabolism. 5th ed. Washington, DC: American Society for Bone and Mineral Research; 2003. p. 495-506.

Smith MR. Diagnosis and management of treatment-related osteoporosis in men with prostate carcinoma. Cancer. 2003 Feb 1;97(3 Suppl):789-95.

Stein E, Shane E. Secondary osteoporosis. Endocrinol Metab Clin N Am. 2003 Mar;32(1):115-34, vii.

Tannenbaum C, Clark J, Schwartzman K, Wallenstein S, Lapinski R, Meier D, Luckey M. Yield of laboratory testing to identify secondary contributors to osteoporosis in otherwise healthy women. J Clin Endocrinol Metab. 2002 Oct;87(10):4431-7.

Thomas J, Doherty SM. HIV infection—A risk factor for osteoporosis. J Acquir Immune Defic Syndr. 2003 Jul 1;33(3):281-91.

Tian E, Zhan F, Walker R, Rasmussen E, Ma Y, Barlogie B, Shaughnessy JD Jr. The role of the Wnt-signaling antagonist DKK1 in the development of osteolytic lesions in multiple myeloma. N Engl J Med. 2003 Dec 25;349(26):2483-94.

Tuzun S, Altintas A, Karacan I, Tangurek S, Saip S, Siva A. Bone status in multiple sclerosis: Beyond corticosteroids. Mult Scler. 2003 Dec; 9(6):600-4.

van Staa TP, Leufkens HGM, Cooper C. The epidemiology of corticosteroid-induced osteoporosis: a meta-analysis. Osteoporos Int. 2002 Oct;13(10):777-87.

Wermers RA, Khosla S, Atkinson EJ, Hodgson SF, O'Fallon WM, Melton LJ 3rd. The rise and fall of primary hyperparathyroidism: A population-based study in Rochester, Minnesota, 1965-1992. Ann Intern Med. 1997 Mar 15;126(6):433-40.

WHO Scientific Group on the Burden of Musculoskeletal Conditions at the Start of the New Millennium. The burden of musculoskeletal conditions at the start of the new millennium: Report of a scientific group. Geneva, Switzerland:World Health Organization technical report series 919; 2003:, p. 57.

Whooley MA, Kip KE, Cauley JA, Ensrud KE, Nevitt MC, Browner WS. Depression, falls, and risk of fracture in older women. Study of Osteoporotic Fractures Research Group. Arch Intern Med. 1999 Mar 8;159(5):484-90.

Whyte, MP. Sclerosing bone disorders. In: Favus, MJ, editor. Primer on the metabolic bone diseases and disorders of mineral metabolism. 5th ed. Washington, DC: American Society for Bone and Mineral Research; 2003. p. 449-66.

Wynne AG, van Heerden J, Carney JA, Fitzpatrick LA. Parathyroid carcinoma: Clinical and pathological features in 43 patients. Medicine. 1992 Jul;71(4):197-205.

Part Two

WHAT IS THE STATUS OF BONE HEALTH IN AMERICA?

To provide an answer to this question, this part of the report describes the magnitude and scope of the problem from two perspectives. The first is the prevalence of bone disease within the population at large, and the second is the burden that bone diseases impose on society and those who suffer from them.

Chapter 4 provides detailed information on the incidence and prevalence of osteoporosis, fractures, and other bone diseases. Osteoporosis is by far the most common bone disease, although other related bone diseases are important as well. Where available, the chapter also provides data on bone disease in men and minorities. While older White women are clearly at risk, bone disease can strike anyone, at any age, including men, premenopausal women, and ethnic minorities. Chapter 4 also offers some chilling projections for the future prevalence of bone disease, citing forecasts of significant increases in the prevalence of both osteoporosis and fractures, and a steep rise in the costs of caring for bone disease.

Chapter 5 examines the costs of bone diseases and their effects on well-being and quality of life both from the point of view of the individual patient and society at large. While bone disease seldom leads directly to death, it can start a downward spiral in physical and mental health that has a dramatic impact on an individual's functional status and quality of life. All too often this downward spiral concludes with premature death. To illustrate the burden of bone diseases, the chapter includes real-life vignettes that describe the terrible impact that osteoporosis, Paget's disease, osteogenesis imperfecta, and other related bone diseases can have on those who suffer from them and their family members.

Chapter 4: Key Messages

- The biggest problem created by bone disease, especially osteoporosis, is fractures, which may be the first visible sign of disease in patients. Each year an estimated 1.5 million individuals suffer a fracture due to bone disease.

- The risk of a fracture increases with age and is greatest in women. Roughly 4 in 10 White women age 50 or older in the United States will experience a hip, spine, or wrist fracture sometime during the remainder of their lives. Looking ahead, the lifetime risk of fractures will increase for all ethnic groups as people live longer.

- Osteoporosis is the most common cause of fractures. Roughly 10 million individuals over age 50 in the United States have osteoporosis of the hip. An additional 33.6 million individuals over age 50 have low bone mass or "osteopenia" of the hip and thus are at risk of osteoporosis and its potential complications later in life.

- Due primarily to the aging of the population, the prevalence of osteoporosis and low bone mass is expected to increase. By 2020, one in two Americans over age 50 is expected to have or be at risk of developing osteoporosis of the hip; even more will be at risk of developing osteoporosis at any site in the skeleton.

- Osteoporosis does not affect everyone to the same degree. Women, especially older women, are more likely to get the disease than are men. An estimated 35 percent of postmenopausal White women have osteoporosis of the hip, spine, or distal forearm. That said, men, especially elderly men, can and do get osteoporosis.

- The age-adjusted prevalence of osteoporosis and the rate of hip fracture are lower in Black women than in White women in the United States. The prevalence of osteoporosis in Hispanic and Asian women is similar to that found in White women, and the incidence of hip fractures among Hispanic women in California appears to be on the rise. However, it is important to remember that osteoporosis is a real risk for *any* aging man or woman.

- Much less is known about the frequency of most other skeletal diseases, due in part to underdiagnosis and underreporting. Some data, however, are available. An estimated one million individuals in the United States have Paget's disease, while roughly 20,000 to 50,000 Americans may have OI.

Chapter 4

THE FREQUENCY OF BONE DISEASE

While they may not get as much attention as heart disease, cancer, and other major diseases, bone diseases are common in the United States, especially among the elderly, and they take a large toll on the Nation's overall health status. Fractures are the biggest problem associated with bone disease; they are common, costly, and become a chronic burden on both individuals and society. Osteoporosis is a leading underlying cause of fractures, especially among the elderly. It affects both sexes and all races, although to varying degrees. The reason for the disease's high prevalence is relatively simple—almost everyone loses bone as they grow older. Other bone disorders, such as Paget's disease of bone, hyperparathyroidism, osteogenesis imperfecta, rickets, and osteomalacia are much less common. Like osteoporosis, these diseases also have adverse effects on bone strength and fracture risk by affecting bone density, bone turnover, or bone structure. Although some bone diseases lead to pain and deformity, most adverse effects relate to fractures.

This chapter reviews the most recent evidence related to the occurrence of fractures and bone diseases in the community. The following chapter deals with the burden caused by these fractures and diseases, including the most common complications that may ensue, such as physical disability, depression, a reduced quality of life, and potentially death. The following chapter also discusses the large costs associated with fractures and bone disease.

Fractures Caused by Bone Disease

Fractures are by far the biggest problem caused by bone disease. They are common and can be quite debilitating. In many cases they are the first sign of the disease in patients.

Incidence of Fractures

An estimated 1.5 million individuals suffer a fracture caused by bone disease annually (Riggs and Melton 1995, Chrischilles et al. 1991). In fact, fractures are the most common musculoskeletal condition requiring hospitalization among Medicare enrollees (who are age 65 and older). Approximately one-third (500,000) of fracture patients are hospitalized (see Table 5-1 in Chapter 5 for more details), while many more suffer fractures that do not require or result in hospitalization.

The risk of fracture increases dramatically with age in both sexes, both because bones become more fragile and the risk of falling increases. Roughly one in four (24 percent) women age 50 or older fall each year, compared to nearly half (48 percent) of women age 85 or older; comparable figures for men are 16 percent and 35 percent (Winner et al. 1989). These falls can result in fractures, and when they do the fracture is almost always caused by low bone mass or osteoporosis. (See next section for more on osteoporosis and low bone mass.)

Another way to examine the frequency of fractures is to consider the chances of experiencing one or more of them during a lifetime of average length. What is clear from this analysis is that a substantial portion of the population faces a serious risk. As illustrated in Table 4-1, roughly 4 in 10 White women age 50 or older in the United States will experience a hip, spine, or wrist fracture sometime during the remainder of their lives; 13 percent of White men in this country will suffer a similar fate (Cummings and Melton 2002). Figures for men are lower due to their shorter life expectancy and lower fracture incidence rates. However, these data do not include other fractures (e.g., of the upper arm, pelvis, lower leg, ribs); if all fractures are included, the overall lifetime risk of fracture is even greater. Hip fractures are the most serious threat, as 17 percent of White women and 6 percent of White men age 50 and older will suffer a hip fracture sometime during the remainder of their life. The lifetime risks of clinically diagnosed spine fractures in these populations are 16 percent and 5 percent, respectively, and 16 percent and 2 percent for wrist fractures (Cummings and Melton 2002). The lifetime risk

for nonwhites is less across all of these fracture types.

Looking ahead, the lifetime risk of fractures will increase for all groups as people live longer. An analysis in Sweden, for example, found that increasing life expectancy significantly increased the lifetime risk of hip fracture, from 14 percent to 23 percent in women and from 5 percent to 11 percent in men (Oden et al. 1998). If incidence rates were to rise by just 1 percent annually in Sweden, the lifetime risk of hip fracture could increase still further, to 35 percent in women and 17 percent in men. Of course, most hip fractures occur in the elderly and thus affect individuals only late in life. Other types of fractures are more likely to strike younger. For example, wrist and other limb fractures are ten times more common than are hip fractures among women who have just gone through menopause (Cooper and Melton 1992).

Although fractures of the upper arm, pelvis, and some other sites are more common in the elderly, the fractures most closely associated with bone disease are those of the hip (proximal femur), spine (vertebrae), and wrist (distal forearm). The annual incidence of hip fractures increases dramatically with age, from just 2 fractures per 100,000 among White women

Table 4–1. Lifetime Risk of Fracture at Age 50 Years

Type of fracture	White women	White men
Hip (%)	17.5	6.0
Vertebra(%)	15.6	5.0
Forearm (%)	16.0	2.5
Any of the three (%)	39.7	13.1

Source: Cummings and Melton 2002.

under age 35 to over 3,000 fractures per 100,000 among White women age 85 and older (Figure 4-1). Hospital discharge rates for hip fractures per 1,000 Medicare enrollees increased by 9.2 percent between 1992 and 1999, and then fell by 5.5 percent from 1999 to 2001 (Dartmouth 2004). Although achieved over a short time interval, this recent decline in hip fracture incidence is consistent with falling hip fracture rates that have been observed among White women in California (Zingmond et al. 2004). While the reasons for this decline are not entirely clear, it could potentially be due to the use of new therapies, e.g., pharmaceuticals, as discussed in Chapter 9. Nevertheless, even with modest reductions in the incidence rate of fractures (i.e., the number of fractures per 1,000 Medicare enrollees), the total number of hip fractures will likely increase significantly over the next 20–50 years due to the aging of the population. In other words, a modest decline in fracture rates per 1,000 Medicare enrollees will be overwhelmed by the growth in (and aging of) the overall Medicare population. The only way to realize meaningful reductions in the absolute number of hip fractures is to significantly reduce hip fracture rates, as outlined in the *Healthy People 2010* goals. These goals call for more than a 50 percent reduction in the hip fracture rates for females and a 20 percent decrease for males (see Table 1-1 for more details). Hip fracture incidence in men is about half that in women at any given age. Since there are fewer elderly men than there are women (due to shorter life expectancy), women account for 80 percent of all hip fractures (Cooper and Melton 2002). The greater risk of hip fractures in elderly women has been attributed both to their lower bone density compared to men as well as to their high risk of falling.

There is no generally accepted definition of a spine fracture (Genant and Jergas 2003), and estimates of the overall prevalence of spine fractures in postmenopausal women vary widely depending on the definition used (Black et al. 1991). Although experts do not always agree with the morphometric classification of specific patients, x-ray readings suggest that an estimated 20–25 percent of postmenopausal White women have at least one moderately deformed vertebra (Grados et al. 2004), while about 10 percent have the more severe spine fractures that are most likely to produce symptoms (see below). Most studies also show that the prevalence of spine fractures is similar in middle-aged women and men, but some of those in men may not be due to osteoporosis but rather to job-related injuries or trauma (O'Neill et al. 1996). It is important to remember, however, that the incidence of clinically diagnosed spine fractures (i.e., those diagnosed by a physician after a patient complains of symptoms) is much less than the incidence rates suggested by vertebral morphometry. In a recent study from Sweden, only 23 percent of vertebral deformities in women were diagnosed clinically (Kanis et al. 2004). In other words, there are many "silent" spine fractures that produce no obvious symptoms to the patient. These silent fractures may involve compression (or flattening or crushing) of the vertebrae, can result in kyphosis (curvature of the spine) and chronic back pain, and may be associated with an increase in morbidity.

Falls account for about one-fourth of the spine fractures that come to clinical attention (Cooper et al. 1992a); the majority of clinically diagnosed spine fractures result from excess stresses on the spine caused by everyday activities (Myers and Wilson 1997). The incidence of clinically recognized spine fractures increases rapidly with age in both sexes (Figure 4-1). Since rates are higher among women, who

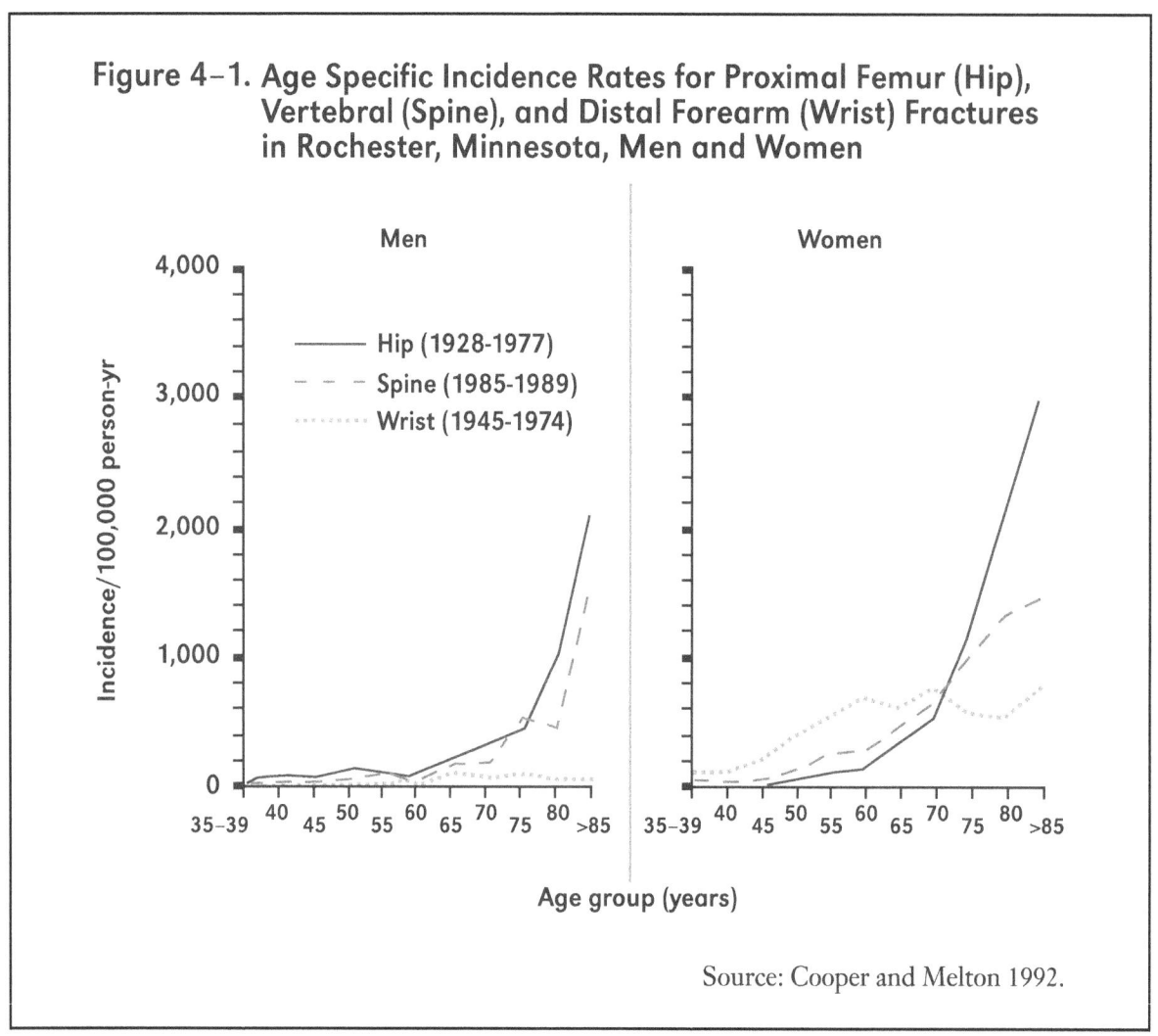

Figure 4–1. Age Specific Incidence Rates for Proximal Femur (Hip), Vertebral (Spine), and Distal Forearm (Wrist) Fractures in Rochester, Minnesota, Men and Women

Source: Cooper and Melton 1992.

also live longer, three-fourths of all spine fractures are diagnosed in women (Cooper et al. 1992a).

Finally, wrist fractures tend to occur among younger individuals with osteoporosis, but these patients are at increased risk of a hip fracture later in life (Klotzbuecher et al. 2000). The incidence of wrist fracture rises little with age among men (Figure 4-1), so most distal forearm fractures are in women.

Variations Across Ethnic Groups and Geographic Regions

Fracture incidence in the United States is usually highest for Whites and lower for other ethnic groups (Melton and Cooper 2001, Lauderdale et al. 1997). The lower incidence of fractures among Blacks has generally been explained by their greater bone mass. But differences in bone mass fail to explain the lower hip fracture rates observed in Hispanics and

Figure 4–2. **A - Hip Fracture Incidence by Race/Ethnicity Among Women 55 Years of Age and Older in California, 1983 to 2000.**

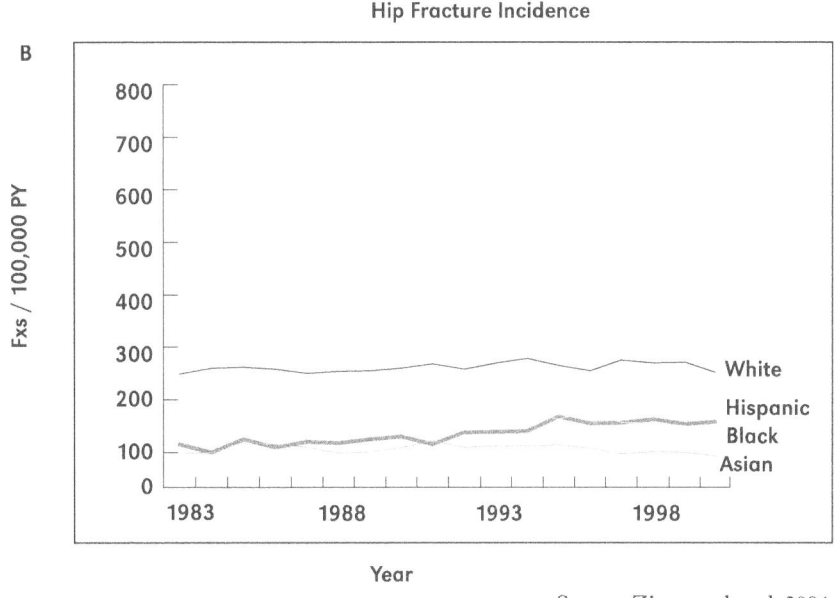

B - Hip Fracture Incidence by Race/Ethnicity Among Men 55 Years of Age and Older in California, 1983 to 2000.

Source: Zingmond et al. 2004.

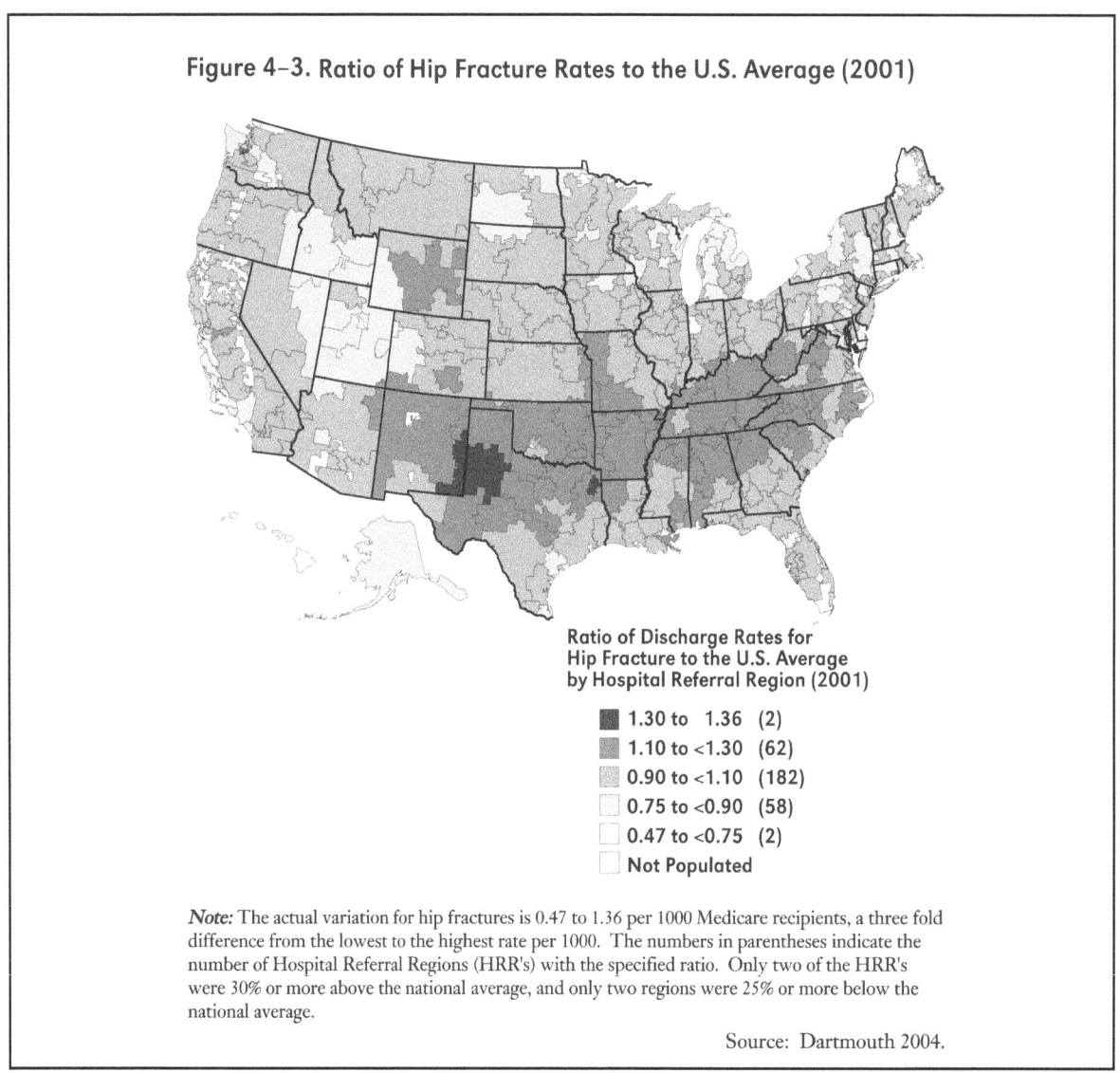

Figure 4-3. Ratio of Hip Fracture Rates to the U.S. Average (2001)

Ratio of Discharge Rates for
Hip Fracture to the U.S. Average
by Hospital Referral Region (2001)

- 1.30 to 1.36 (2)
- 1.10 to <1.30 (62)
- 0.90 to <1.10 (182)
- 0.75 to <0.90 (58)
- 0.47 to <0.75 (2)
- Not Populated

Note: The actual variation for hip fractures is 0.47 to 1.36 per 1000 Medicare recipients, a three fold difference from the lowest to the highest rate per 1000. The numbers in parentheses indicate the number of Hospital Referral Regions (HRR's) with the specified ratio. Only two of the HRR's were 30% or more above the national average, and only two regions were 25% or more below the national average.

Source: Dartmouth 2004.

Asians. One hypothesis for these lower fracture rates is that Asians are less likely to fall (Davis et al. 1999). Hip fracture hospitalization rates for male and female non-Hispanic Whites, Blacks, Hispanics, and Asians over age 50 were tracked in New York City from 1988 to 2002. Females were more likely to fracture than males across all ethnic and racial minorities, and the risk of a hip fracture in these minority groups was one-third to one-half that of their White counterparts (Fang et al. 2004). This finding is consistent with recent data from California, which also shows a lower risk of fractures in minorities and men (see Figure 4-2). However, in California, the State with the largest population of Hispanic residents in the United States, hip fracture incidence increased among Hispanic women and men from 1983 to 2000, while it fell among non-Hispanic White women during the same time period. The magnitude of the decrease—almost 1 percent per year—is similar to rates observed in White women in Rochester, MN (Zingmond et al. 2004). As a consequence of these trends, although the majority of hip fracture patients continue to be non-Hispanic Whites, ethnic minorities are an increasing proportion of all cases encountered in California.

Spine fractures among Asians are about as frequent as they are in Whites (Ross et al. 1995). Few data are available for other ethnic groups. Hospital admissions for spine fractures in the United States are about four times greater for elderly Whites than for Blacks (Jacobsen et al. 1992). Hospital admissions, however, may not be a very accurate marker of spine fractures, as few patients are actually admitted for spine fractures. Also, African Americans and other underserved groups may not have ready access to hospital care. Likewise, spine fractures are less frequent among Mexican-Americans as compared to non-Hispanic White women (Bauer and Deyo 1987). Forearm fractures are also less common in Black and Asian populations (Chung and Spilson 2001). Lower rates for Blacks than Whites have also been reported for most other types of fractures. Finally, although limited data are available on the prevalence of osteoporosis in the American Indian and Alaska Native (AIAN) population, one study suggests that fracture risk in AIAN women is similar to that in White women (Siris et al. 2001).

Fracture rates tend to vary across countries and regions within countries (Cummings and Melton 2002). For example, wrist and hip fracture rates in the United Kingdom are around 30 percent lower than in the United States. However, hip fracture rates vary more than sevenfold from one country to another within Europe (Melton and Cooper 2001), and similar variation has been observed for spine fractures

(O'Neill et al. 1996). Differences in the frequency of falls in different parts of Europe may explain in part the difference in limb fractures (Roy et al. 2002). Likewise, hip fracture incidence differs among various Asian countries (Lauderdale et al. 1997). Marked variation in fracture incidence is seen even within specific countries. As shown in Figure 4-3, hip fractures in the United States are most prevalent in the South (where hip bone density is lowest [Looker et al. 1998]), with two areas of Texas having the highest rates of fracture (Dartmouth 2004). However, the incidence of arm fractures is higher in the East and lower in the West (Karagas et al. 1996).

Osteoporosis

Osteoporosis and osteopenia (see box) are by far the most common causes of the fractures discussed in the previous section (although other bone diseases can cause fractures as well). In fact, decreased bone density is an important risk factor for fractures both in postmenopausal women (Stone et al. 2003) and older men (Nguyen et al. 1996). A panel of experts judged that skeletal fragility might be responsible for 80–95 percent of hip and spine fractures in White women, depending on age, along with 70–80 percent of distal forearm fractures and 45–60 percent of fractures at other skeletal sites (Melton et al. 1997). The comparable figures were less for women of other races and for men. While the risk of fracture is highest in those who have osteoporosis, many more individuals with osteopenia (low bone mass) are at increased risk as well. In fact, an analysis of peripheral bone mineral density (BMD) and fractures in over 200,000 women (The National Osteoporosis Risk Assessment, or NORA, study) suggests that at least half of all fragility fractures occur in this low bone mass group (Siris et al. 2001).

Figure 4–4. Projected Prevalence of Osteoporosis and/or Low Bone Mass of the Hip in Women, Men, and Both Sexes, 50 Years of Age or Older

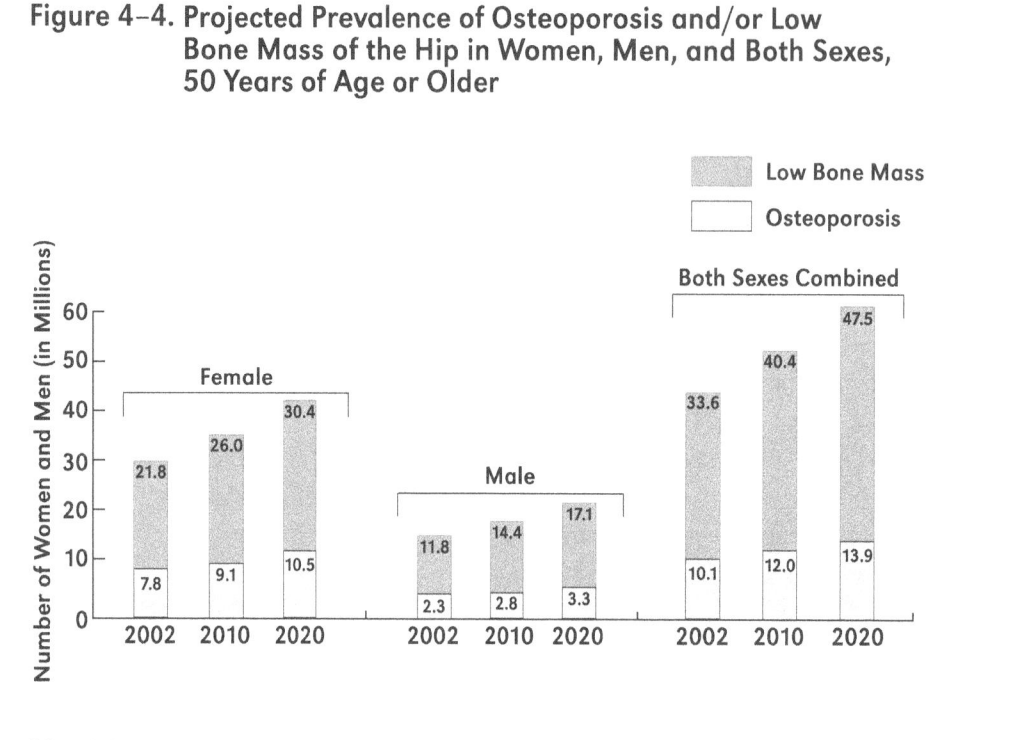

Note: The National Health and Nutrition Examination Survey (NHANES) is conducted by the National Center for Health Statistics, a part of the Centers for Disease Control and Prevention. This survey is conducted on a nationally representative sample of Americans. As a part of NHANES, bone mineral density of the hip was measured in 14,646 men and women over 20 years of age throughout the United States from 1988 until 1994. These values were compared with the WHO definitions to derive the percentage of individuals over the age of 50 who have osteoporosis and low bone mass. These percentages were then applied to the total population of men and women over the age of 50 to estimate the absolute number of males and females in the United States with osteoporosis and low bone mass. Projections for 2010 and 2020 are based on population forecasts for these years; they are significantly higher than current figures due to both the expected growth in the overall population and the expected aging of the population.

Source: NOF 2002.

Prevalence

As noted in the previous chapter, the World Health Organization has defined osteoporosis, for practical purposes, as a bone mineral density(BMD) value more than 2.5 standard deviations below the mean for normal young White women. Based on this definition, it has been estimated that roughly 10 million individuals over age 50 in the United States have osteoporosis of the hip, as shown in Figure 4-4 (NOF 2002, Looker 1997, Looker 1998). (The precise number suffering from the disease is difficult to determine, since bone loss varies in the different parts of the skeleton where bone mass is measured and definitions of osteoporosis have not been developed for all subpopulations.) An additional 33.6 million individuals over age 50 have low bone mass or "osteopenia" of the hip and they are at risk of osteoporosis and its potential complications later in life (NOF 2002, Looker 1997, Looker 1998).

Due primarily to the aging of the population, the prevalence of osteoporosis and low bone mass is expected to increase to 12 million cases of osteoporosis and 40 million cases of low bone mass among individuals over the age of 50 by 2010, and to nearly 14 million cases of osteoporosis and over 47 million cases of low bone mass in individuals over that age by 2020 (NOF 2002). In other words, **by 2020 one in two Americans over age 50 is expected to have or to be at risk of developing osteoporosis of the hip**; even more will be at risk of developing osteoporosis at any site in the skeleton.

One problem in estimating the frequency of osteoporosis is that many individuals may have the disease but not know it. The National Health and Nutrition Examination Survey (NHANES) revealed that only 1 percent of men and 11 percent of women age 65 and older reported that they had osteoporosis; testing at the hip showed that four times as many men (4 percent) and 2.5 times as many women (26 percent) actually had the disease (Table 4-2). In fact, more men (2 percent) reported a history of hip fracture than reported a prior diagnosis of osteoporosis (1 percent); for women the figures were reversed, 6.1 percent and 11.1 percent, respectively. These data for both men and women reveal not only the underdiagnosis of osteoporosis but also the failure to recognize that most hip fractures are due, at least in part, to osteoporosis. The likelihood of experiencing most other bone diseases is lower. In fact, only about 1 percent of the population age 45 and older has evidence of Paget's disease of bone and probably less than 1 percent has hyperparathyroidism (see below).

Variations Across Gender, Race, and Ethnicity

Osteoporosis does not affect everyone to the same degree. Women, especially older women, are much more likely to get the disease than are

What Is Osteopenia?

The term "osteopenia" is used to define individuals who have low bone mass and some increased risk of fracture. Their bone mass is not so low that they are deemed to have osteoporosis. This classification is similar to that used for people with high levels of LDL (or so-called "bad") cholesterol, where individuals with values over 160 mg/dl are deemed "high risk" and those between 130 and 160 mg/dl are deemed "moderate risk." The range defining osteopenia or low bone mass is quite large, ranging from -1 to -2.5 T-scores (that is, bone density levels that are 1 to 2.5 standard deviations below the average for young adults who have achieved normal peak bone mass), which translates into bone mass that is 10–30 percent below this average level. Thus, osteopenia is not a disease but rather a way of describing the results of a measurement. Obviously, given the wide range in this measurement, not everyone with osteopenia is at the same risk of fracture. Since individuals who are told they have osteopenia may become excessively concerned, providers should be sure to frame the bone health issue in terms of fracture risk. As emphasized elsewhere in this report (see Chapter 8), BMD T-scores are only one component of that risk, and fracture risk may actually be quite low for many people with osteopenia, particularly younger individuals. To avoid causing unnecessary alarm among patients, many health care professionals prefer to avoid the term "osteopenia," instead telling patients that they have "somewhat low bone mass" and then explaining what that means in terms of fracture risk and how the problem can best be dealt with to minimize that risk.

Table 4–2. Prevalence (per 100 persons) of Osteoporosis and Hip Fracture in Persons 65 Years of Age and Older, by Gender and Age: United States, 1988-1994

	Self-reported		Tested
Gender and age	Hip fracture %	Osteoporosis %	Osteoporosis %
Male	2.3	1.3	3.8
65–74 years	2.1	1.3	2.0
75–84 years	2.4	1.3	6.4
85 years and over	4.1	1.6	13.7
Female	6.1	11.1	26.1
65–74 years	4.5	10.9	19.0
75–84 years	7.3	12.1	32.5
85 years and over	11.8	9.7	50.5

Source: Praemer et al. 1999. Published with permission from the American Academy of Orthopaedic Surgeons.

men. In fact, women over age 50 accounted for over 75 percent (7.8 million) of the total cases of osteoporosis at the hip in 2002 (NOF 2002). Women are more susceptible than men to osteoporosis because they begin with less bone mass and lose it at a somewhat faster rate. As shown in Figure 4-5 (Looker et al. 1998), White women lose one-third of their hip BMD between the ages of 20 and 80, while White men lose only a quarter during this time. These data on hip BMD are from NHANES III, where a large representative sample of the U.S. population was assessed at a single point in time (cross-sectional data). Bone loss in other parts of the body, however, does not necessarily follow the same pattern. For example, while bone loss from the hip is approximately linear across adult life, bone loss in other parts of the skeleton begins around the time of menopause in women and at a comparable age or later in men (Melton et al. 2000).

Using the World Health Organization's definition, an estimated 35 percent of postmenopausal White women have osteoporosis of the hip, spine, or distal forearm (Melton et al. 1998) and are at increased risk of future fractures. Since bone mass decreases slowly over time, it is no surprise that the prevalence of osteoporosis (the proportion of the population within a certain age range affected at any given time) increases with age. NHANES data show that the prevalence of osteoporosis at the hip increases over tenfold among postmenopausal White women, from 4 percent in those between the ages of 50 and 59 to 52

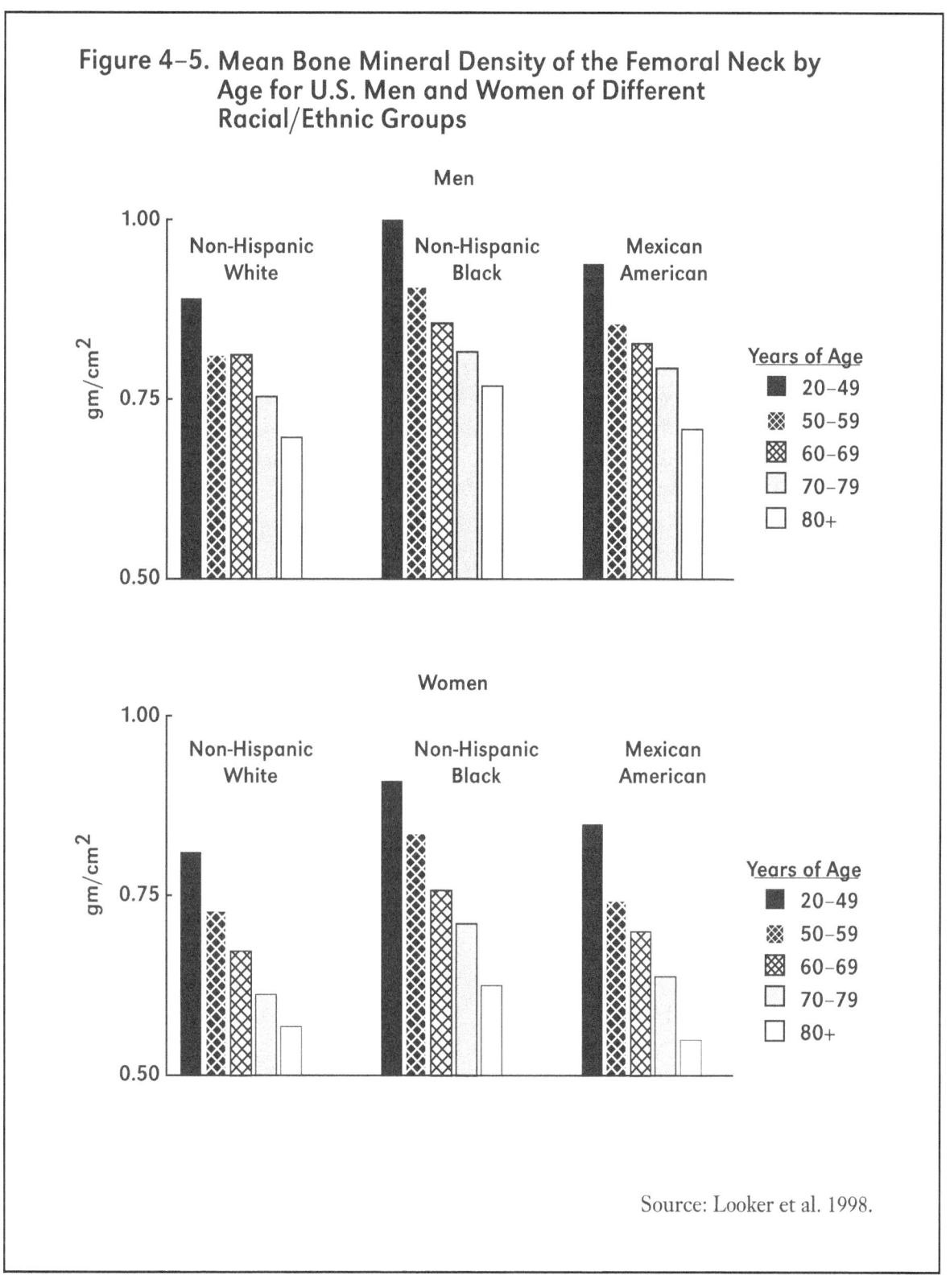

Figure 4–5. Mean Bone Mineral Density of the Femoral Neck by Age for U.S. Men and Women of Different Racial/Ethnic Groups

Source: Looker et al. 1998.

percent among those age 80 and older (Looker et al 1997). The overall prevalence of osteoporosis of the hip among postmenopausal White women is 17 percent in NHANES, compared to 21 percent in Sweden (Kanis et al. 2000) and only 8 percent in Canada (Tenenhouse et al. 2000). These variations may explain the differences in hip fractures among women in these various countries, with Swedish women being the most likely to suffer fractures and Canadian women the least (Melton and Cooper 2001).

While NHANES did not assess bone density at the spine or wrist (and consequently more such data are needed), other studies suggest that the prevalence of osteoporosis at these sites follows a somewhat similar pattern. For example, the prevalence of osteoporosis at the wrist increases thirteenfold, from 6 percent among women age 50–59 to 78 percent among those age 80 and older, yielding an overall prevalence of osteoporosis of the wrist among postmenopausal White women of 33 percent (Melton et al. 2000). Due to increasing difficulty in accurately assessing bone loss from the spine as individuals age (because of artifacts that mask bone loss; see Chapter 8 for more details), the diagnosed prevalence of osteoporosis in White women age 80 and older is only twice that among those between the ages of 50 and 59 (Melton et al. 2000). Thus, just 8 percent of postmenopausal women appear to have osteoporosis of the spine. The comparable figure in Canadian women is 12 percent (Tenenhouse et al. 2000).

There is some lack of agreement about how osteoporosis should be defined in men and non-Whites. Since aging men of all races also lose bone from the hip (Figure 4-1), one would expect the prevalence of osteoporosis to increase with age in men as it does in women. However, due to the limited data available at the time, the World Health Organization did not propose a specific definition of osteoporosis for men. Based on the same absolute cut-off value for men as for women (0.56 g/cm2 for femoral neck BMD), the prevalence of osteoporosis among White, Mexican-American, and Black men age 50 and older is 4 percent, 2 percent, and 3 percent, respectively, according to NHANES III (Looker et al. 1997). When the normal values for a young adult male are used as the cut-off point, the estimated prevalence of osteoporosis in these men increases substantially to 7 percent, 3 percent, and 5 percent, respectively. The comparable figure for Canadian men is about 4 percent (Tenenhouse et al. 2000). The fact that many fewer men than women develop very low levels of bone density, where fracture risk is greatest, helps explain the lower incidence of hip fractures in men.

With respect to non-White women, comparisons of BMD to normal values for non-Hispanic White women suggest that the age-adjusted prevalence of osteoporosis at the hip among Black women in the United States is 6 percent, compared to 17 percent for postmenopausal White women. This is consistent with the much lower fracture rates observed in Blacks (Melton and Cooper 2001). Mexican-American women in the United States have an estimated prevalence of hip osteoporosis of 14 percent (Looker et al. 1997), which is consistent with the somewhat lower risk of hip fractures in most populations of Spanish heritage compared to those of Northern European extraction. It has generally been presumed that Asians have a prevalence of osteoporosis similar to that in Whites. Japanese data indicate that the prevalence of osteoporosis at the lumbar spine is as high or higher than in White women while the prevalence of osteoporosis at the hip (12 percent) is lower (Iki et al. 2001). This goes along with the fact that spine fractures are almost as common among Asian women as they are in White women, while hip fractures are considerably less common (Melton and Cooper 2001).

Other Metabolic Bone Diseases

Much less is known about the frequency of most other skeletal diseases. This is because many of them, such as Paget's disease of bone and primary hyperparathyroidism, appear to be underdiagnosed. Others, such as osteomalacia and renal osteodystrophy, may in some cases be complications of some other condition and thus they are not counted separately. For example, the U.S. Renal Data System reports that almost 325,000 Americans are being treated for chronic renal failure by dialysis or renal transplantation (USRDS 2000). Over a third of those are Black, and their dialysis rate is five times greater than that of Whites. Although fracture rates are increased in these individuals (Alem et al. 2000), there appear to be no estimates of the actual prevalence of renal bone disease (see Chapter 3). By contrast, Black Americans are at a lower risk of primary hyperparathyroidism than are White Americans (Melton 2002). The condition is more common in women than men, and its prevalence increases with age in both sexes. Although there are indications that up to 1 percent of the population may be affected at any given time (Melton 2002), the annual incidence of diagnosed primary hyperparathyroidism has been estimated at only 21 per 100,000 (Wermers et al. 1997). However, the frequency of diagnosis of primary hyperparathyroidism is affected by how often blood calcium levels are measured and acted upon in clinical practice.

Paget's Disease of Bone

Based on an x-ray survey of the hip, pelvis, and spine by the first National Health and Nutritional Examination Survey, the prevalence of Paget's disease of bone has been estimated at 1.3 per 100 women and men age 45–74 (Siris 1999). This would represent over one million affected individuals in this country today. However, just as for spine fractures, many Pagetic bone lesions are asymptomatic and consequently undetected by health care professionals, meaning that the prevalence of clinically diagnosed cases of Paget's disease is much less. The incidence of the disease rises with age but is generally less than one per 1,000 per year, even among elderly individuals. The incidence is about twice as great in men as it is in women, and most patients are of Northern European heritage. Indeed, Paget's disease is most common in North America and Western Europe, except Scandinavia (Siris 1999). There is some evidence that the incidence of Paget's disease may be falling, but this may be the result of a decrease in the frequency of routine screening procedures (Tiegs et al. 2000).

Developmental Skeletal Disorders

There are many congenital disorders of the skeleton, but most are quite rare. Two of the more common conditions are osteopetrosis and the various forms of osteogenesis imperfecta (see Chapter 3). Altogether, 20,000 to 50,000 Americans may have osteogenesis imperfecta according to the Osteogenesis Imperfecta Foundation. The Paget's Foundation estimates that about 14,000 people in the United States (equivalent to one out of every 20,000 individuals) have osteopetrosis.

Acquired Skeletal Disorders

There are no estimates of the incidence of aseptic necrosis, despite its being a not uncommon complication of hip fracture and glucocorticoid therapy (see Chapter 3). Primary bone neoplasms, such as osteosarcoma, are less common. The most frequent malignancy arising in bone is multiple myeloma, which was described in Chapter 3. This malignancy affects men more than women and Blacks more than Whites. Altogether, there are about 2,400 new cases and 1,300 deaths each year in this country from cancer of the bones and joints, compared to 14,600 new cases and 10,900 deaths annually from multiple myeloma (ACS 2001). Of the more than 560,000 people who die of cancer each year, most will have had skeletal complications of their malignancy (bone metastases) at some point during their illness. Bone metastases most commonly occur in individuals with breast, prostate, kidney, lung, pancreatic, colorectal, stomach, thyroid, and ovarian cancers. People dying of breast and prostate cancer almost always experience bone metastases, causing a great deal of the pain in the last days of life. Bone metastases most commonly occur in the spine; other common sites include the pelvis, hip, upper leg bones, and the skull (ACS 2004).

Prospects for the Future

The prevalence of bone diseases is going to increase significantly as the population ages. In the United States, the number of people age 65 and older is expected to rise from 35 to 86 million between 2000 and 2050, while the number age 85 and older will increase from 4 to 20 million (US Census Bureau 2004). Much of this increase will occur in the next 25 years as the "baby boomers" reach their 70s and 80s. Unless prevention activities are greatly enhanced, this demographic change alone will cause a substantial increase in the number of people with bone diseases. For example, based on data from NHANES, it is estimated that 7.8 million women and 2.3 million men in the United States already have osteoporosis at the hip. These figures could rise to 10.5 million women and 3.3

million men (an increase of 35 percent in women and 43 percent in men, respectively) by 2020 (Figure 4-4) (NOF 2002). These trends make reaching the *Healthy People 2010* goal (which is to reduce the overall prevalence of osteoporosis at the hip among adults from 10 percent to 8 percent) all the more difficult (USDHHS 2000).

In fact, these demographic changes could cause the number of hip fractures in the United States to double or triple by 2040 (Schneider and Guralnik 1990). Any such increase will also make it very difficult to achieve another *Healthy People 2010* goal of reducing the annual incidence of hip fractures by 60 percent (from 1,056 to 416 per 100,000) among women age 65 or older, and by 20 percent (from 593 to 474 per 100,000) among elderly men (USDHHS 2000). History does not offer much optimism that these goals will be reached, either. In fact, *Healthy People 2000* called for a nearly 15 percent reduction in the overall incidence of hip fractures among men and women age 65 and older (from 714 per 100,000 in 1988 to 607 per 100,000 by 2000) (USDHHS 1991). The annual incidence among this population actually increased by over 17 percent, to 840 per 100,000, in 2000.

The aging phenomenon and its potential impact on bone disease are not unique to the United States. Across the globe, the number of individuals age 65 and older is expected to increase nearly fivefold between 1990 and 2050, from 323 million to 1.55 billion. This trend alone could result in a 3.7-fold increase in the number of hip fractures worldwide, from an estimated 1.7 million in 1990 to a projected 6.3 million in 2050 (Cooper et al. 1992b). Even this figure may prove conservative, as it assumes that the incidence of hip fractures among individuals of a given age remains constant. If, instead, incidence rates remain constant in Europe and North America (they have stabilized in these areas recently) but increase by 3 percent annually elsewhere (as is occurring in some parts of the world), the total worldwide number of hip fractures each year could exceed 21 million by 2050 (Gullberg et al. 1997).

Key Questions for Future Research

Research questions for Chapter 4 have been merged with those for Chapter 5 because of the close relationship between frequency and burden of disease issues. (See Chapter 5, page 103.)

References

Alem AM, Sherrard DJ, Gillen DL, Weiss NS, Beresford SA, Heckbert SR, Wong C, Stehman-Breen C. Increased risk of hip fracture among patients with end-stage renal disease. Kidney Int. 2000 Jul;58(1):396-9.

American Cancer Society. Cancer facts & figures 2001. Atlanta (GA): American Cancer Society; 2001.48 p.

American Cancer Society. Cancer reference information Web site [homepage on the Internet]. Washington (DC): American Cancer Society [cited 2004 Apr 14]. Available from: http://www.cancer.org/docroot/CRIcontentCRI_2_2_1X_How_many_people_get_bone_metastasis_66.asp?sitearea=

Bauer RL, Deyo RA. Low risk of vertebral fracture in Mexican American women. Arch Intern Med. 1987 Aug;147(8):1437-9.

Black DM, Cummings SR, Stone K, Hudes E, Palermo L, Steiger P. A new approach to defining normal vertebral dimensions. J Bone Miner Res. 1991 Aug;6(8):883-92.

Chrischilles EA, Butler CD, Davis CS, Wallace RB. A model of lifetime osteoporosis impact. Arch Intern Med. 1991 Oct; 151(10):2026-32.

Chung KC, Spilson SV. The frequency and epidemiology of hand and forearm fractures in the United States. J Hand Surg [AM]. 2001 Sep;26(5):908-15.

[a]Cooper C, Atkinson EJ, O'Fallon WM, Melton LJ 3rd. Incidence of clinically diagnosed vertebral fractures: A population-based study in Rochester, Minnesota, 1985-1989. J Bone Miner Res. 1992 Feb;7(2):221-7.

[b]Cooper C, Campion G, Melton LJ 3rd. Hip fractures in the elderly: A world-wide projection. Osteoporosis Int. 1992 Nov;2(6):285-9.

Cooper C, Melton LJ 3rd, Epidemiology of osteoporosis. Trends Endocrinol Metab 1992;3:224-229.

Cummings SR, Melton LJ 3rd. Epidemiology and outcomes of osteoporotic fractures. Lancet. 2002 May 18;359(9319):1761-7.

Dartmouth Atlas of Health web site [homepage on the Internet]. Dartmouth (NH): Center for the Evaluative Clinical Sciences at Dartmouth Medical School; [cited 2004 Apr 12]. Available from: http://www.dartmouthatlas.org/.

Davis JW, Nevitt MC, Wasnich RD, Ross PD. A cross-cultural comparison of neuromuscular performance, functional status, and falls between Japanese and white women. J Gerontol A Biol Sci Med Sci. 1999 Jun;54(6):M288-92.

Fang J, Freeman R, Jeganathan R, Alderman MH. Variations in hip fracture hospitalization rates among different race/ethnicity groups in New York City. Ethn Dis. 2004 Spring;14(2):280-4.

Genant HK, Jergas M. Assessment of prevalent and incident vertebral fractures in osteoporosis research. Osteoporos Int. 2003;14 Suppl 3:S43-55.

Grados F, Marcelli C, Dargent-Molina P, Roux C, Vergnol JF, Meunier PJ, Fardellone P. Prevalence of vertebral fractures in French women older than 75 years from the EPIDOS study. Bone 2004 Feb;34(2):362-7.

Gullberg B, Johnell O, Kanis JA. World-wide projections for hip fracture. Osteoporos Int. 1997;7(5):407-13.

Iki M, Kagamimori S, Kagawa Y, Matsuzaki T, Yoneshima H, Marumo F. Bone mineral density of the spine, hip and distal forearm in representative samples of the Japanese female population: Japanese Population-Based Osteoporosis (JPOS) Study. Osteoporosis Int. 2001;12(7):529-37.

Jacobsen SJ, Cooper C, Gottlieb MS, Goldberg J, Yahnke DP, Melton LJ 3rd. Hospitalization with vertebral fracture among the aged: A national population-based study, 1986-1989. Epidemiology. 1992 Nov;3(6):515-8.

Kanis JA, Johnell O, Oden A, Jonsson B, De Laet C, Dawson A. Risk of hip fracture according to the World Health Organization criteria for osteopenia and osteoporosis. Bone. 2000 Nov;27(5):585-90.

Kanis JA, Johnell O, Oden A, Borgstrom F, Zethraeus N, De Laet C, Jonsson B. The risk and burden of vertebral fractures in Sweden. Osteoporos Int. 2004 Jan;15(1): 20-6.

Karagas MR, Baron JA, Barrett JA, Jacobsen SJ. Patterns of fracture among the United States elderly: Geographic and fluoride effects. Ann Epidemiol. 1996 May;6(3):209-16.

Klotzbuecher CM, Ross PD, Landsman PB, Abbott TA 3rd, Berger M. Patients with prior fractures have an increased risk of future fractures: A summary of the literature and statistical synthesis. J Bone Miner Res. 2000 Apr;15(4):721-39.

Lauderdale DS, Jacobsen SJ, Furner SE, Levy PS, Brody JA, Goldberg J. Hip fracture incidence among elderly Asian-American populations. Am J Epidemiol. 1997 Sep 15;146(6):502-9.

Looker AC, Orwoll ES, Johnston CC Jr, Lindsay RL, Wahner HW, Dunn WL, Calvo MS, Harris TB, Heyse SP. Prevalence of low femoral bone density in older U.S. adults from NHANES III. J Bone Miner Res. 1997 Nov;12(11):1761-8.

Looker AC, Wahner HW, Dunn WL, Calvo MS, Harris TB, Heyse SP, Johnston CC Jr, Lindsay R. Updated data on proximal femur bone mineral levels of US adults. Osteoporosis Int. 1998;8(5):468-9.

Melton LJ 3rd, Thamer M, Ray NF, Chan JK, Chesnut CH 3rd, Einhorn TA, Johnston CC, Raisz LG, Silverman SL, Siris ES. Fractures attributable to osteoporosis: Report from the National Osteoporosis Foundation. J Bone Miner Res. 1997 Jan;12(1):16-23.

Melton LJ 3rd, Atkinson EJ, O'Connor MK, O'Fallon WM, Riggs BL. Bone density and fracture risk in men. J Bone Miner Res. 1998 Dec;13(12):1915-23.

Melton LJ 3rd, Khosla S, Achenbach SJ, O'Connor MK, O'Fallon WM, Riggs BL. Effects of body size and skeletal site on the estimated prevalence of osteoporosis in women and men. Osteoporos Int. 2000;11(11):977-83.

Melton, LJ 3rd; Cooper, C. Magnitude and Impact of Osteoporosis and Fractures. In: Marcus, R; Feldman, D; Kelsey, J, editors. Osteoporosis, 2nd ed. Vol. 1. San Diego: Academic Press; 2001; pp. 557-67.

Melton LJ 3rd. The epidemiology of primary hyperparathyroidism in North America. J Bone Miner Res. 2002 Nov; 17 Suppl 2:N12-17.

Myers ER, Wilson SE. Biomechanics of osteoporosis and vertebral fracture. Spine. 1997 Dec 15;22(24 Suppl):25S-31S.

National Osteoporosis Foundation. America's bone health: The state of osteoporosis and low bone mass in our nation. Washington (DC): National Osteoporosis Foundation; 2002.

Nguyen TV, Eisman JA, Kelly PJ, Sambrook PN. Risk factors for osteoporotic fractures in elderly men. Am J Epidemiol. 1996 Aug 1;144(3):255-63.

Oden A, Dawson A, Dere W, Johnell O, Jonsson B, Kanis JA. Lifetime risk of hip fractures is underestimated. Osteoporos Int. 1998;8(6):599-603.

O'Neill TW, Felsenberg D, Varlow J, Cooper C, Kanis JA, Silman AJ. The prevalence of vertebral deformity in European men and women: The European Vertebral Osteoporosis Study. J Bone Miner Res. 1996 Jul;11(7):1010-8.

Praemer A, Furner S, Rice DP. Musculoskeletal conditions in the United States Rosemont, IL: American Academy of Orthopaedic Surgeons; 1999. 182 p.

Riggs BL, Melton LJ 3rd. The worldwide problem of osteoporosis: Insights afforded by epidemiology. Bone. 1995 Nov;17(5 Suppl):505S-511S.

Ross PD, Fujiwara S, Huang C, Davis JW, Epstein RS, Wasnich RD, Kodama K, Melton LJ 3rd. Vertebral fracture prevalence in women in Hiroshima compared to Caucasians or Japanese in the US. Int J Epidemiol. 1995 Dec;24(6):1171-7.

Roy DK, Pye SR, Lunt M, O'Neill TW, Todd C, Raspe H, Reeve J, Silman AJ, Weber K, Dequeker J, et al. Falls explain between-center differences in the incidence of limb fracture across Europe. Bone. 2002 Dec;31(6):712-7.

Schneider EL, Guralnik JM. The aging of America: Impact on health care costs. JAMA. 1990 May 2;263(17):2335-40.

Siris ES. Paget's disease of bone. In: Favus MJ, editor. Primer on the Metabolic Bone Diseases and Disorders of Mineral Metabolism. 4th ed. Philadelphia: Lippincott Williams & Wilkins; 1999. p. 415-425.

Siris ES, Miller PD, Barrett-Connor E, Faulkner KG, Wehren LE, Abbott TA, Berger ML, Santora AC, Sherwood LM. Identification and fracture outcomes of undiagnosed low bone mineral density in postmenopausal women: Results from the National Osteoporosis Risk Assessment. JAMA. 2001 Dec 12;286(22):2815-22.

Stone KL, Seeley DG, Lui LY, Cauley JA, Ensrud K, Browner WS, Nevitt MC, Cummings SR; Osteoporotic Fractures Research Group. BMD at multiple sites and risk of fracture of multiple types: Long-term results from the Study of Osteoporotic Fractures. J Bone Miner Res. 2003 Nov;18(11):1947-54.

Tenenhouse A, Joseph L, Kreiger N, Poliquin S, Murray TM, Blondeau L, Berger C, Hanley DA, Prior JC; CaMos Research Group. Canadian Multicentre Osteoporosis Study. Estimation of the prevalence of low bone density in Canadian women and men using a population-specific DXA reference standard: The Canadian Multicentre Osteoporosis Study (CaMos). Osteoporosis Int. 2000;11(10):897-904.

Tiegs RD, Lohse CM, Wollan PC, Melton LJ 3rd. Long-term trends in the incidence of Paget's disease of bone. Bone. 2000 Sep;27(3):423-7.

U.S. Census Bureau [homepage on the Internet]. U.S. Interim Projections by Age, Sex, Race, and Hispanic Origin. Washington (DC): U.S. Census Bureau, Population Division, Populations Projection Branch; c2004 [revised May 18, 2004; cited 2004 Jul 9]. Available at http://www.census.gov/ipc/www/usinterimproj/.

U.S. Department of Health and Human Services, Public Health Service. Healthy People 2000. Washington (DC): U.S. Government Printing Office; 1991. USDHHS Publication No. (PHS)91-50212.

U.S. Department of Health and Human Services. Healthy People 2010. Washington (DC): January 2000.

U.S. Renal Data System. USRDS 2000 annual data report. Bethesda (MD): National Institutes of Health (NIH), USDHHS; 2000. Available at www.usrds.org.

Wermers RA, Khosla S, Atkinson EJ, Hodgson, SF, O'Fallon WM, Melton LJ 3rd. The rise and fall of primary hyperparathyroidism: A population-based study in Rochester, Minnesota, 1965-1992. Ann Intern Med. 1997 Mar;126(6):433-40.

Winner SJ, Morgan CA, Evans JG. Perimenopausal risk of falling and incidence of distal forearm fracture. BMJ. 1989 Jun 3;298(6686):1486-8.

Zingmond DS, Melton LJ 3rd, Silverman SL. Increasing hip fracture incidence in California Hispanics, 1983 to 2000. Osteoporos Int. 2004 Mar 4 [Epub ahead of print].

Chapter 5: Key Messages

- Bone diseases have a major impact on the population as a whole and especially on affected individuals and their families. Although some bone diseases lead directly to pain and deformity, bone disease often is a "silent" disorder until it causes fractures.

- The 1.5 million osteoporotic fractures in the United States each year lead to more than half a million hospitalizations, over 800,000 emergency room encounters, more than 2,600,000 physician office visits, and the placement of nearly 180,000 individuals into nursing homes. Hip fractures are by far the most devastating type of fracture, accounting for about 300,000 hospitalizations each year.

- Caring for these fractures is expensive. Studies show that annual direct care expenditures for osteoporotic fractures range from $12 to $18 billion per year in 2002 dollars. Indirect costs (e.g., lost productivity for patients and caregivers) likely add billions of dollars to this figure. These costs could double or triple in the coming decades.

- From an individual's perspective, bone disease has a devastating impact on patients and their families. While few die directly from bone disease, for many individuals a fracture can lead to a downward spiral in physical and mental health that for some ultimately results in death. In fact, hip fractures are associated with a significantly increased risk of death, especially during the first year after the fracture.

- Bone diseases dramatically affect functional status. Many individuals who suffer fractures experience significant pain and height loss, and may lose the ability to dress themselves, stand up, and walk. These individuals are also at risk of complications such as pressure sores, pneumonia, and urinary tract infections. Nearly one in five hip fracture patients ends up in a nursing home, a situation that a majority of participants in one study compared unfavorably to death.

- Fractures can also have a negative impact on self-esteem, body image, and mood, which may lead to psychological consequences. Individuals who suffer fractures may be immobilized by a fear of falling and suffering additional fractures. Not surprisingly, they may begin to feel isolated and helpless.

- Many bone disorders other than osteoporosis add greatly to the burden of bone disease in the population, although the impact varies enormously and is largely dependent upon the severity of the disease.

Chapter 5

THE BURDEN OF BONE DISEASE

Bone diseases have a major impact on the population as a whole and especially on affected individuals and their families. Osteoporosis, in particular, is an important public health problem that affects a large segment of the community. Although some bone diseases lead directly to pain and deformity, bone disease more commonly is a "silent" disorder until it causes one or more fractures. The many individuals with bone disease who suffer fractures must deal with the complications that may ensue, including ill health (morbidity), disability, a reduced quality of life, and possibly even death. The care of patients with these fractures is also very expensive, and costs will continue to rise as the frequency of bone disease increases in the future with the anticipated growth of the elderly population. These aspects of the problem are reviewed in the sections that follow, focusing first on the effects of bone disease on society as a whole and then on the problems that bone diseases pose for individuals. What these statistics make clear is that the burden of bone disease is enormous.

Most of the statistics that follow relate to osteoporosis, the most common and perhaps most "burdensome" bone disease from society's perspective. While the burden of osteoporosis has been well documented, there is relatively little information on the burden imposed by other disorders that affect bone health, even though they can cause marked impairment of health and even death in those who are affected. Recognizing the limits on available information, this chapter nonetheless provides some general descriptions on the burden of these other bone diseases on page 102.

Impact on Society

Mortality

Despite the large numbers affected, very few people die as a direct result of bone disease, although bone disease may be under-appreciated as an indirect cause of death. Bone diseases accounted directly for only a tiny fraction of the 2.4 million deaths reported nationally in 1999 (NCHS 1999). Other diseases, such as heart disease and cancer, are much more likely to directly cause an individual's death. Even hip fractures, which represent one of the most serious consequences of bone disease, seldom directly result in death. In fact, in 1999 hip fractures were listed as the cause of death on only 12,661 death certificates (NCHS 1999), representing less than 4 percent of the number of patients who were hospitalized for hip fractures in that year (Popovic 2001). Bone disease can indirectly lead to death, as fractures and their associated complications can in some cases trigger a downward spiral in health. In one population sample, the risk of mortality was four times greater among hip fracture patients during the first 3 months after the fracture than was the comparable risk among fracture-free individuals

The Real-Life Burden of Osteoporosis

Osteoporosis has a significant impact on the everyday lives of those who suffer from the disease, as the following story clearly illustrates.

This 73-year-old wife and grandmother suffered her first fracture 18 years ago and has had eight additional fractures since that time. Each caused tremendous pain and required long hospital stays and extended periods on medication. Unfortunately, however, because she does not tolerate osteoporosis medications well, her primary treatment has consisted of estrogen, vitamin D, and calcium supplements. As bad as the actual fractures have been, it is the fear of additional fractures that may well have the largest impact on her life. As a result of this fear, she limits the time she spends with her grandchildren, as well as the types of activities she enjoys with them (three of her fractures occurred while playing with her grandchildren). She finds it impossible to lie down on her back or right side and difficult to get in and out of bed or a chair. She has had to give up dancing, one of her favorite

> *"I had planned to spend these years enjoying my grandchildren, but I've really had to curtail my activities with them. I've fractured my back three times while playing with them."*
> *—Long-time osteoporosis sufferer*

activities, and feels she has become a "drag" on family members who must slow down to accommodate her limitations.

A Parent's Perspective on the Burden of Bone Disease

This story illustrates the devastating impact that bone disease can have in those rare instances when it strikes children.

This mother has two children with bone disease. Her daughter, now in her mid-20s, suffers from osteoporosis. Yet it is her son's battle with severe OI that is most tragic. Now in his late 20s, he suffered nearly a dozen bone fractures at birth. When he was two months old, the mother endured the horrible sound of hearing her son's arm break as she turned him over in his crib. To date, he has suffered 140 fractures, some caused by acts as simple as sneezing or being startled. Fractures, however, are not the only health problems he faces. Like many OI sufferers, he also must live with scoliosis, broken teeth, hernias, kidney stones, and hearing loss. He presently requires full-time oxygen. Only 3 feet tall, he has never slept through the night.

Like many OI patients, he is highly intelligent and engaging, a true joy to be around. He spoke in complete sentences by the age of 1 and was reading at the age of 2. He showed an interest in politics by age 5, querying his mother on whom she was going to vote for in the presidential election and why. His tremendous intellectual abilities and engaging personality are as much or more a part of him as are his disabilities. His personality and story make him an excellent spokesperson for the disease.

of similar gender and age. Approximately 20 percent of the hip fracture patients died within a year of the fracture (Leibson et al. 2002). These overall rates may overstate the increased risk of death that is attributable to the fracture, as some of these patients were already in a nursing home and may have died even in the absence of the fracture. Another study, which included only patients who were ambulatory and not living in nursing homes at the time of their hip fracture, found that hip fracture patients had a 2.8-fold increased risk of dying during the 3 months following the fracture, although this risk also depended on their pre-fracture health. Those with poor pre-fracture health had higher mortality rates (Richmond et al. 2003). A recent analysis of NHANES I found that, over a follow-up period of 8–22 years, each standard deviation decrease in bone density was associated with a 10–40 percent increase in mortality (Mussolino et al. 2003). A prospective study of women over 65 (which was part of the Study of Osteoporotic Fractures) showed that each standard deviation of bone loss at the hip was associated with a 30 percent increase in total mortality (Kado et al. 2000). Recent studies from Sweden have shown increased mortality after spine fractures as well as hip fractures (Kanis et al. 2004, Johnell et al. 2004).

Morbidity

Bone diseases are much more likely to lead to poor health (i.e., morbidity) than they are to cause death. Most bone diseases disproportionately affect the elderly, who may already have substantial problems with frailty and reduced functional capacity. Fractures are the biggest problem facing most individuals with bone disease, especially those with osteoporosis. The cumulative impact of these fractures is quite devastating. As shown in Table 5-1, osteoporotic fractures in the United States in 1995 led to more than half a million hospitalizations, over 800,000 emergency room encounters, more than 2.6 million physician office visits, and the placement of nearly 180,000 individuals into nursing homes. Based on a statistical model, it has been estimated that over a 10-year period White women age 45 and older in the United States could experience 5.2 million fractures of the hip, spine, or forearm, resulting in 2 million person-years of disability related to the fractures (Chrischilles et al. 1994). Unfortunately, comparable estimates are not available for other diseases of the skeleton.

Hip fractures are by far the most devastating type of fracture, accounting for about 300,000 hospitalizations each year. Almost all hip fracture patients are hospitalized, and they represent nearly half of all hospitalizations for osteoporotic fractures in the United States (Table 5-1). Hip fractures frequently lead to disability. More than one in four (26 percent) individuals suffering a hip fracture becomes disabled in the following year because of the fracture (i.e., this figure represents disabilities that are in addition to those resulting from the functional losses that would ordinarily occur in frail older persons) (Magaziner et al. 2003). Due primarily to dementia and the inability to walk independently, nearly one out of five requires long-term nursing home care (Table 5-2). In aggregate, hip fractures were responsible for nearly 140,000 nursing home admissions in 1995 (Ray et al. 1997). Spine fractures are less devastating, with only 1 in 10 patients requiring hospitalization and less than 2 percent requiring nursing home care (Chrischilles et al. 1991). They account for nearly 66,000 physician office visits and at least 45,000—and perhaps as many as 70,000—hospital admissions each year (Table 5-1). Half of these patients require some continuing care in a skilled nursing facility

Table 5–1. Resource Utilization Attributable to Osteoporotic Fractures Among Persons ≥ 45 Years of Age in the United States in 1995, by Type of Service and Type of Fracture

Type of service	Total	Type of fracture			
		Hip%	Forearm%	Spine%	Other sites%†
Inpatient hospitalizations	547,000	49	3	8	39
Nursing home residents	179,000	77	1	3	20
Physician Visits	2,634,000	14	20	3	63
Emergency room encounters	807,000	21	9	4	66
Physical therapy sessions	194,000	23	39	1	38
Diagnostic radiology	1,902,000	18	17	4	62
Medications	2,358,000	13	13	3	71
Home health care visits	2,250,000	60	2	3	35
Ambulance encounters	220,000	36	0	10	55
Orthopedic/other supplies	492,000	28	0	9	63

† These include fractures of the arm, lower leg, pelvis, ribs, ankle, and foot. The role of osteoporosis in fractures at other sites depends on age, race, and gender. There is disagreement about how many of these are osteoporotic-related fractures, although estimates range from 15% to 60%.

Source: Modified from Ray et al. 1997. Reproduced from J Bone Miner Res 1997: Jan; 12(1): 24–35 with permission of the American Society for Bone and Mineral Research.

(Gehlbach et al. 2003). Fractures of the wrist (also known as the distal forearm) are the least debilitating. Only about one-fifth of patients suffering a wrist fracture are hospitalized, and they rarely require nursing home care (Tables 5-1, 5-2). Yet even this relatively less traumatic event still accounts for nearly 20,000 hospital admissions and over 530,000 physician visits each year (Table 5-1). Surprisingly, these fractures consume more outpatient physical therapy services than do hip fractures.

Cost

Bone diseases are expensive, in terms of direct health care expenditures and indirect expenditures as well as lost productivity/workdays for patients and caregivers. While the figures cited below are large, it is important to remember that they represent today's costs. Given health care inflation and the projections for significant increases in the number of fractures (see Chapter 4), it is not unreasonable to assume that the direct and indirect costs of bone disease will more than double or triple in the coming decades (Burge et al. 2003).

Direct Costs

Studies show that annual direct care expenditures for osteoporotic fractures range from $12.2–$17.9 billion per year in 2002 dollars (Tosteson 1999). While women account for the majority of these costs, White men also incur substantial overall costs for osteoporotic fracture care (representing 18 percent of the total costs of osteoporosis, or $3.2 billion). In addition, non-White women and men of all ages account for $1 billion annually in total direct care expenditures on osteoporotic fractures (Ray et al. 1997).

Although large, expenditures related to osteoporosis represent just 7 percent of total heath care costs among women age 45 and older (Hoerger et al. 1999). This is more than double the amount spent for gynecological cancers but only a fraction of the cost of cardiovascular disease. However, osteoporosis accounts for nearly 14 percent of all nursing home days, due to the late age at which expenses are incurred for osteoporosis relative to other diseases (Hoerger et al. 1999).

Table 5-2. Disability Resulting From Osteoporotic Fractures

	Functionally dependent† (%)	Nursing home (%)
Hip fracture	10	19
Spine fracture	4	2
Forearm fracture	2	—
Any of these	7	8

† Community dwelling but requiring human assistance or unable to perform one or more activities of daily living.

Source: Chrischilles et al. 1991.

Hospital care accounts for more than half of the total direct costs, with nursing home care also responsible for a large portion of the total. As noted, hip fractures are the most devastating complication of osteoporosis, and therefore it is no surprise that they account for the largest proportion (63 percent or $11.3 billion) of medical care costs (Table 5-3). This is because hip fractures are very expensive to treat, with per-fracture costs estimated to range from $30,100–$43,400 in 2002 dollars (Tosteson 1999). The costs of caring for hip fractures are not limited to this initial treatment, however, as those suffering hip fractures require follow-up care as a direct result of their injury. A recent study estimated that hospital and outpatient care (excluding nursing home care) due to a hip fracture adds $14,600 to direct medical expenditures in the year following the fracture (Gabriel et al. 2002). The overall lifetime cost attributable to a hip fracture could exceed $81,000 (Braithwaite et al. 2003).

Although hip fractures account for the majority of costs, more than $6.5 billion is spent annually to treat those suffering from other types of osteoporotic fractures (Ray et al. 1997).

The direct costs of osteoporotic fractures are typically borne by society, primarily through Medicare and Medicaid. Among women over age 45, the government pays for most of the costs of osteoporotic fractures: Medicaid covers almost a fourth of the expense and Medicare pays nearly half (Hoerger et al. 1999). This is to be expected since nearly three-quarters of

Table 5-3. **Direct Health Care Expenditures for Care of Osteoporotic Fractures Among Persons ≥ 45 Years of Age in the United States by Type of Service and Type of Fracture, 1995**

Type of fracture	Type of service (millions of $)						
	Inpatient hospital	Emergency room	Outpatient physician	Outpatient hospital	Other outpatient*	Nursing home	Total
Hip	5576	130	67	9	90	2811	8682
Forearm	183	55	93	8	4	41	385
Spine	575	20	13	3	10	126	746
All other sites†	2259	3632	297	45	91	899	3953
Total	8594	567	470	65	194	3875	13,764

*Includes home health care, ambulance services, and medical equipment.
† Depending on age, race, and gender, from 15% to 60% of all other fractures were attributed to osteoporosis

Source: Ray et al. 1997. Reproduced from J Bone Miner Res 1997: Jan; 12(1): 24–25 with permission of the American Society for Bone and Mineral Research.

all hip, spine, and distal forearm fractures occur among patients 65 years and over.

Indirect Costs

In addition to imposing direct medical costs on society, osteoporosis also results in indirect costs, primarily related to reduced productivity due to disability and premature death. Indirect costs are inherently difficult to measure, and much more needs to be done in this area. One method judges lost productivity on the basis of reduced earnings. For bone diseases, which affect a large number of retired persons, indirect costs are underestimated by this approach. Nonetheless, assuming that people are worth what they earn, one study estimates that the cost of premature death and of restricted activity resulting from fractures accounts for 26 percent of total fracture costs and 12 percent of hip fracture costs (Praemer et al. 1999). A recent study from California (where 12 percent of the US population resides) found that the indirect cost to society (based only on lost earnings from premature deaths) accounted for 17 percent of the total cost related to osteoporosis (Max et al. 2002).

Impact on the Individual

While the statistics cited in the previous section relate to the impact of bone disease on society, it is important to remember that these "global" statistics really take on meaning when examining what they mean for individuals. In fact, osteoporosis and other bone diseases have a profound impact on those individuals who suffer from them and on their families. This section examines that impact, highlighting the very real burden that bone disease can place on the physical health, mental well-being, and financial stability of those individuals and family members affected by the disease.

The Chance of Dying From Bone Disease

While the chance of dying varies by fracture type, the vast majority of individuals suffering from osteoporosis and osteoporotic-related fractures do not die directly as a result of their disease. As noted previously, hip fractures are among the most devastating type of fracture; it has been estimated that approximately 20 percent of all patients die within a year (Leibson et al. 2002). The oldest hip fracture patients are most likely to die, and survival rates are lower for men (both White and Black) than for women, although Black women are more likely to die from a hip fracture than are White women. These differences may be due in part to the older age at which men and Black women are likely to suffer a hip fracture as well as to differences in their medical care (Figure 5-1). It is important to note, however, that the typical hip fracture patient is about 80 years old, and thus their risk of death from any cause is not trivial. Thus, it is more accurate to say that a hip fracture decreases the chance of survival in the first year by about 12–20 percent in this already at-risk population. Another way to look at this statistic is that 9 out of every 100 women with a hip fracture will die as a result of the fracture (Magaziner et al. 1997). The increased risk of death is especially high (10 times more than the expected death rate) in the first few weeks following a hip fracture. While the excess risk of death due to hip fractures diminishes with time, there may still be some additional risk for a number of years. For example, roughly 5 percent of hip fracture patients experience a severe medical complication, causing an increase in their risk of death (Lawrence et al. 2002). In addition, as noted previously, most hip fracture patients have other serious medical problems (comorbidities that more directly contribute to death) (Browner et al. 1996). Even so, with any given amount of preexisting comorbidity, the occurrence of a hip fracture substantially increases the likelihood of dying (Poór et al. 1995).

Other types of fractures are less likely to result in death. For example, patients suffering a wrist fracture are no more likely to die than anyone else (Melton 2003). Other limb fractures have been linked to an increased risk of death (Browner et al. 1996), although only a few of these deaths are related directly to the fracture. Most of the deaths seem to result from the presence of some other serious disease. For example, the death rate following a fracture of the spine is 1.2 to 1.9 times greater than expected (Melton 2003), but most of the deaths occur long after the fracture and appear to be due to serious underlying medical conditions that not only increase the risk of dying but also are likely the cause of the bone loss and associated fractures.

As noted in Chapter 3, inherited bone diseases have been found to increase the risk of death; in fact, in some cases these diseases are so severe that they are incompatible with life. Likewise, survival is much reduced among patients with bone cancer and multiple myeloma (Praemer et al. 1999). It is unclear whether or not patients with primary hyperparathyroidism face an increased risk of death, although survival does appear to be worse for the most severely affected patients, including those with the highest blood calcium levels and those with other serious diseases (Vestergaard et al. 2003).

Impact on Morbidity, Levels of Disability, and Functional Status

Bone diseases dramatically affect the functional status of those who get them. Many individuals who suffer fractures as a result of osteoporosis suffer significant pain, height loss, and may lose the ability to dress themselves, stand up, and walk. These patients are also at risk of acute complications such as pressure sores,

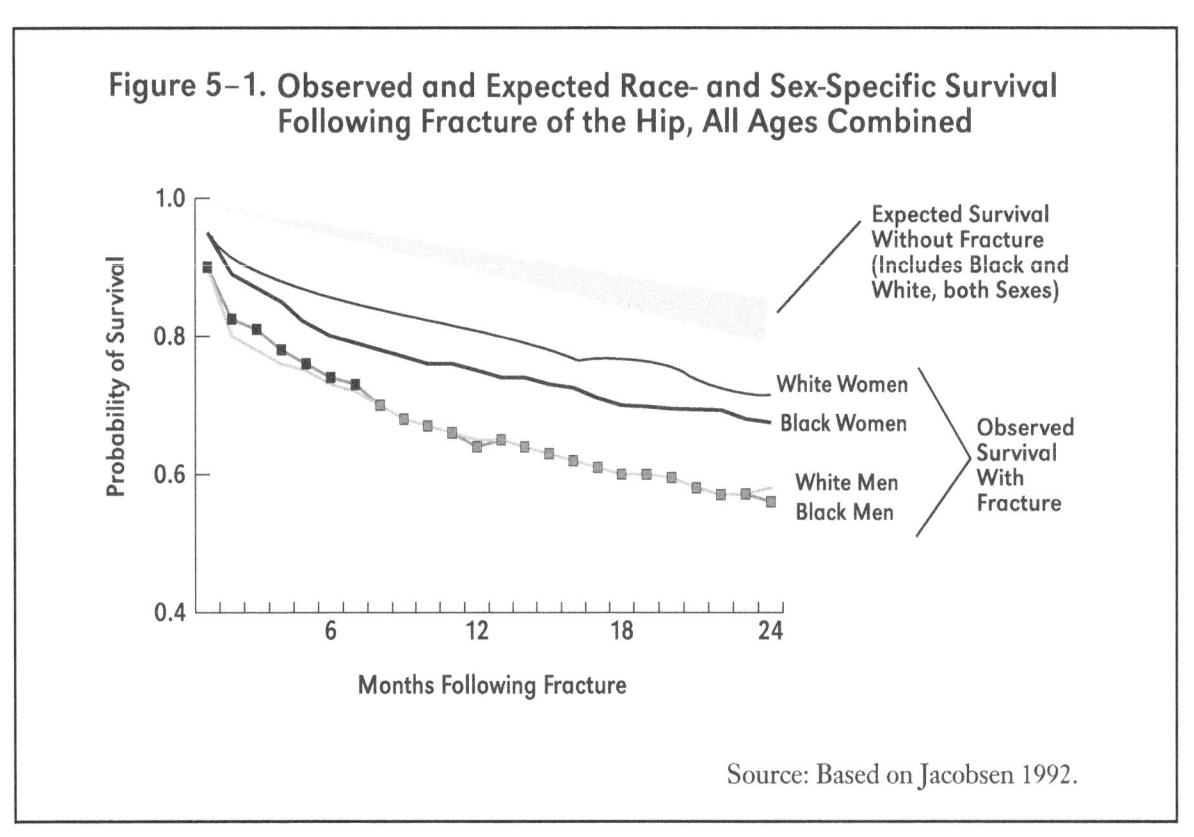

Figure 5–1. Observed and Expected Race- and Sex-Specific Survival Following Fracture of the Hip, All Ages Combined

Source: Based on Jacobsen 1992.

pneumonia, and urinary tract infections. Nearly one in five ends up in a nursing home, a situation that a majority of participants in one study compared unfavorably to death (Salkeld et al. 2000). As illustrated in Figure 5-2, different types of osteoporotic fractures have a different impact on the patients who suffer them. Wrist fractures commonly occur in women in their mid-50s and usually have only a short-term impact, whereas spine fractures typically occur at a later age and may give rise to permanent morbidity. By contrast, hip fractures occur later in life (around age 80 on average) and usually result in permanent disability (Kanis and Johnell 1999). Each of these fracture types will be discussed in more detail below.

Two-thirds of hip fracture patients do not return to the level of function they enjoyed before the fracture (OTA 1994), particularly those who become depressed (Magaziner et al. 2003). Many lose their ability to walk. In fact, only 40–79 percent of patients regain their previous ambulatory function a year after the fracture, and less than half return to their prefracture status with respect to the activities of daily living (Greendale and Barrett-Connor 2001). For example, data from the Established Populations for Epidemiologic Studies of the Elderly (EPESE) project show that 86 percent of patients could dress by themselves before the fracture, but only 49 percent afterwards. Similarly, 90 percent could move from chair to

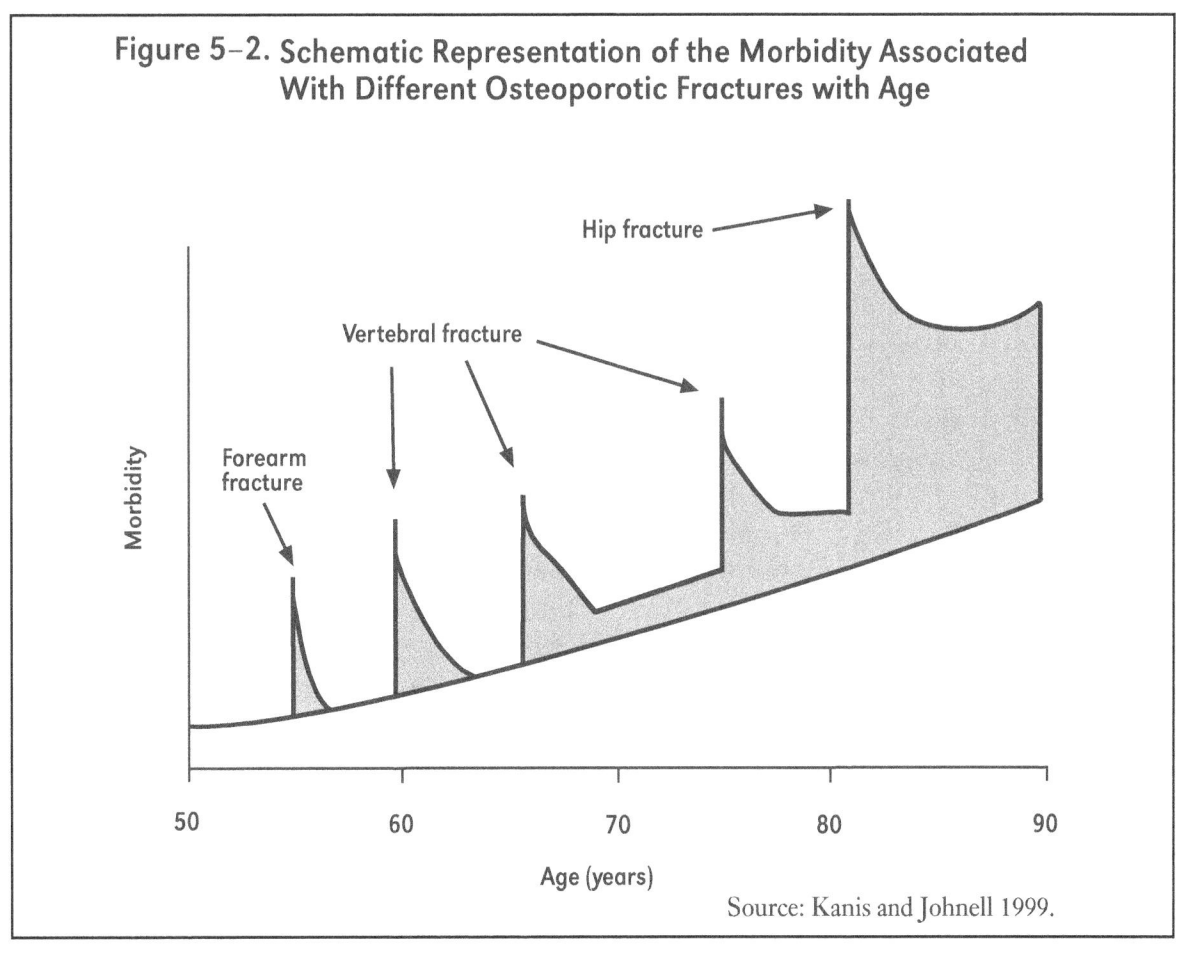

Figure 5–2. Schematic Representation of the Morbidity Associated With Different Osteoporotic Fractures with Age

Source: Kanis and Johnell 1999.

standing before the fracture and only 32 percent after. Comparable figures for walking across the room are 75 percent and 15 percent (Marottoli et al. 1992). Indeed, hip fracture patients are as likely to have impaired ambulation and other functional deficits as are those who suffer a stroke (Lieberman et al. 1999). Even among people who were previously independent, many activities cannot be carried out independently following a hip fracture (Table 5-4). Hip fractures cause an "extra" 10 percent of women to become functionally dependent (i.e., 10 percent more women become dependent than would have in the absence of the fractures), and 19 percent of women who suffer hip fractures require long-term nursing home care (Chrischilles et al. 1991).

Other types of fractures, while somewhat less devastating than hip fracture, nevertheless take a toll on those who suffer them. For example, while spine fractures rarely cause institutionalization (Chrischilles et al. 1991), their adverse influence on most activities of daily living is almost as great as that seen for hip fractures (Greendale et al. 1995).

This loss in functional status is mainly the result of the pain caused by spine fractures. New spine fractures may produce severe back pain that lasts for weeks or months (Ross 1997). Ettinger and colleagues found that 50 percent of elderly women had a mild or moderate spine deformity on x-ray, yet they were only slightly more likely to have constant or severe back pain, back disability, or substantial height loss than those with no evidence of a spine fracture (Ettinger et al. 1992). Ten percent of the elderly women in this study had a severe spine deformity, and this group showed a significantly increased risk of these problems, especially in those individuals with fractures in multiple vertebrae. Not surprisingly, the more severe fractures are also the most likely to be diagnosed,

and thus they represent the vast majority of spine fractures that are recognized clinically. However, even spine fractures that escape diagnosis can cause an increase in back pain and limited activity (Nevitt et al. 1998).

Wrist fractures seldom cause long-term disability, but they nonetheless are painful, requiring repositioning of the bones to their normal position and stabilization in a cast for 4–6 weeks. Recent studies suggest that wrist fractures may cause a number of short-term problems, including persistent pain, loss of function, nerve impairments (such as carpal tunnel syndrome), bone deformities, and arthritis (Greendale and Barrett-Connor 2001). In fact, nearly half of all patients report only fair or poor functional outcomes 6 months following a wrist fracture. Women and the elderly are the most likely to report such outcomes. There is no question that the overall impact of wrist fractures on a patient's functional status is much less than that of a hip fracture. In fact, less than 1 percent of wrist fracture patients become completely dependent as a result of the fracture (Chrischilles et al. 1991). These fractures may be as disabling as hip fractures with respect to some specific activities of daily living such as meal preparation.

Finally, while they are less devastating than hip fractures, spine, wrist, and the other limb fractures are more common, and they are the main contributors to osteoporosis-related morbidity in middle-aged women and men (Kanis et al. 2001). In addition, the occurrence of one of these fractures is a strong risk factor for additional fractures (see Chapter 8).

Impact on Emotional State

In addition to functional impairments, fractures from bone disease can have a negative impact on self-esteem, body image, and mood (Ross 1997), which may lead to psychological

Table 5–4. Postfracture Dependency† at 12 and 24 Months Among Patients Who Were Independent Prior to Hip Fracture

	12 months %	24 months %
Lower extremity physical activity of daily living		
Climbing five stairs	90	91
Getting in/out of bath/shower	83	83
Walking one block	55	53
Getting into a car	45	50
Rising from an armless chair	50	54
Walking 10 feet	40	37
Taking a shower/bath/sponge bath	38	44
Getting on/off the toilet	66	63
Putting socks and shoes on	33	33
Getting in/out of bath	31	33
Putting on pants	20	20
Instrumental activities of daily living		
Housecleaning	62	43
Getting places out of walking distance	53	53
Shopping	42	41
Cooking	24	23
Handling money	31	31
Taking medications	28	29
Using the telephone	22	23

† Dependency is defined as the need for either human or equipment assistance or inability to perform the activity due to health reasons.

Source: Magaziner et al. 2000.

consequences (Gold et al. 2001). Individuals who suffer fractures may be immobilized by a fear of falling and suffering additional fractures. Not surprisingly, they may begin to feel isolated and helpless. In a survey conducted by the National Osteoporosis Foundation, 89 percent of women who had already had an osteoporotic fracture said they feared breaking another bone; 80 percent were afraid that they would be less able to perform their daily activities; 80 percent feared losing their independence; 73 percent were concerned that they would have to reduce activities with family and friends; and 68 percent worried that another fracture would result in their having to enter a nursing home. If not addressed, fear about the future and a sense of helplessness can produce significant anxiety and depression. These problems may be compounded by an inability to fulfill occupational, domestic, or social duties (Table 5-5), thus leading to further social isolation.

Impact on Quality of Life

Not surprisingly, the increased levels of morbidity and disability and the declines in functional status and mental health that are typically associated with bone disease and fractures can have a profound impact on an individual's quality of life. Some studies have begun to address these intangible aspects of osteoporosis and other bone diseases by having individuals rate their quality of life in a given year, using a measure known as quality-adjusted life years (QALYs). When estimating QALYs, each year of life is assigned a preference weight between 1 and 0, where 1 represents perfect health and 0 represents death. Different individuals with similar health status may rate the quality of their life very differently, depending upon how they personally value that health status compared to being in perfect health and to dying. While results vary depending on the type of fracture being measured, patient age, and the assessment technique used, individuals suffering osteoporotic-related fractures consistently report significant reductions in QALYs; these reductions range from 0.05–0.55 on the 0 to 1 scale mentioned above (Tosteson and Hammond 2002). For example, spine

---

Table 5-5. Clinical Consequences of Spine Fractures

Symptoms	Signs	Function	Future risks
Back pain (acute, chronic)	Height loss	Impaired activities in daily living (e.g., bathing, dressing)	Increased risk of fracture
Sleep disturbance	Kyphosis		Increased risk of death
Anxiety	Decreased lumbar lordosis	Difficulty fitting clothes due to kyphosis, protuberant abdomen	
Depression	Protuberant abdomen		
Decreased self-esteem	Reduced lung function	Difficulty bending, lifting, descending stairs, cooking	
Fear of future fracture and falling	Weight loss		
Reduced quality of life			
Early satiety			

Source: Papaioannou et al. 2002. Reprinted from The American Journal of Medicine, Diagnosis and management of vertebral fractures in elderly adults. 113(3): 220–228 (2002), with permission from Excerpta Medica, Inc.

---

fractures are associated with a 20 percent reduction in the quality of life in the first 12 months and a 15 percent reduction after two years (Tosteson et al. 2001). Even those who manage to remain independent following a fracture typically experience a substantially reduced quality of life. For example, relatively healthy survivors of a hip fracture report a 52 percent reduction in quality of life in the first 12 months and a 21 percent reduction after two years (Tosteson et al. 2001). Similar differences were seen in a recent study comparing function and quality of life in Belgian women with a hip fracture compared to age-matched controls (Boonen et al. 2004). Health-related quality of life is also decreased in patients with spine fractures, particularly those who have had repeated episodes (Cockerill et al. 2004). Quality of life is also reduced in patients with other bone diseases. For example, patients with Paget's disease report a high frequency of hearing loss and boney deformities, but many also report depression (53.4 percent), sleep problems (51.5 percent), and poor quality of life (42.1 percent report poor or fair QOL). In the only published study to explore factors related to QOL in Paget's disease (Gold et al. 1996), the authors found that the psychological factors (including depression and loss of self-esteem) were the most important contributors to reduced QOL in these patients; they explained more of the variance (19 percent) in QOL than did biomedical (3 percent), social (2 percent), or cost (1 percent) factors. They also found that QOL was significantly decreased in patients with more extensive or symptomatic Paget's disease. These data, combined with similar data from studies of osteoporosis, suggest that the negative impact of bone disease is substantial.

Impact on Financial Well-Being

In addition to a decline in physical and mental health, patients with bone disease also bear significant financial expenses. Although better information is needed, these patients often must pay for a variety of expenses out of their own pockets (Table 5-6), creating a financial burden for many patients and their families. Hoerger and colleagues estimated that 17 percent of the cost of managing osteoporosis is not covered by insurance (i.e., Medicare, Medicaid, or private coverage) (Hoerger et al. 1999). Patients and/or family members may be responsible for some proportion of the average $2,000 increase in direct medical expenses that occur in the year following a fracture (Gabriel et al. 2002). They may also have to pay a portion of the cost of any drug therapy to prevent additional fractures (these costs are not included in the $2,000 figure cited above) and to bear the costs associated with disability during the recovery period and over the long term. Furthermore, younger family members may experience reductions in earning power as they take time away from work to assist older patients during the convalescence period (Brainsky et al. 1997); few studies to date have accounted for this type of lost productivity among individuals who must care for those who sustain fractures. Even if the hours of care provided by family and friends (informal care) are valued at the minimum wage, they represent a substantial proportion of the overall costs of care in the first 6 months following a hip fracture (Table 5-6). While the proportion of total care costs represented by informal care actually drop following a fracture (due to the high expenses of treating the fracture), the absolute dollar value of these costs more than doubles in the first 6 months after the fracture.

The Burden of Other Bone Diseases

As indicated in Chapter 4, thousands of Americans are affected by other bone diseases such as rickets and osteomalacia, renal osteodystrophy, primary hyperparathyroidism, Paget's disease, osteogenesis imperfecta, bone cancer, and other developmental and acquired skeletal disorders. Estimates of the societal burden of these conditions are not readily available. The impact of these conditions on individuals, moreover, varies enormously, and is largely dependent upon the severity of the disease.

The majority of patients with primary hyperparathyroidism are asymptomatic, but a small number suffer from kidney stones, fractures, or rarely dangerously high blood calcium levels that can lead to severe impairment of kidney function, coma, and death. Most Paget's disease patients suffer from pain, but some also develop nerve damage, fractures, or osteosarcoma (a type of bone cancer). Few patients with Paget's disease die from the condition, although, as discussed earlier, they often find their QOL to be reduced significantly because of the disease. Some patients with

Table 5–6. Costs Per Month Per Patient, Before and After Hip Fracture, Adjusted for Death and Excluding the Cost of the Initial Hospitalization

	($/month/patient)	
	Before fracture	After fracture
	Previous 6 months	First 6 months
Other hospitalizations	255	1015
Nursing home stays	6	864
Rehabilitation	4	681
Physician visits	24	103
Nurse/aide visits	10	77
Home aide services	133	445
Physical therapy	8	58
Durable equipment	11	111
Meals-on-wheels	4	9
Arranging services	1	5
Transportation	17	43
Emotional support	27	132
Informal care	1244	2517
Total per month	1744	6060

Source: Brainsky et al. 1997.

chronic renal disease who are on dialysis develop a severely debilitating bone disorder that results in pain and fractures. Others lose bone rapidly after renal transplantation and, despite the successful improvement of their kidney function, have poor health because of fractures.

Among the genetic skeletal disorders, the dense bones associated with osteopetrosis and the fragile bones associated with osteogenesis imperfecta (OI) can both cause severe illness. While some patients with osteopetrosis can be treated by bone marrow transplantation and others with stimulators of bone breakdown, success has been limited and many patients die from these conditions. OI often causes severe crippling and in its most severe form is fatal, although treatment with inhibitors of bone breakdown appears to be effective and is being explored further. (See box on page 90 for an example of OI's impact on an individual patient.) Cancer in bone often causes severe symptoms and frequently leads to death. Myeloma causes severe pain and bone loss with multiple fractures. Other types of cancer, including breast and prostate, can spread (metastasize) to bone, although (as discussed in Chapter 9) this can be reduced by treatments that block bone breakdown (Ross et al. 2004, Rosen et al. 2004).

In summary, there are a number of disorders other than osteoporosis that add greatly to the burden of bone disease in our population. Fortunately, the ability to diagnosis and treat many of these disorders has improved in recent years (see Chapters 8 and 9), thus making it possible to reduce this burden substantially in the future.

Key Questions for Future Research

Much more information on the frequency and burden of osteoporosis and other bone diseases is needed if plans to prevent the projected "epidemic" are to be successful. Careful collection of national and local data on all osteoporotic-related fracture types is needed so that progress in meeting prevention goals can be measured. Specific research questions that need to be answered include the following:

- How common are fractures in the community? Better data on fractures identified in physician's offices as well as in hospitals are needed.
- How common are hip fractures among the Medicare and non-Medicare population? What are the trends over time and across geographic regions and racial and ethnic groups?
- What is the true incidence and burden of spine fractures, given that many are "silent"? Surveys using dual x-ray absorptiometry (DXA) to assess spine deformities may help to answer this question.
- What is the impact of non-hip fragility fractures on morbidity, mortality, and quality of life?
- What is the impact on quality of life of asymptomatic spine fractures? These fractures may cause deformity and musculoskeletal symptoms such as low back pain, and may negatively affect cardiopulmonary and gastrointestinal function.
- What are the economic costs of osteoporosis and fragility fractures? While some data are presented in this chapter, more detail is needed, including information on non-Medicare patients, men, and racial and ethnic minorities.
- What is the prevalence and burden of osteoporosis and the incidence and burden of fractures in men and racial and ethnic minorities, including Blacks, Asians, and Hispanics?

- What environmental factors are responsible for geographic variations in fracture rates?
- What is the prevalence and burden of bone diseases and disorders other than osteoporosis, including hyperparathyroidism, osteomalacia, renal osteodystrophy, osteogenesis imperfecta, and congenital disorders affecting bone such as osteopetrosis? This examination of other bone diseases should include a review of their impact on racial and ethnic minorities.
- What impact do the skeletal implications of malignancy have on morbidity, mortality, and quality of life?
- What is the projected incidence and burden of bone disease if current practice is maintained and how much could these be changed by various levels of improvement in awareness, diagnosis, prevention, and treatment of bone disease?

References

Boonen S, Autier P, Barette M, Vanderschueren D, Lips P, Haentjens P. Functional outcome and quality of life following hip fracture in elderly women: A prospective controlled study. Osteoporos Int. 2004 Feb;15(2): 87-94.

Brainsky A, Glick H, Lydick E, Epstein R, Fox KM, Hawkes W, Kashner TM, Zimmerman SI, Magaziner J. The economic cost of hip fractures in community-dwelling older adults: A prospective study. J Am Geriatr Soc. 1997 Mar;45(3):281-7.

Braithwaite RS, Col NF, Wong JB. Estimating hip fracture morbidity, mortality and costs. J Am Geriatr Soc. 2003 Mar;51(3):364-70.

Browner WS, Pressman AR, Nevitt MC, Cummings SR. Mortality following fractures in older women. The Study of Osteoporotic Fractures. Arch Intern Med 1996 Jul 22;156(14):1521-5.

Burge RT, King AB, Balda E, Worley D. Methodology for estimating current and future burden of osteoporosis in state populations: Application to Florida in 2000 through 2025. Value Health. 2003 Sep-Oct;6(5);574-83.

Chrischilles EA, Butler CD, Davis CS, Wallace RB. A model of lifetime osteoporosis impact. Arch Intern Med 1991 Oct;151(10):2026-32.

Chrischilles E, Shireman T, Wallace R. Costs and health effects of osteoporotic fractures. Bone. 1994 Jul-Aug;15(4):377-86.

Cockerill W, Lunt M, Silman AJ, Cooper C, Lips P, Bhalla AK, Cannata JB, Eastell R, Felsenberg D, Gennari C, et al. Health-related quality of life and radiographic vertebral fracture. Osteoporos Int. 2004 Feb;15(2):113-9.

Ettinger B, Black DM, Nevitt MC, Rundle AC, Cauley JA, Cummings SR, Genant HK, Genant HK. Contribution of vertebral deformities to chronic back pain and disability. The Study of Osteoporotic Fractures Research Group. J Bone Miner Res. 1992 Apr;7(4):449-56.

Gabriel SE, Tosteson AN, Leibson CL, Crowson CS, Pond GR, Hammond CS, Melton LJ 3rd. Direct medical costs attributable to osteoporotic fractures. Osteoporosis Int. 2002;13(4):323-30.

Gehlbach SH, Burge RT, Puleo E, Klar J. Hospital care of osteoporosis-related vertebral fractures. Osteoporos Int. 2003 Jan;14(1):53-60.

Gold DT, Boisture J, Shipp KM, Pieper CF, Lyles KW. Paget's disease of bone and quality of life. J Bone Miner Res. 1996 Dec;11(12):1897-904.

Gold, DT; Lyles, KW; Shipp, KM; Drezner, MK. Osteoporosis and its nonskeletal consequences: Their impact on treatment decisions. In: Marcus, R; Feldman, D; Kelsey, J, editors. Osteoporosis, 2nd ed. Vol. 2. San Diego: Academic Press; 2001; pp. 479-84.

Greendale GA, Barrett-Connor E, Ingles S, Haile R. Late physical and functional effects of osteoporotic fracture in women: The Rancho Bernardo Study. J Am Geriatr Soc. 1995 Sep;43(9):955-61.

Greendale, GA; Barrett-Connor, E. Outcomes of osteoporotic fractures. In: Marcus, R; Feldman, D; Kelsey, J, editors. Osteoporosis, 2nd ed. Vol. 1. San Diego: Academic Press; 2001; pp. 819-29.

Hoerger TJ, Downs KE, Lakshmanan MC, Lindrooth RC, Plouffe L Jr, Wendling B, West SL, Ohsfeldt RL. Healthcare use among U.S. women aged 45 and older: Total costs and costs for selected postmenopausal health risks. J Womens Health Gend Based Med. 1999 Oct;8(8):1077-89.

Jacobsen SJ, Goldberg J, Miles TP, Brody JA, Stiers W, Rimm AA. Race and sex differences in mortality following fracture of the hip. Am J Public Health 1992;82(8):1147-50.

Johnell O, Kanis JA, Oden A, Sernbo I, Redlund-Johnell I, Petterson C, De Laet C, Jonsson B. Mortality after osteoporotic fractures. Osteoporos Int. 2004 Jan;15(1):38-42.

Kado DM, Browner WS, Blackwell T, Gore R, Cummings SR. Rate of bone loss is associated with mortality in older women: A prospective study. J Bone Miner Res. 2000 Oct;15(10):1974-80.

Kanis JA, Johnell O. The burden of osteoporosis. J Endocrinol Invest. 1999 Sep;22(8):583-8.

Kanis JA, Oden A, Johnell O, de Laet C, Dawson A. The burden of osteoporotic fractures: A method for setting intervention thresholds. Osteoporos Int. 2001;12(5):417-27.

Kanis JA, Oden A, Johnell O, De Laet C, Jonsson B. Excess mortality after hospitalisation for vertebral fracture. Osteoporos Int. 2004 Feb;15(2):108-12.

Lawrence VA, Hilsenbeck SG, Noveck H, Poses RM, Carson JL. Medical complications and outcomes after hip fracture repair. Arch Intern Med. 2002 Oct 14;162(18):2053-7.

Leibson CL, Tosteson AN, Gabriel SE, Ransom JE, Melton LJ. Mortality, disability, and nursing home use for persons with and without hip fracture: A population-based study. J Am Geriatr Soc. 2002 Oct; 50(10):1644-50.

Lieberman D, Friger M, Fried V, Grinshpun Y, Mytlis N, Tylis R, Galinsky D, Lieberman D. Characterization of elderly patients in rehabilitation: Stroke versus hip fracture. Disabil Rehabil. 1999 Dec;21(12):542-7.

Magaziner J, Lydick E, Hawkes W, Fox KM, Zimmerman SI, Epstein RS, Hebel JR. Excess mortality attributable to hip fracture in white women aged 70 years and older. Am J Public Health. 1997 Oct;87(10):1630-6.

Magaziner J, Hawkes W, Hebel JR, Zimmerman SI, Fox KM, Dolan M, Felsenthal G, Kenzora J. Recovery from hip fracture in eight areas of function. J Gerontol A Biol Sci Med Sci 2000;55(9):M498-507.

Magaziner J, Fredman L, Hawkes W, Hebel JR, Zimmerman S, Orwig DL, Wehren L. Changes in functional status attributable to hip fracture: A comparison of hip fracture patients to community-dwelling aged. Am J Epidemiol. 2003 Jun 1;157(11):1023-31.

Marottoli RA, Berkman LF, Cooney LM Jr. Decline in physical function following hip fracture. J Am Geriatr Soc. 1992 Sep;40(9):861-6.

Max W, Sinnot P, Kao C, Sung HY, Rice DP. The burden of osteoporosis in California, 1998. Osteoporos Int. 2002;13(6):493-500.

Melton LJ 3rd. Adverse outcomes of osteoporotic fractures in the general population. J Bone Miner Res 2003 Jun;18(6):1139-41.

Mussolino ME, Madans JH, Gillum RF. Bone mineral density and mortality in women and men; The NHANES I epidemiologic follow-up study. Ann Epidemiol. 2003 Nov;13(10);692-697.

National Center for Health Statistics (US), Data Warehouse. GMWK I: Total deaths for each cause by 5-year age groups. Hyattsville (MD): U.S. Department of Health and Human Services; 1999.

Nevitt MC, Ettinger B, Black DM, Stone K, Jamal SA, Ensrud K, Segal M, Genant HK, Cummings SR. The association of radiographically detected vertebral fractures with back pain and function: A prospective study. Ann Intern Med. 1998 May 15;128(10):793-800.

Office of Technology Assessment, U. S. Congress. Hip fracture outcomes in people age 50 and over — Background paper. Washington (DC): U.S. Government Printing Office;1994 Jul. OTA-BP-H-120.

Papaioannou A, Watts NB, Kendler DL, Yuen CK, Adachi JD, Ferko N. Diagnosis and management of vertebral fractures in elderly adults. Am J Med 2002;113(3):220-8.

Poór G, Atkinson EJ, O'Fallon WM, Melton LJ 3rd. Determinants of reduced survival following hip fractures in men. Clin Orthop. 1995 Oct;(319):260-5.

Popovic JR. 1999 National Hospital Discharge Survey: Annual summary with detailed diagnosis and procedure data. Vital Health Stat 13. 2001 Sep;(151):i-v, 1-206.

Praemer A, Furner S, Rice D. Musculoskeletal Conditions in the United States. Rosemont, IL: American Academy of Orthopaedic Surgeons; 1999.

Ray NF, Chan JK, Thamer M, Melton LJ 3rd. Medical expenditures for the treatment of osteoporotic fractures in the United States in 1995: Report from the National Osteoporosis Foundation. J Bone Miner Res. 1997 Jan;12(1):24-35.

Richmond J, Aharonoff GB, Zuckerman JD, Koval KJ. Mortality risk after hip fracture. J Orthop Trauma. 2003 Sep;17(8 Suppl):S2-5.

Rosen LS. New generation of bisphosphonates: Broad clinical utility in breast and prostate cancer. Oncology (Huntingt). 2004 May; 18(5 Suppl 3):26-32.

Ross JR, Saunders Y, Edmonds PM, Patel S, Wonderling D, Normand C, Broadley K. A systematic review of the role of bisphosphonates in metastatic disease. Health Technol Assess. 2004;8(4):1-176.

Ross PD. Clinical consequences of vertebral fractures. Am J Med. 1997 Aug 18;103(2A):30S-42S; discussion 42S-43S.

Salkeld G, Cameron ID, Cumming RG, Easter S, Seymour J, Kurrle SE, Quine S. Quality of life related to fear of falling and hip fracture in older women: A time trade off study. BMJ. 2000 Feb 5;320(7231):341-6.

Tosteson ANA. Economic impact of fractures. In: Orwoll ES, editor. Osteoporosis in men: The effects of gender on skeletal health. San Diego: Academic Press; 1999. pp. 15-27.

Tosteson AN, Gabriel SE, Grove MR, Moncur MM, Kneeland TS, Melton LJ 3rd. Impact of hip and vertebral fractures on quality-adjusted life years. Osteoporos Int. 2001 Dec;12(12):1042-9.

Tosteson AN, Hammond CS. Quality-of-life assessment in osteoporosis: Health-status and preference-based measures. Pharmacoeconomics. 2002;20(5):289-303.

Vestergaard P, Mollerup CL, Frøkjaer VG, Christiansen P, Blichert-Toft M, Mosekilde L. Cardiovascular events before and after surgery for primary hyperparathyroidism. World J Surg. 2003 Feb;27(2):216-22.

Part Three

WHAT CAN INDIVIDUALS DO TO IMPROVE THEIR BONE HEALTH?

Part Three of the report is the first of three sections that address the question of what can be done to improve the bone health status of Americans. This part of the report approaches the issue from the perspective of the individual, examining those factors that determine bone health and describing lifestyle approaches that individuals can take to improve their personal bone health.

Chapter 6 highlights the critical role that lifestyle factors such as nutrition and physical activity play in overall bone health status. It also provides a thorough review of the evidence on precisely how these factors influence bone health, including those behaviors that promote it (e.g., physical activity, adequate calcium and vitamin D intake) and those that can impair it (e.g., smoking, excessive alcohol consumption). The chapter emphasizes the fact that many Americans do not currently get enough exercise and consume enough calcium and vitamin D to achieve optimal bone health. The chapter also reviews evidence on the impact of other factors on bone health, including the presence of other diseases; the use of certain medications; weight and weight loss; and reproductive issues such as pregnancy, lactation, amenorrhea, oophorectomy, and contraceptive use.

Chapter 7 provides practical, real-world guidance on lifestyle approaches that individuals can take to improve their own bone health, including the following: what foods are the best sources of calcium and vitamin D; how to calculate daily calcium intake; when calcium and/or vitamin D supplementation should be considered; and what types of physical activity can contribute to bone health and overall health. The good-news message of this chapter is that it is surprisingly easy to meet recommended guidelines for nutrition and physical activity, and that following these guidelines not only promotes bone health, but it also enhances overall health and well-being and helps to avoid the onset of other chronic diseases.

Chapter 6: Key Messages

- While genetic factors play a significant role in determining bone mass, controllable lifestyle factors such as diet and physical activity can mean the difference between a frail and strong skeleton.

- Calcium has been singled out as a major public health concern today because it is critically important to bone health and the average American consumes levels of calcium that are far below the amount recommended for optimal bone health.

- Vitamin D is important for good bone health because it aids in the absorption and utilization of calcium. There is a high prevalence of vitamin D insufficiency in nursing home residents, hospitalized patients, and adults with hip fractures.

- Physical activity is important for bone health throughout life. It helps to increase or preserve bone mass and to reduce the risk of falling. All types of physical activity can contribute to bone health, albeit in different ways.

- Maintaining a healthy body weight is important for bone health throughout life. Being underweight raises the risk of fracture and bone loss. Weight loss is associated with bone loss as well, although adequate diet and physical activity may reduce this loss.

- Fractures are commonly caused by falls, and thus fall prevention offers another opportunity to protect bones, particularly in those over age 60. Several specific approaches have demonstrated benefits, including muscle strengthening and balance retraining, professional home hazard assessment and modification, and stopping or reducing psychotropic medications.

- Reproductive issues can affect bone health. Pregnancy and lactation generally do not harm the skeleton of healthy adult women. Amenorrhea (cessation of menstrual periods) after the onset of puberty and before menopause is a very serious threat to bone health and needs to be attended to by individuals and their health care providers.

- Several medical conditions and prescription medications can affect bone health through various mechanisms, and health care professionals should treat the presence of such conditions and the use of such medications as a potential red flag that signals the need for further assessment of bone health and other risk factors for bone disease.

- Smoking can reduce bone mass and increase fracture risk and should be avoided for a variety of health reasons. Heavy alcohol use has been associated with reduced bone mass and increased fracture risk.

Chapter 6

DETERMINANTS OF BONE HEALTH

As discussed in Chapter 2, bone is a remarkable tissue with a functional structure (the skeleton) that is strong enough to withstand intense physical activity, adaptive enough to respond to changes in activity, and lightweight enough to allow efficient movement. Bone is resilient because of its intrinsic material characteristics (mass, density, mineral composition, strength) and its dimensions (size, shape, and structure). Throughout life, bone must adapt to the stresses imposed upon it, and its ability to do so depends on both lifestyle and genetic factors. A variety of studies indicate that genetic factors are responsible for determining 50–90 percent of bone mass and other qualitative aspects of bone (Recker and Deng 2002). Heredity not only sets limits on how much bone a person acquires, but also on bone structure, the rate of bone loss, and the skeleton's response to environmental stimuli like nutrients and physical activity. Normal bone mass and strength is controlled by many genetic elements working in concert. The tendency to develop bone diseases like osteoporosis and Paget's disease also appears to be due to genetic factors, although this tendency may also be influenced by environmental factors that are not yet completely understood. Osteogenesis imperfecta (OI), a condition in which bones break easily, often for little or no apparent cause, is clearly determined by the malfunction of specific collagen genes that have been identified. The search for the particular genes that control bone mass and affect the tendency to develop bone diseases is a very active area of research. Finding these elements may lead to new therapeutic strategies and prevention tools for osteoporosis.

While genetic factors play an important role in determining bone mass, it is critical not to underestimate the important role that individuals can play in promoting their own bone health status. In fact, controllable lifestyle factors such as diet and physical activity are responsible for 10–50 percent of bone mass and structure. These influences are illustrated in Figure 6-1.

Controlling these factors can literally mean the difference between a frail and a strong skeleton. This is because even relatively small changes in bone mass can have a significant impact on overall bone health. In fact, it has been estimated that a 10 percent increase in bone mass could reduce fracture risk by as much as 50 percent (Cummings et al. 1993). In other words, paying attention to lifestyle factors such as diet and physical activity throughout life can yield bone health benefits that are equal to or greater than those offered by the most powerful drugs currently used to treat osteoporosis.

While good nutrition and regular physical activity are important to bone health throughout life, the optimal type of nutrition and activity will vary across the life span, as will the impact

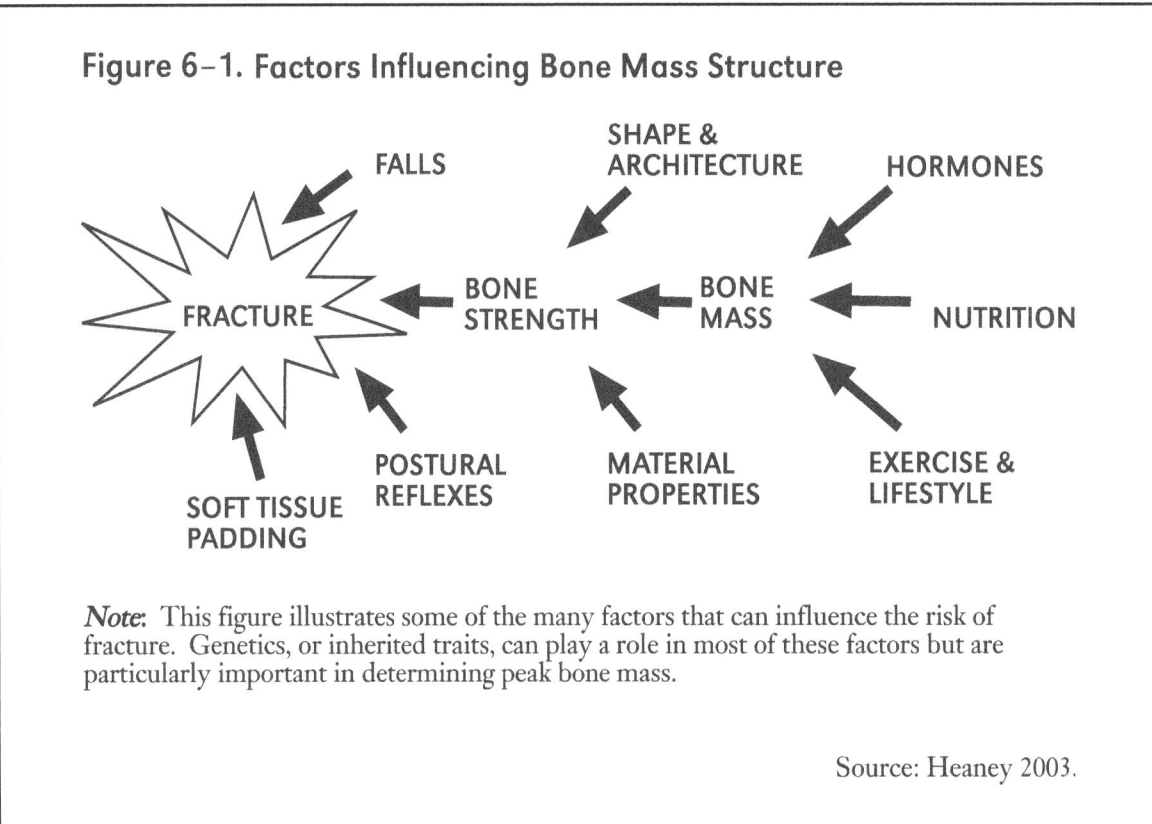

Figure 6-1. Factors Influencing Bone Mass Structure

Note: This figure illustrates some of the many factors that can influence the risk of fracture. Genetics, or inherited traits, can play a role in most of these factors but are particularly important in determining peak bone mass.

Source: Heaney 2003.

that each will have on bone. As a result, this chapter will analyze the evidence about the key determinants of bone health. It uses a life span approach, considering the following phases: a) the growth phase that occurs during childhood and adolescence; b) the maintenance phase that occurs during young to middle adulthood; c) the mid-life bone loss phase that typically occurs in adults between age 50–70; and d) the frailty phase that typically occurs in adults over age 70. These phases are general and do not correspond to a specific chronological age in an individual. Additional information on the various kinds of evidence and studies that are cited in this chapter can be found in Appendix B, "How We Know What We Know: The Evidence Behind the Evidence."

The goal of this chapter is to discuss the evidence related to these controllable factors that affect bone health throughout the different stages of life. Most of the information in this chapter focuses on osteoporosis and fracture; unfortunately, there are no known preventive regimens to address other bone diseases. Early recognition and intervention is the optimal strategy for these other bone diseases at the present time, as described in Chapters 8, 9, and 10.

A Review of the Critical Life Stages of Bone

As discussed in Chapter 2, bone tissue continues to renew itself, or remodel, throughout life by breaking down old bone (bone resorption) and replacing it with new bone (bone formation). Figure 6-2 illustrates how the skeleton changes over the life span. Because lifestyle changes made during the acquisition phase affect the achievement of peak bone mass, these lifestyle changes are critically important to bone health throughout life.

Adolescence is a particularly critical period for bone health because the amount of bone mineral gained during this period typically equals the amount lost throughout the remainder of adult life (Bailey et al. 2000). As illustrated in Figure 6-2, failure to achieve an optimized bone mass at the end of adolescence leaves an individual with much less reserve to withstand the normal losses during later life. Most gains in bone mass during puberty are due to an increase in bone length and size rather than bone density (Katzman et al. 1991). Fracture rates go up during this period of extremely rapid growth, possibly because the bone is temporarily weaker because bone mineralization lags behind growth in bone length (Khosla et al. 2003).

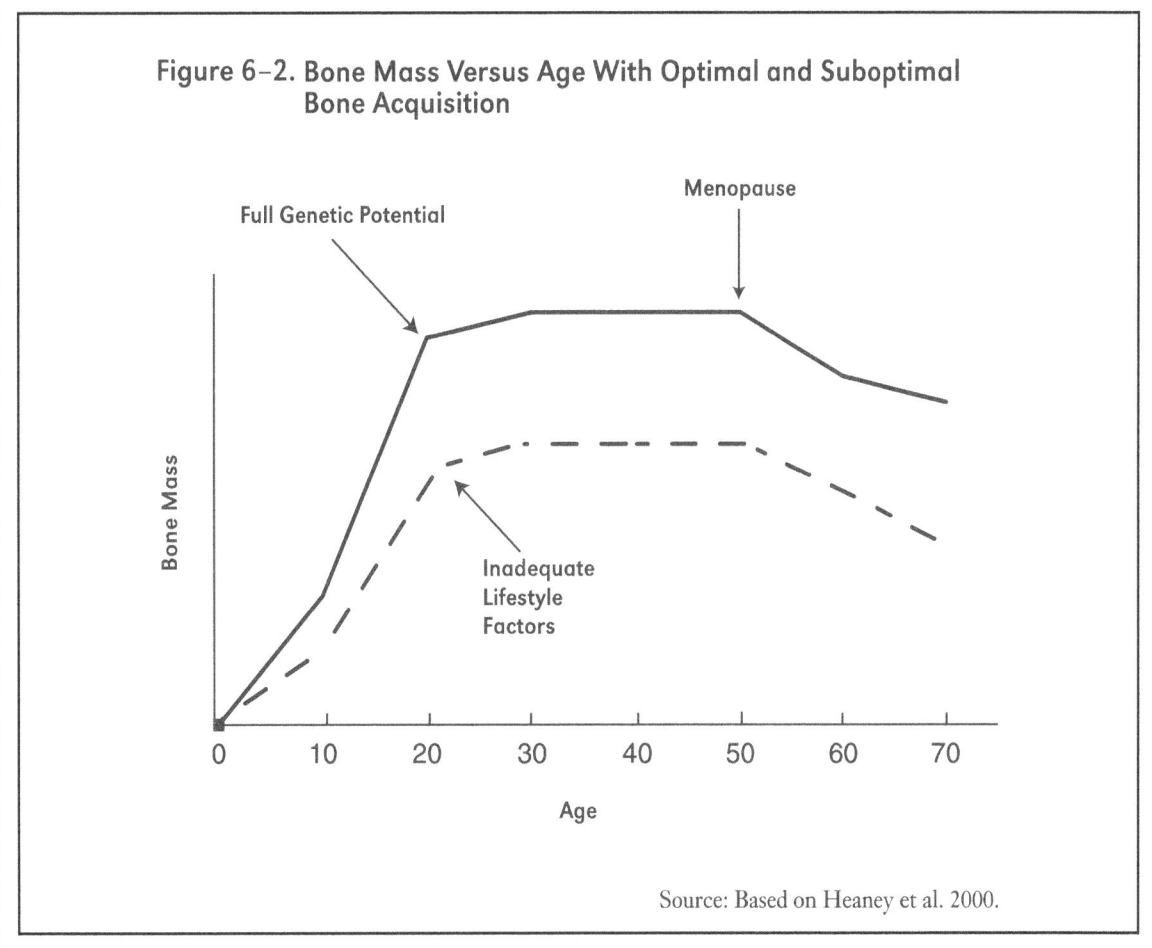

Figure 6–2. Bone Mass Versus Age With Optimal and Suboptimal Bone Acquisition

Source: Based on Heaney et al. 2000.

Review of the Life Stages of Bone, continued

After individuals achieve peak bone mass in late adolescence, bone health is optimized by maintaining as much of this bone mass as possible throughout adulthood. Bone formation and resorption are generally in balance with each other during the young to mid-adult years, so optimally bone mass is maintained at many skeletal sites. There is bone loss at some skeletal sites, such as the hip, before age 50, but it does not normally compromise strength. Bone loss begins or accelerates at midlife for both men and women (Riggs et al. 2002), meaning that the goal during this time of life is to keep bone loss to a minimum and to recognize and avoid both bone-specific and non-specific threats to bone health, such as other illnesses and falls. After age 40–50, bone loss may progress slowly in both sexes, with a period of more rapid loss in women surrounding the menopausal transition. During this period of age–related bone loss, both sexes may lose a total of 25 percent of bone. Bone loss continues in both men and women after age 70 (Riggs et al. 2002).

These later stages in bone life are depicted in Figure 6-3, which shows three women with increasingly severe bowing of the spine (kyphosis) due to osteoporotic fractures of the spine. But fractures are not a natural consequence of aging. Rather, they can be avoided, to some extent, by focusing on controllable factors such as diet and physical activity.

Figure 6-3. The Progression of Osteoporosis

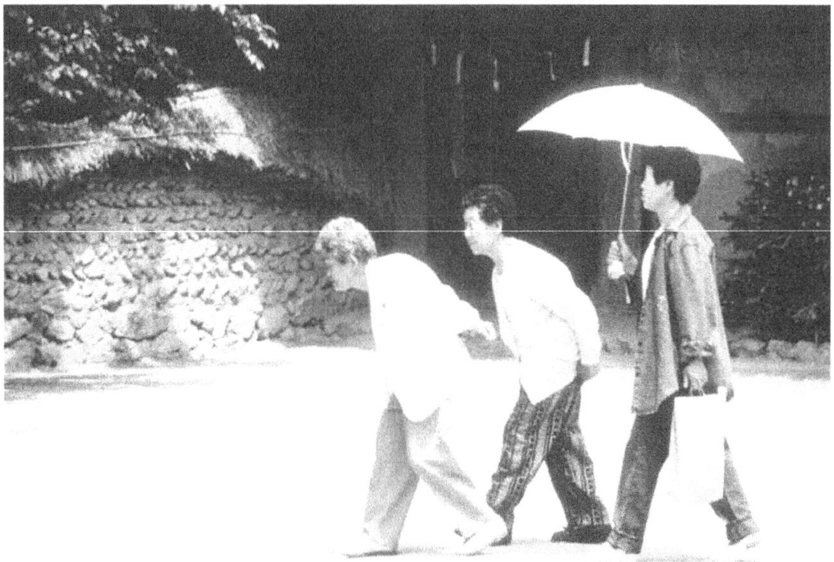

Note: Three women demonstrate increasingly severe bowing of the spine (kyphosis) due to osteoporotic fractures of the spine.

Source: Higgs and AAOS 2001.

Nutrition's Impact on Bone Health: A Review of the Evidence

Nutrition and Bone Health: What the Evidence Tells Us

- Research suggests that a well-balanced diet is important for bone health throughout life. Depending on age, it may help increase or preserve bone mass.
- Much of the research to date has focused on calcium and vitamin D. Calcium and vitamin D play crucial roles in bone health, although other nutrients are also important.
- The Institute of Medicine recommends a steady increase in calcium intake as children age, beginning with 210 mg per day in infants and rising to 1,300 mg per day in those age 9–18. Recommended levels drop to 1,000 mg per day in those age 19–50, and then increase to 1,200 mg per day for those over age 50. The same age-dependent recommendations for calcium apply to pregnant or nursing women. Recommended levels of vitamin D intake are 200 IU per day for those under age 50, 400 IU per day for those 50–70, and 600 IU per day for those over age 70.

The evidence suggests that the composition of the diet can play an important role in building and maintaining bone mass throughout life, primarily by providing bone-building nutrients and by influencing absorption and retention of these nutrients. In addition, diet provides calories (energy input), which together with physical activity (energy output), determines body weight. Maintenance of an adequate body weight can help promote optimal bone health, as discussed later in this chapter.

Background: Why Focus on Vitamin D and Calcium?

As discussed later in this chapter, consuming adequate levels of calcium and vitamin D throughout life are critically important to an individual's bone health. The Institute of Medicine conducted a major review of bone-related nutrients in 1997 (IOM 1997) and developed a set of evidence-based recommendations for calcium and vitamin D intake. The goal of this effort was to determine the level of nutrient intake for normal, healthy individuals that would prevent the development of a chronic condition associated with that nutrient. While many nutrients play a role in bone health, calcium has been singled out as a major public health concern today not only because it is a critical nutrient for bone but also because of national surveys that suggest that the average calcium intake of individuals is far below the levels recommended for optimal bone health (Figure 6-4). One reason for these low levels of calcium intake relates to current lifestyle and food preferences, which have resulted in reduced intake of dairy products and other naturally calcium-rich foods. For some individuals lactose intolerance may play a role in not consuming adequate levels of calcium. Lactose intolerance is a condition in which individuals cannot metabolize lactose, the main sugar found in milk and other calcium-rich dairy products. An estimated 30–50 million Americans (about 25 percent of the U.S. population) are affected by lactose intolerance, although to varying degrees. While least common among Whites (it affects about 15 percent of White adults), lactose

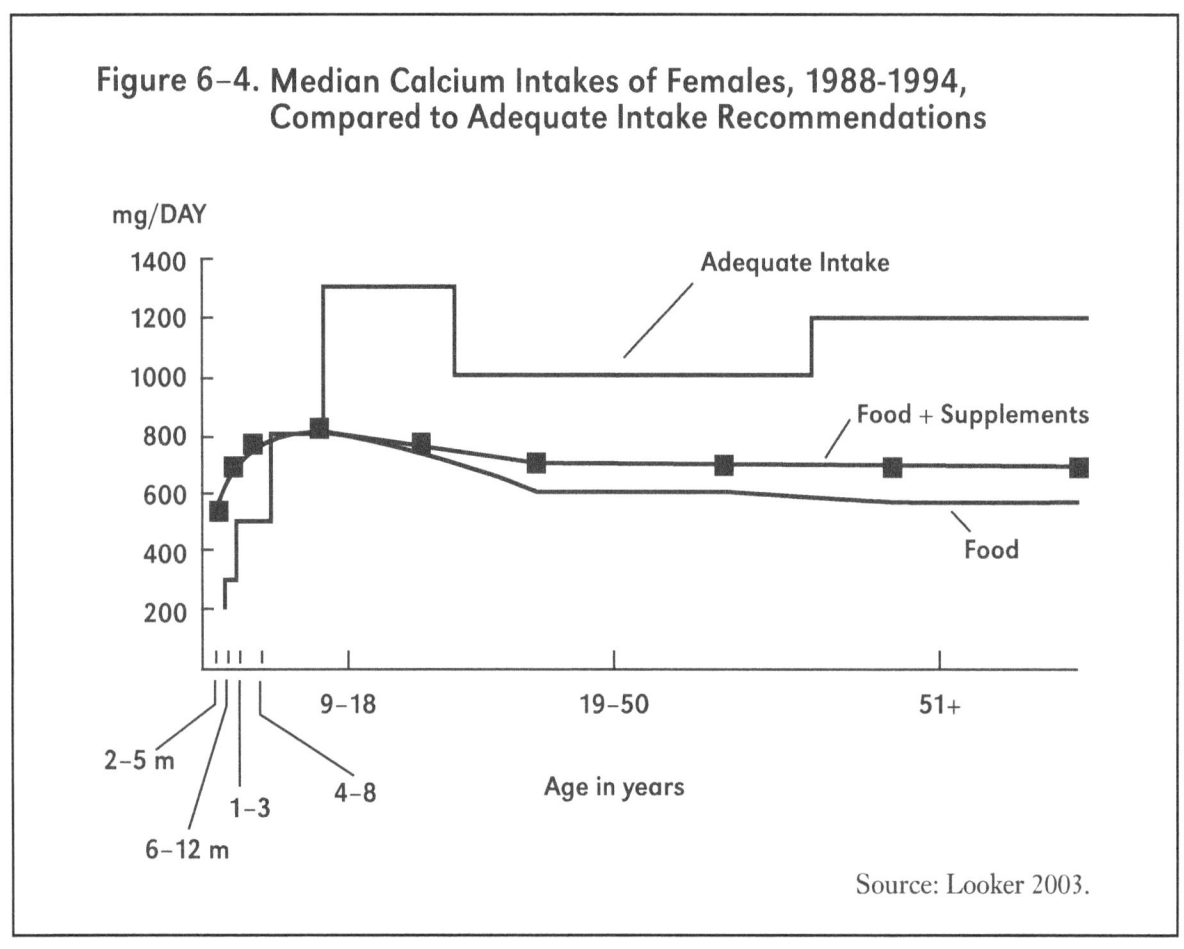

Figure 6–4. Median Calcium Intakes of Females, 1988-1994, Compared to Adequate Intake Recommendations

Source: Looker 2003.

intolerance is widespread among other ethnic groups. Among the adult population, an estimated 70 percent of African-Americans, 74 percent of Native Americans, 53 percent of Mexican-Americans, and 90 percent of Asian-Americans are affected (Jackson and Savaiano 2001, National Women's Health Information Center 2001).

Lactose intolerance has been shown to be associated not only with low milk intake, but also with low bone mass and increased risk of fracture (Obermayer-Pietsch et al. 2004). Thus, these individuals may experience a detrimental effect on their bone health if they avoid consuming dairy products and do not replace them with

other good sources of calcium. Strategies to cope with lactose intolerance are described in more detail in Chapter 7.

While for most individuals the problem is too little calcium, it is important to remember that too much calcium does not have any additive benefit, and can have negative effects in some individuals. For this reason, the Institute of Medicine set a tolerable upper limit for calcium of 2,500 mg per day.

Vitamin D is important for good bone health because it aids in the absorption and utilization of calcium. The main source of vitamin D is sunlight, and most people throughout the world get their supply of vitamin D by the conversion of precursors in the skin to active vitamin D, a process caused by exposure to sunlight. Several factors can limit the production of vitamin D by the skin, including where one lives (those who live in northern latitudes during the winter months do not get adequate exposure to sunlight (Webb et al. 1988)), how much body surface is covered by clothing or sunscreen, the degree of skin pigmentation (darker skin takes longer to make active vitamin D), and age (older individuals are less efficient in making vitamin D). Strategies for overcoming some of these limitations are discussed in Chapter 7.

Due to concerns that individuals do not get enough vitamin D through sunlight, recommendations for intake are set at a level to be adequate for individuals having no sun exposure. The most accurate way to tell if an individual or population group is getting enough vitamin D is by measuring levels of serum 25-hydroxy vitamin D. These levels have been measured in various populations, and they indicate a high prevalence of vitamin D insufficiency in nursing home residents, hospitalized patients, and adults with hip fractures (Webb et al.1990, LeBoff et al. 1999, Thomas et al. 1998). Vitamin D levels commonly deteriorate in older adults, and thus the requirement for vitamin D increases with age. But inadequate vitamin D levels can be a problem at any age. Exclusively breast-fed infants, particularly non-Whites or infants with decreased sunlight exposure, are at greatest risk. As a result, the American Academy of Pediatrics (Gartner and Greer 2003) recommends supplementing breast-fed infants with vitamin D, since breast milk may be a poor source of vitamin D. Infant formulas are fortified with appropriate levels of the vitamin.

Finally, as with calcium, too much vitamin D can be harmful to the skeleton as well. Vitamin

Absorption of Calcium

To reach the skeleton, calcium eaten in the diet must first be absorbed into the body. In fact, much of the calcium consumed in the diet does not make its way to the skeleton; studies indicate that in adults only about 30 percent of calcium intake is actually absorbed by the body (IOM 1997). Moreover, some calcium is excreted from the body into the intestine so that the actual net absorption is even lower (Heaney and Abrams 2004).

Several factors can affect the body's ability to absorb dietary calcium, including vitamin D and estrogen. Deficiencies in either can reduce calcium absorption. The problem of reduced calcium absorption is more acute in older persons, who absorb less dietary calcium because their intestines are no longer as responsive to the action of 1,25-dihydroxy vitamin D (Heaney et al. 1989). Poor absorption of calcium can be overcome by increasing overall calcium intake and maintaining adequate levels of vitamin D.

D is a fat-soluble vitamin, so it can be stored in the body. Excess vitamin D can be toxic, leading to hypercalcemia, kidney failure, and calcification of soft tissue (IOM 1997). As a result, the Institute of Medicine has established a tolerable upper limit for dietary vitamin D intake of 2,000 IU per day. Physicians will often use much higher levels, however, to correct deficiencies.

The Evidence Supporting the Effect of Calcium and Vitamin D on Bone

Individuals who consume adequate amounts of calcium and vitamin D throughout life should enjoy better overall bone health for two reasons. First, they are more likely to achieve optimal skeletal mass early in life, and second, they are less likely to lose bone later in life. The net result should be higher bone mass and fewer fractures. Selected evidence to support the relationship between these nutrients and bone health during different stages of life is summarized below.

The Growth Stage (Children and Adolescents)

The role of calcium and other minerals in achieving peak bone mass begins before birth. Premature infants tend to have lower bone mineral content later in life, although this may in part be due to their tendency to be light and short for their age (Fewtrell et al. 1999, Bowden et al. 1999). Low birth weight is also associated with low bone mass later in life (Yarbrough et al. 2000, Antoniades et al. 2003). As discussed in Chapter 10, providing premature and low birth-weight infants with supplemental calcium, phosphorus, and protein may help them to "catch up."

Many observational studies make it clear that the role of calcium in achieving optimal peak bone mass continues into childhood and adolescence (Heaney et al. 2000). Perhaps the most often cited study is that of Matkovic et al., who compared two regions of Croatia with different intakes of calcium (Matkovic et al. 1979). Although the high-calcium region had lower fracture rates, the populations differed in other variables such as exercise that could partially explain the different fracture rates. This study spurred further research into the role of childhood and lifetime calcium consumption on the risk of osteoporosis and fracture.

Several randomized clinical trials have examined the effect of calcium supplements or calcium-rich foods in children and adolescents (Lee et al. 1994, Lee et al. 1995, Lloyd et al. 1993, Nowson et al. 1997, Bonjour et al. 2001, Johnston et al. 1994, Dibba et al. 2000, Cadogan et al. 1997, Merrilees et al. 2000, Chan et al. 1995). These studies have been combined and summarized in

a meta-analysis (Wosje and Specker 2000), which concluded that higher calcium intake increases bone mineral density (BMD) in children and adolescents in certain circumstances. Increases in BMD were more likely in cortical bone sites and among populations with low baseline calcium intakes, and in most studies the increase did not persist beyond the calcium supplementation period. A few studies have examined the impact of higher calcium intake over time. Results from most of these studies suggest that the intake must be maintained for the positive effects on bone to persist (Bonjour et al. 2001, Slemenda et al. 1997, Lee et al. 1996).

Adequate levels of calcium intake may also be important in maximizing the positive effect of physical activity on bone during the growth period. Two recent studies found that physical activity was more beneficial to bone health in infants or young children consuming higher amounts of calcium (Specker et al 1999, Specker and Binkley 2003).

There have been no randomized clinical trials to measure the impact of vitamin D supplements alone on bone health in children and adolescents. However, vitamin D deficiency is known to cause inadequate mineralization of the growing skeleton, leading to rickets (Goldring et al. 1995). In addition, one small observational study found higher bone density in prepubertal girls who took vitamin D supplements during infancy (Zamora 1999).

The Maintenance Stage (Adults)

Eating adequate amounts of nutrients continues to be important during the young adult years when bone formation and bone resorption are balanced. Unfortunately, most studies of diet and supplement use and bone health have focused on either younger or older individuals.

A meta-analysis of calcium and bone density in premenopausal women indicated that calcium had a positive effect on BMD in this group, as the supplemented groups lost less bone per year (Welten et al. 1995). However, only one of the four intervention studies in this meta-analysis used a double-blinded, placebo-controlled design. In addition, these studies focused on premenopausal women between the age of 30 and 55, not on younger adult women. There have not been many studies of vitamin D in young adults. One study did find that even young men may experience low vitamin D levels in the winter, and that these low levels were associated with lower BMD (Valimaki et al. 2004). More information is needed about the role of calcium, vitamin D, and other nutrients in maintaining bone in this age group of women and in men.

The Early Bone Loss and Frailty Stages (Older Adults)

Most randomized clinical trials examining the effect of calcium and vitamin D on bone health have focused on postmenopausal women and the elderly, so the role of these nutrients in promoting bone health is more clearly established for this age group. In fact, a carefully conducted meta-analysis of randomized clinical trials on the effects of calcium supplementation for the prevention of postmenopausal osteoporosis was recently published (Shea et al. 2002). The investigators performed a thorough search to identify all trials (including unpublished ones) examining the effect of calcium (with minimal vitamin D) on bone density and fractures in postmenopausal women since 1966. Of the 66 trials that were identified and screened, 15 met the inclusion criteria. After analyzing these trials, the investigators concluded that calcium supplements reduced bone loss by approximately 2 percent after two

or more years of use. More importantly, their results suggested that calcium supplements led to a significant (roughly 23 percent) reduction in the risk of spine fractures.

Just as with children, moreover, it appears that there may be a positive interaction between the effects of physical activity and calcium on bone health in older adults. (This relationship is discussed further in the section on physical activity.) Calcium may also help enhance the effect of drugs that reduce bone loss, such as estrogen and bisphosphonates (e.g., drugs that restrict the action of cells that resorb bone) (Heaney 2001).

A carefully conducted meta-analysis of randomized trials on the effect of vitamin D on bone density and fracture risk has also been recently conducted (Papadimitropoulos et al. 2002). All trials, including unpublished studies, conducted since 1966 were evaluated, with 25 meeting the criteria for inclusion. While the results from the different trials tended to vary somewhat, the authors concluded that vitamin D supplements reduced the risk of spine fractures by approximately 37 percent. This decline in fracture risk may be due in part to vitamin D's ability to reduce the risk of falls. Vitamin D may reduce falls by acting directly on muscle. There are vitamin D receptors in human muscle that may play a role in increasing muscle strength and thereby enhancing stability (Bischoff et al. 2001). While elderly individuals who are vitamin D deficient face an increased risk of falls (Flicker et al. 2004), studies have shown that vitamin D supplementation in these individuals may negate this effect (Bischoff et al. 2003, Latham et al. 2003, Dukas et al. 2004). It is important to note that the design of many of the randomized, controlled trials examining the effect of vitamin D supplements on bone loss or fracture incidence also called for participants to use a calcium supplement. Thus, it is not possible to isolate the benefits of calcium and/or vitamin D alone in these studies. While a few studies have simultaneously evaluated the effects of the two nutrients separately, the results are mixed. For example, one study found that calcium prevented hip bone loss in most elderly men and women, but vitamin D only modestly lowered bone loss (Peacock et al. 2000). In a different study, annual vitamin D injections did not prevent hip fractures (Heikenheimo et al. 1992). However, in a third randomized, controlled trial, 400 IUs of vitamin D per day prevented hip bone loss over 2 years in elderly women (Ooms et al. 1995). In a recent study, vitamin D supplementation was found to have more beneficial effects when used in combination with calcium supplementation in women who had suffered a hip fracture (Harwood et al. 2004). Thus, the question of the role of vitamin D alone in promoting bone health remains unresolved. Vitamin D can probably be most effective in populations with an underlying deficiency and in those individuals for whom other components of bone health, such as adequate levels of calcium and physical activity, are optimized.

It may not be realistic, however, to try to dissect the individual contributions of calcium, vitamin D, and physical activity on bone health, since they all need to be optimized. As a result, some studies have looked at the impact of combinations of the three on bone health. The most promising study of a combination of calcium and vitamin D on bone fractures was conducted in France in the early 1990s (Chapuy et al. 1992). Over 3,000 elderly women received supplements with calcium and vitamin D or placebo pills. Hip fractures were reduced by 43 percent among the women treated with vitamin D and calcium compared to those who received placebo. This is the only large trial to date to show a reduction in hip fractures due to supplements. The women in the study were quite elderly (average age 83) and vitamin D deficient, so it is possible that correcting the deficiency led to the dramatic drop in fractures. In a smaller study of elderly individuals in New England, Dawson-Hughes and colleagues showed that supplementation with calcium and vitamin D moderately reduced bone loss and the incidence of non-spine fractures (Dawson-Hughes et al. 1997). Tests of calcium and vitamin D supplementation to prevent hip fractures are currently being conducted in a large population of healthy postmenopausal women in the Women's Health Initiative; these results should be available in late 2005 (Jackson et al. 2003).

Other Nutrients With a Role in Bone Health

Bone health requires more than just attention to calcium and vitamin D. In fact, data suggest that many other nutrients can affect bone in positive or negative ways. (For more information, see Table 7-5, which lists some of the other nutrients that can affect bone.) The roles of many of these nutrients with respect to bone health have not been as well established as for calcium and vitamin D. Since the vast majority of individuals consume an appropriate amount of these nutrients (i.e., not too much or too little), they have not become a target for special attention.

Nevertheless, the Institute of Medicine recently considered other bone-related nutrients, including phosphorus, magnesium, and fluoride (IOM 1997). Phosphates make up more than half the mass of bone mineral. About 85 percent of the body's phosphorus and 60 percent of the body's magnesium are found in the skeleton. Both phosphorus deficiency and excess have been considered as having adverse effects on bone health (Heaney 2004), but both can be avoided with a healthy diet. Magnesium may enhance bone quality by influencing growth of crystals of hydroxyapatite, the mineral compound found in bone. Fluoride is known to reduce cavities in teeth, a hard tissue that is similar to bone, but its role in maintaining skeletal health is less clear (IOM 1997). Other nutrients/dietary components that appear to play a positive role in bone health include vitamin K, vitamin C, copper, manganese, zinc, and iron. These micronutrients are essential to the function of enzymes and local regulators and therefore are important to forming the optimal bone matrix.

Potassium also appears to play an important role in bone health. Diets abundant in potassium-rich fruits and vegetables may reduce the need for calcium to be mobilized from the skeleton. Epidemiologic and short-term intervention studies suggest higher intakes of alkaline potassium salts reduce urine calcium excretion and markers of bone resorption and have been associated with increased bone density (Barzel 1995, Sellmeyer et al. 2002, New et al. 2000, New et al. 2004, Tucket et al. 1999, Sebastian et al. 1994).

It is important to remember that some dietary components may negatively affect calcium balance. While their effects tend to be small, these include caffeine, protein, and excess phosphorus intake (i.e., more than 3-4 grams per day) (Fitzpatrick and Heaney 2003; Kerstetter et al. 2003). Sodium also affects calcium balance by increasing its excretion, and high-salt diets are fairly common in the United States. But unlike with these other nutrients, the effects of sodium on calcium balance are more pronounced. Results of two studies in adult women suggest that each additional gram of sodium eaten per day increases bone loss by 1 percent per year, unless the extra calcium lost in the urine is replaced by more calcium in the diet

(Devine et al. 1995, Shortet al. 1988). The negative effects of sodium and these other dietary components can be countered by consuming an adequate amount of calcium in the diet. Diets high in sodium are associated with hypertension. Therefore, lowering intake of sodium in concert with meeting calcium requirements is prudent (USDA 2000). Finally, although protein causes some loss of calcium from the body, only very high protein diets that are not compensated for by extra calcium are a concern (Dawson-Hughes 2003). In fact, higher protein intakes may be associated with higher levels of IGF-1, a marker of bone formation, and lower levels of urinary n-telopeptide crosslinks, a marker of bone breakdown (Dawson-Hughes et al. 2004). Far more serious is the low protein intake of many older persons (Rizzoli and Bonjour 2004). Inadequate protein intake negatively affects bone health in the elderly (Kerstetter et al. 2003) and may diminish the ability to repair and recover from fractures (Schurch et al. 1998). Nutritional supplementation has been recommended as a means of boosting protein intake in elderly individuals recovering from a hip fracture (Schurch et al. 1998), although the evidence to support this approach is limited (Avenell and Handoll 2004). Finally, excess dietary vitamin A (as retinol) may also negatively affect bone health by increasing bone resorption (Sheven and Hamilton 1990).

Since many nutrients in addition to calcium and vitamin D play a role in bone health, it is important to consume a well-balanced diet containing a variety of food, rather than just focusing on one or two bone-related nutrients. This approach can have positive effects on other aspects of health as well. For example, the DASH diet (Dietary Approach to Stop Hypertension), which encourages fruit and vegetable intake in addition to more calcium and less sodium intake, has been linked to lower bone turnover and better cardiovascular status (Lin et al. 2003). In a recent study of young girls a high intake of fruits and vegetables was associated with increased bone mineral content (Tylavsky et al. 2004). Fruit and vegetables also provide vitamins, minerals, and fiber, and should be encouraged for overall good nutrition. As alluded to above, abundant potassium intake via increased fruit and vegetable intake may be particularly beneficial for skeletal health. Specific suggestions for selecting a well-balanced diet are provided in Chapter 7.

Physical Activity

Physical Activity, Body Weight, and Bone Health: What the Evidence Tells Us

- Physical activity is important for bone health throughout life.
  - ~ Depending on age, it may help increase or preserve bone mass.
  - ~ It may also help reduce the risk of falling.
- All types of physical activity can contribute to bone health.
  - ~ Activities that are weight bearing or involve impact are most useful for increasing or maintaining bone mass.
  - ~ Some activities that are not weight bearing or are low impact may help improve balance and coordination and maintain muscle mass, which can help prevent falls.
  - ~ Specific recommendations are given in Chapter 7.

Physical activity of all kinds has overall benefits to health and weight maintenance. Regular physical activity lowers risk factors for cardiovascular disease, colon cancer, and type 2 diabetes, and helps to control blood pressure (USDA 2000). Physical activity plays an important role in skeletal health because, as discussed in Chapter 2, bone mass is responsive to the mechanical loads placed on the skeleton.

Background: Why Focus on Physical Activity?

As discussed in Chapter 2, the body constantly monitors the strain on bones caused by muscle action, and any substantial increase in these forces signals the need to build more bone. Conversely, reductions in biomechanical forces from lower activity levels or loss of muscle mass (sarcopenia) signals less need for bone, which leads to the elimination of bone. The latter process may be worsened by estrogen deficiency, which appears to reduce the sensing of biomechanical strains by bone cells (Riggs et al. 2002).

Physical activity has been identified as one of the Leading Health Indicators in the *Healthy People 2010* health objectives for the Nation during the next decade. It is one of the most important controllable lifestyle changes to help prevent (or reduce the risk of) a number of chronic conditions, including heart disease, diabetes, and some cancers. It also helps with weight control and the lessening of symptoms related to arthritis (USDHHS 1996).

Many adult Americans do not engage regularly in leisure-time physical activity. As shown in Figure 6-5, the participation by both men and women declines with age, with women being consistently less active than men (Schiller et al. 2004). The same problem exists for children. Many children become far less active as they pass through adolescence. Only half of those age 12–21 exercise vigorously on a regular basis and 25 percent report no exercise at all (Gordon-Larsen et al. 1999). Children may find

Figure 6-5. Percent of Adults Aged 18 Years and Over Who Engaged in Regular Leisure Time Physical Activity, by Age Group and Sex: United States, January–September 2003

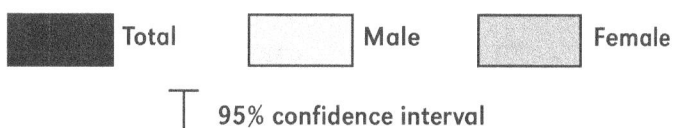

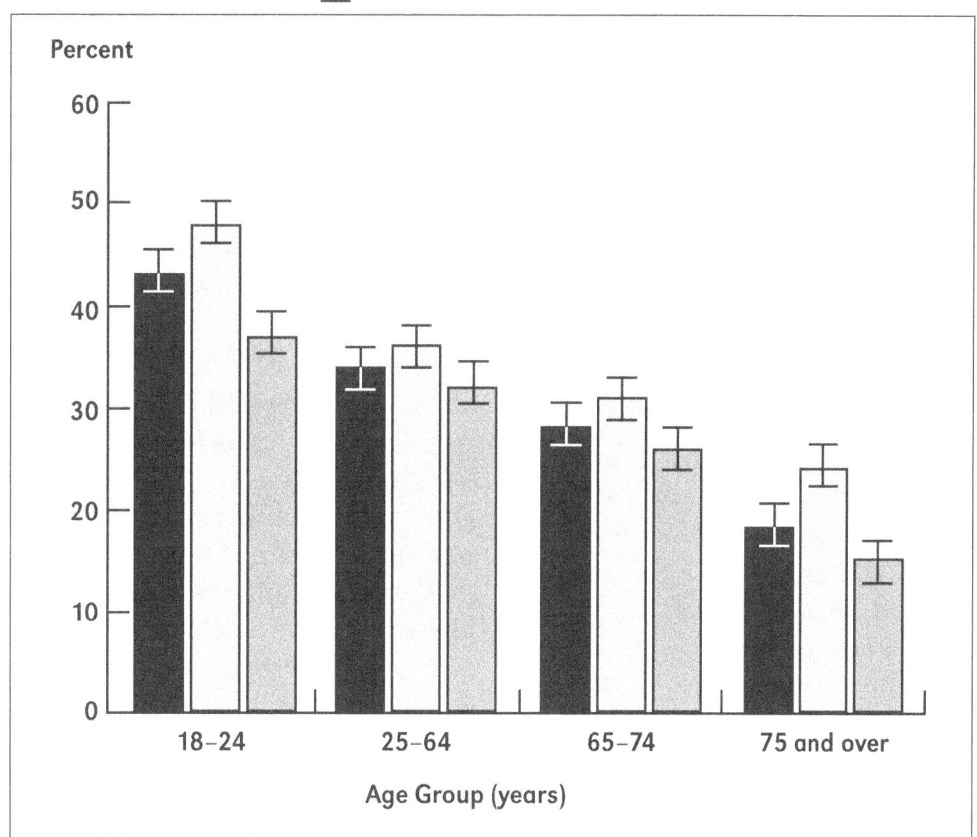

Note: This measure reflects the definition used for the physical activity leading health indicator in Healthy People 2010. Regular leisure-time physical activity is defined as engaging in light-moderate leisure-time physical activity for greater than or equal to 30 minutes at a frequency greater than or equal to five times per week, or engaging in vigorous leisure-time physical activity for greater than or equal to 20 minutes at a frequency greater than or equal to three times per week. The analyses excluded 697 persons (3.0%) with unknown physical activity participation. For both sexes combined, the percent of adults who engaged in regular leisure-time physical activity decreased with age. For all age groups, women were less likely than men to engage in regular leisure-time physical activity.

Source: Ni et al. 2004.

it difficult to get daily physical activity in schools. While most schools have requirements for physical activity of some kind, only 8 percent of elementary schools, 6.4 percent of middle/junior high school, and 5.8 percent of senior high schools provide physical education on a daily basis (SHPPS 2001). At the other extreme, some girls and young women, especially those training for elite athletic competition, exercise too much, eat too little, and as a result develop delayed puberty or amenorrhea (cessation of menstrual periods). These girls are at risk for low bone mass and fractures (Warren 1999). One of the national health objectives for 2010 is to increase to 30 percent the proportion of adults who perform, more than 2 days per week, physical activities that enhance and maintain muscular strength and endurance (USDHHS 2000). Only 12 percent of people age 65–74 and 10 percent of those over age 75 meet that objective, underscoring the need for programs that encourage older adults to incorporate strength training and regular physical activity into their lives (Kruger et al. 2004).

To encourage increased levels of physical activity among all age groups, "Physical Activity and Health: A Report of the Surgeon General" recommends a "minimum of 30 minutes of physical activity of moderate intensity (such as brisk walking) on most, if not all, days of the week" (USDHHS 1996). Children and adolescents should aim for at least 60 minutes of physical activity per day (USDA 2000). In addition to helping achieve healthy weight and avoid chronic diseases like heart disease and diabetes, this type of physical activity can benefit skeletal health by building muscle mass and promoting balance and coordination, which may help individuals avoid falls and/or minimize the impact if a fall does occur. But the skeleton responds preferentially to strength training and short bouts of high-load impact activity (such as skipping or jumping), both of which improve bone mass and strength, as discussed below. In light of this, "Physical Activity and Health: A Report of the Surgeon General" also recommended that adults supplement their cardiorespiratory endurance activity with strength-developing exercise at least two times per week (USDHHS 1996). Chapter 7 will address some specific ways to incorporate strength and loading activities into an overall habit of physical activity.

Physical Activity and Bone Health: A Review of the Evidence

This section will discuss the evidence of the impact of exercise and physical activity on fractures and on bone mass and other bone qualities.

Impact of Physical Activity on Fractures

Although no randomized intervention trials have addressed the issue, data from longitudinal observational studies have shown a link between physical activity and reduced fracture risk. In these studies, subjects are asked about their physical activity habits and then followed for some period of time to determine if they fracture. As suggested earlier, this study design cannot prove that physical activity causes a reduction in risk, since there is an inherent bias in the study—i.e., that healthy people are able to be more active. A number of risk factors for osteoporosis and fracture (e.g., health, diet, body size) may be unequally distributed between those who choose to be physically active and those who do not. Nevertheless, recent reviews of the epidemiologic evidence suggests that physical activity is associated with reduction in the risk of hip fracture in both men and women and that there is a "dose-response" effect, i.e., risk goes down as physical activity level goes up (Gregg et al. 2000, Karlsson 2002). In a large

Challenges in Studying the Impact of Physical Activity on Bone Health

One of the biggest challenges to researchers in determining the effect of physical activity on bone is to have an accurate and measurable outcome. Fracture would be the best outcome to study, but there are no large studies that have determined the effect of physical activity on the risk of fracture using a randomized clinical trial design. Most physical activity studies have had small sample sizes and have used BMD, as measured by dual-energy x-ray absorptiometry (DXA), as the outcome. As described in Chapter 8, DXA measurements of bone-mineral content (measured in grams) and areal bone-mineral density (g/cm^2 [grams per centimeter squared]) do not directly measure bone size or reflect bone geometry, and thus they can significantly underestimate the effect of physical activity on overall bone strength (Jarvinen et al. 1999). Thus, while a convenient measure, BMD may not be sensitive to the multiple effects of physical activity on the musculoskeletal system.

study of older women (Gregg et al. 1998), higher levels of leisure time physical activity and household chores were associated with an overall 36 percent reduction in hip fractures. The effect varied with the level of the activity, with very active women having greater reductions in risk compared with inactive women. However, even walking, the most common leisure time physical activity for women, can have a positive effect on bone health. For example, the Nurses Health Study concluded that walking at least 4 hours per week was associated with a 41 percent lower risk of hip fracture compared with walking less than an hour per week, even among women who

did no other exercise (Feskanich et al. 2002). Several other longitudinal observational studies have confirmed a similar reduction in hip fracture risk in men who exercise regularly compared to inactive men (Paganini-Hill et al. 1991, Kujala et al. 2000).

Impact on Bone Mass, BMD, and Other Bone Qualities

Randomized intervention trials that focused on the effects of physical activity on bone mass (either bone mineral density or bone mineral content) have identified some important points about physical activity and skeletal health.

- First, these studies show that bone mass is improved, but only at the skeletal sites that received the impact. In other words, lifting weights with arms will not improve bone density of the hips.
- Second, the effects of physical activity on bone health will vary by age, and thus younger individuals should be studied separately from older individuals.
- Third, the effect of physical activity on bone does not persist if the activity level is stopped or reduced (an exception may be the effect of physical activity on bone that occurs during childhood and adolescence). Thus, as with intake of dietary calcium, physical activity levels need to be maintained for optimal bone health to be achieved.
- Fourth, the effect of physical activity on bone appears to be greater in those who are less active than in those who are already active, e.g., bone gains will be greater in a sedentary person who becomes physically active than in an active person who increases his or her level of physical activity.

More specific evidence supporting these points is presented on the following pages.

Children and Adolescents. As noted earlier, physical activity appears to increase the positive effects of calcium. A randomized trial of physical activity with or without supplemental calcium in young children (3–5 years old) indicated that calcium intake can modify the bones' response to physical activity (Specker and Binkley 2003). In this study, bone mineral density was not the most sensitive indicator of physical activity effects on bone; rather it was primarily the shape and size of bone that was being affected. The combination of both increased activity and 1,000 mg of supplemental calcium increased the width of the cortical bone and the entire diameter of the bone in the leg more than did exercise alone. Both of these changes suggest greater bone strength, and they are particularly important if they represent permanent differences. The study results also suggest that high calcium is necessary to realize the full potential benefits of physical activity on the bone of children. A different study of tennis players found that loading exercises before puberty increased bone size and bone's resistance to bending (Bass et al. 2002).

The pubertal phase of adolescence is a particularly valuable time to improve bone mass via physical activity. As noted previously, the period of puberty represents a 2- to 3-year window when, on average, 25–30 percent of total body adult bone mass is gained (Bailey et al. 2000). During this period, bone may be especially responsive to activity-induced loading (MacKelvie et al. 2002). Hormone levels may also influence the amount of bone gained during this period. In a trial with prepubertal and early pubertal girls, greater gains in bone mass with physical activity were seen in the girls in early puberty, possibly because of their increasing estrogen levels (MacKelvie et al. 2001).

A study conducted in Finland provided even more evidence of the benefits of physical activity during puberty. This study compared the bone mineral content of the playing arm of adult woman tennis and squash players with their non-dominant arm. In other words, each woman in the study served as her own control (Kannus et al. 1995). Most people have about a 3–5 percent difference in their dominant and non-dominant arm, which reflects greater use of the dominant arm in everyday life. In the racquet players, the difference in bone content between the two arms was much greater (12–16 percent), due to their training regimen. But the difference was twofold greater when the comparison was restricted to women who began training before puberty versus those who took up the sport later (Figure 6-6). This observation underscores the importance of the timing of physical activity and supports the concept that there is a "window of opportunity" during childhood and adolescence for building bone (Khan et al. 2000).

Exercise-intervention studies in girls (Morris et al. 1997) suggest that relatively short periods of appropriate exercise can stimulate bone gain at trabecular bone sites (hip and spine). Jumping activities appear to be particularly effective, and the greatest gains occur in early or mid-puberty (MacKelvie et al. 2003). High-intensity jumping improves both hip and lumbar spine bone mass and increases bone area in pre-pubertal children (Fuchs et al. 2001). Moreover, the bone mass gains at the hip that accrue from high-impact jumping are retained for at least a short period of time (an equivalent period of detraining) (Fuchs and Snow 2002). Thus, jumping from a moderate height (roughly 20 inches is a safe, effective, and simple method of improving bone mass and size in children, and these activities could easily be incorporated into physical education classes) (Figure 6-7). What is not clear, however, is whether or not early gains in bone mass and geometry confer a long-lasting reduction in

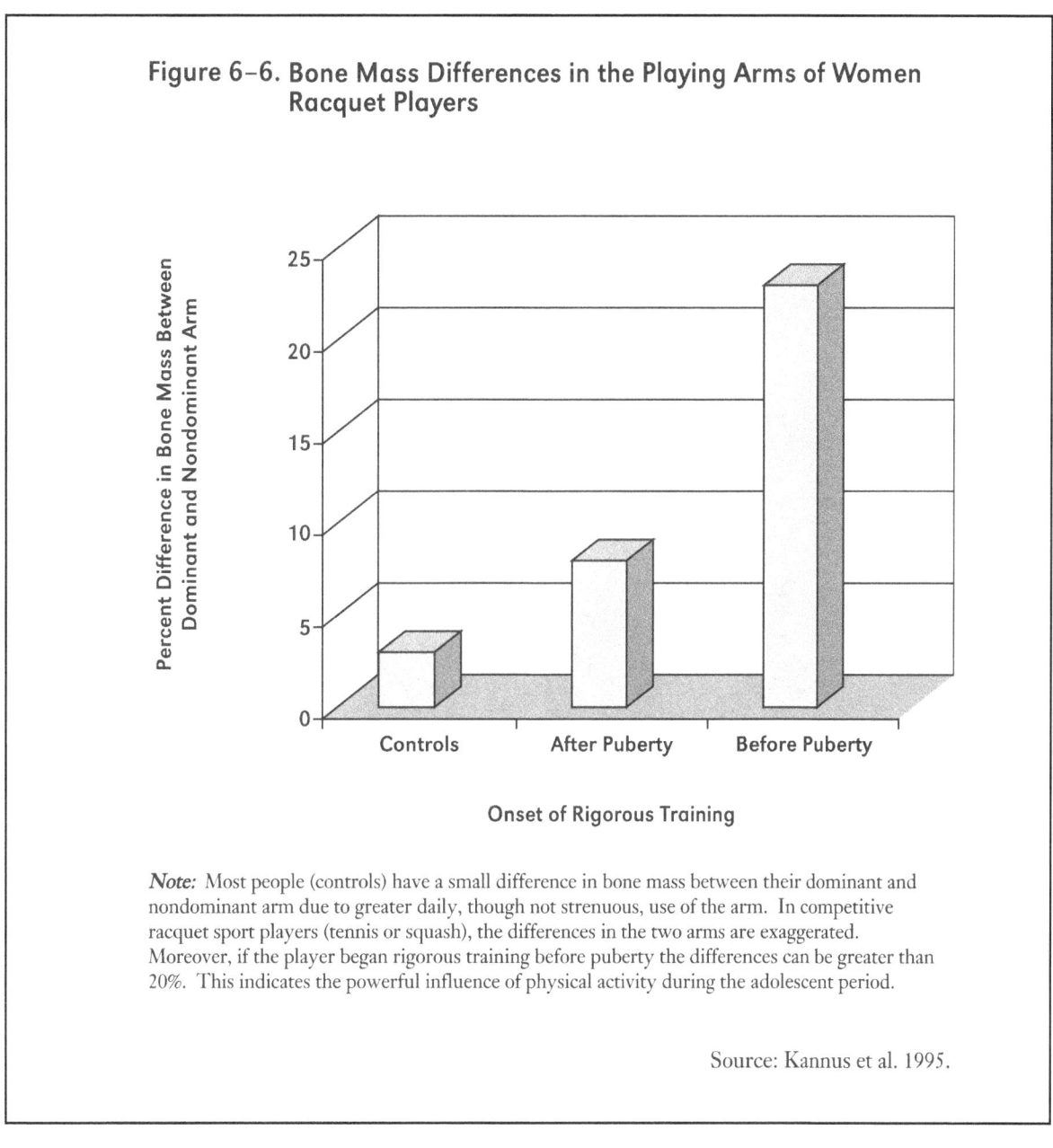

Figure 6-6. Bone Mass Differences in the Playing Arms of Women Racquet Players

Note: Most people (controls) have a small difference in bone mass between their dominant and nondominant arm due to greater daily, though not strenuous, use of the arm. In competitive racquet sport players (tennis or squash), the differences in the two arms are exaggerated. Moreover, if the player began rigorous training before puberty the differences can be greater than 20%. This indicates the powerful influence of physical activity during the adolescent period.

Source: Kannus et al. 1995.

fracture rate. Although some evidence supports a lasting beneficial effect of early sports training and exercise on bone (Kontulainen et al. 2001, Bass et al. 1998), this area remains controversial and it may be that stopping exercise or reducing its intensity over time may lessen its benefit in old age (Seeman 2001). For example, Karlsson et al. (2000) found little residual protection in soccer players who had been retired for more than 20 years. So the benefits of physical activity in reducing fracture risk, even if started in youth when bone is most malleable, may be attenuated if an individual becomes sedentary later in life.

Adults. Because adulthood is a time of bone conservation—not bone building—the primary impact of physical activity is to maintain bone mass

Figure 6–7. High-Intensity Jumping Improves Hip and Lumbar Spine Bone Mass and Size in Pre-Pubertal Children

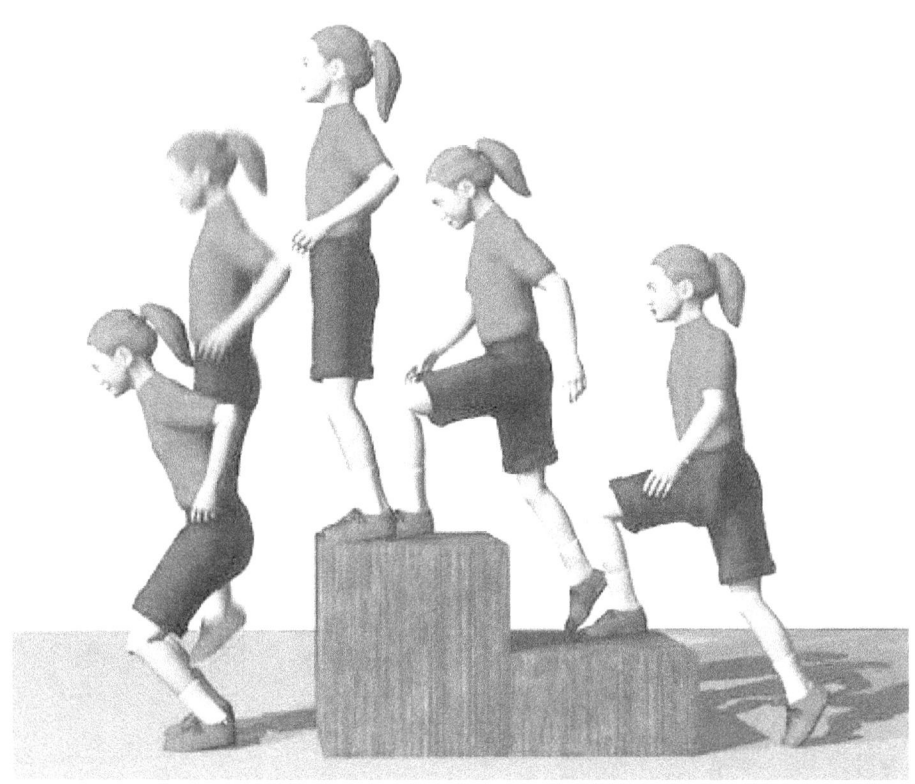

Note: Jumping from a moderate height of approximately 20 inches is safe and effective in increasing bone mass and size in children, with the greatest gains occurring in early or mid-puberty.

Source: Fuchs et al. 2001. Reproduced from J Bone Miner Res 2001: Jan; 16(1): 148–56 with permission of the American Society for Bone and Mineral Research.

during this stage. While it is not possible to assign a specific age range to this period of bone maintenance, it would optimally last from the end of puberty until age- or menopause-related bone loss begins. Very little research has focused on the impact of physical activity on bone mass in this age range. However, several reviews and meta-analyses have included pre-menopausal women (Wolff et al. 1999, Wallace and Cumming 2000, Kelley et al 2001) and they have generally found a modest but consistent positive effect (approximately 1 percent) from exercise on BMD; a similar effect was found in postmenopausal women. The effect is more clear at the spine than the hip, and no optimal types of exercise could be discerned from these analyses.

The Cochrane Collaboration has reviewed the trials of exercise for preventing or treating osteoporosis in postmenopausal women specifically (Bonaiuti et al, 2002). These analyses indicated that aerobic, weight-bearing, and resistance exercises were all effective in increasing BMD at the spine, while walking (as an exercise intervention) was effective in increasing BMD at both the hip and spine.

As alluded to earlier, there is a synergistic effect between physical activity and calcium intake. A meta-analysis of 17 randomized and nonrandomized intervention trials in peri- and postmenopausal women suggests that physical activity is more beneficial in increasing BMD in individuals with high calcium intakes (1,000 mg per day) than in those with lower calcium intakes (Specker 1996). Not all of the studies, however, reported on the calcium intake of participants.

In postmenopausal women, physical activity programs also serve the all-important role of maintaining bone mass. Maintaining bone at a time when bone loss typically increases provides important benefits for the skeleton. Although results may vary, studies suggest that high-impact loading such as jumping, strength-training exercises, or a combination of these can slightly increase or conserve spine bone mass in healthy postmenopausal women and also has a positive effect at the hip (Bassey and Ramsdale 1994, Kohrt et al 1995, Going et al 2003).

One of the few studies to date that included men over age 60 showed significant increases in bone mass among exercisers after 4–8 months (Blumenthal et al 1991). These results are consistent with those found for adult women. In addition, one meta-analysis found that site-specific exercise may help to improve and maintain BMD in men over age 30 (Kelley et al, 2000).

Older Adults (Frailty). Regular physical activity is particularly important for frail older persons, because it delays the onset of functional limitations and loss of independence that are common in this population, especially those over age 75 (Singh 2002). Thus, the substantial reduction in physical activity that is typically seen in individuals as they get older (which was documented earlier in this chapter) represents another important threat to bone health. Maintaining, or preferably increasing, customary physical activity can mitigate some of the musculoskeletal problems of aging and can also provide many other health benefits. Although physical activity must be maintained to preserve bone mass in this age group, the biomechanical strains from enhanced physical activity may promote increases in bone size that can help preserve bone strength even in the face of bone loss (Kaptoge et al. 2003). This protective expansion of bone area is more pronounced in men, possibly because of their higher testosterone levels.

One of the biggest bone-related problems facing the frail elderly relates to the loss of muscle strength and function (Doherty 2003). Sarcopenia is the involuntary loss of skeletal muscle mass and function that occurs as people age. On average, 5 percent of muscle mass is lost per decade after age 30 and this loss may accelerate after age 65. This muscle loss results in impaired functional performance and increased risk for falls. It is unclear whether the age-related decrease in muscle size and strength is related to the age-related decrease in BMD, or whether both contribute to increased fracture risk independently.

The mechanisms that underlie sarcopenia are just beginning to be understood. As people age, their ability to synthesize certain proteins decreases in comparison to their ability to break down protein. This leads to loss of type II, or fast-twitch, muscle fibers. Several other age-related changes are also thought to contribute to sarcopenia, including declines in: a) enzyme activity in the muscle cell mitochondria; b) hormones important in muscle turnover, such as testosterone and growth hormone; and c) muscle blood flow and nerve function (Greenlund and Nair 2003). Sarcopenia occurs in all individuals to some degree as they age, but it can be accelerated by a variety of factors, including chronic illness, inactivity, and poor nutrition, especially inadequate protein and caloric intake. Although physical activity cannot completely reverse the effects of aging, it can increase mitochondrial enzyme activity. Muscle-strengthening exercises and activities appear to improve strength and performance even in frail nursing home residents (Morris et al.1999). Thus it appears that physical activity and muscle strengthening may be useful for treating or preventing sarcopenia.

The response of elderly individuals' muscles to physical activity may have greater significance to bone health than does the response of BMD. Muscle strengthening reduces the risk of fractures by improving balance, mobility, and speed of movement, each of which helps to prevent or reduce the severity of falls. In fact, muscle strength seems highly adaptable to physical activity in the elderly, with increases of over 100 percent being reported in men in their 80s and 90s who exercise (Fiatarone et al. 1990). This increase is far greater than the corresponding increase in muscle volume and BMD. A training program for 21 men over 60 resulted in a 39 percent increase in upper body and a 38 percent increase in lower body strength, as well as a 3 percent increase in femoral neck BMD (Ryan et al. 1994). Generally, strength, flexibility, balance, and reaction time—the factors most amenable to modification—can be addressed in exercise intervention programs to prevent falls in the elderly (Lord et al. 2002). Several large

studies have reported that exercise leads to 10 percent fewer falls, while balance training leads to 17 percent fewer falls (Province et al. 1995). In a series of key studies, lower limb strength and balance exercises reduced the rate of falls among women age 80 and older (Robertson et al. 2002).

Weight

Weight: What the Evidence Tells Us
- Very low body weight in children and adolescents may limit peak bone mass.
- Low body weight increases the risk of hip fracture in older women.
- Weight loss of 10 percent or more in older women also increases the risk of hip fracture.

Maintaining a healthy body weight is one of the goals of *Healthy People 2010* (USDHHS 2000). Although overweight and obesity are the focus of most health campaigns that focus on weight, low body weight can be a problem for bone health. A higher body weight may influence BMD through a variety of mechanisms, including higher mechanical loading, more muscle mass, higher levels of sex hormones and their precursors, and lower bone turnover (Nelson et al. 2002). Body weight may also be related to the level of fat padding, which can provide a cushion during a fall on the hip.

Body weight and pubertal development are the most consistent predictors of bone mass in adolescents (Bachrach 2001, Heaney et al. 2000). Fear of fat and obsession with thinness among pre-teen and teenage girls frequently translates into diets that fail to meet their caloric, calcium, and protein needs. Young women who repeatedly diet to lose weight also have lower bone density, even if they are not underweight (Van Loan and Keim 2000).

Both low body weight and weight loss have been associated with reductions in bone mass and increases in fracture risk in epidemiologic studies. In a follow-up to the first NHANES, women who were relatively thin in middle age (age 50-64) and had lost at least 10 percent of their body weight had the highest risk of hip fracture (Langlois et al. 2001). Although body weight is very strongly associated with BMD (Reid 2002), the relationship of body weight to bone mass is confounded by the fact that smaller people tend to have smaller bones and lower bone mass. Nevertheless, they can have a perfectly adequate skeleton.

Low body weight and weight loss are a particular problem for the elderly, as they may signal a variety of medical problems. Older women who are thin have a higher risk of hip fracture (Farmer et al. 1989, Kiel et al. 1987). Although "thin" has been defined variably in different studies and may be open to clinical interpretation, a large prospective study of older women found a roughly twofold increased risk of hip fracture in women who were below 127 pounds (Ensrud et al. 1997). This study also found no protective effect from increasing weight in these thin women. The increased risk was entirely attributable to hip bone density, which has led to the suggestion that low body weight be used as a surrogate for increased fracture risk when bone density measurements are unavailable. As discussed in Chapters 8 and 10, weight is used in some assessment instruments as an aid in deciding whether BMD testing is necessary.

Older women who experience weight loss in later years have also been found to have a twofold greater risk of subsequent hip fracture, irrespective of current weight or intention to lose weight. These findings indicate that even voluntary weight loss in overweight elderly women increases hip fracture risk (Ensrud et al. 2003).

Whether being overweight reduces fracture risk is less clear. Some older studies have reported a lower risk of fracture in overweight women (Farmer et al. 1989), but a more recent study reported that women of average weight had a risk of hip fracture that was similar to that of heavier women (Ensrud et al. 1997). Of course, being overweight raises the risk of many other health problems, including heart disease and diabetes. The epidemic of overweight and obesity in the United States is well documented (Flegal et al. 2002). As a result, public health efforts should continue to focus on weight reduction in overweight or obese individuals and maintenance of body weight in normal weight individuals, especially at older ages. For overweight individuals, achieving weight loss while maintaining skeletal integrity is the goal. The key may be to increase physical activity in addition to restricting caloric intake. For example, Salamone (1999) found that women who lost weight did lose more bone than weight-stable women, but this bone loss was lessened among those who increased their physical activity. Consuming adequate calcium during weight loss may also help prevent bone loss, at least in postmenopausal women (Ricci et al. 1998). If these results are confirmed in other studies, weight loss recommendations should include physical activity, preferably weight bearing, and adequate calcium to help protect the skeleton.

Finally, the relationship between weight and weight loss, bone density, and fracture risk in men has not been thoroughly addressed.

Falls and Fall Prevention

Falls and Bone Health: What the Evidence Tells Us

- Falls contribute to most fractures.
- There are a number of identifiable risk factors for falls in the elderly.
- Interventions targeted at multiple risk factors can reduce the number of falls and possible the number of fractures as well.

Background: Why Focus on Falls?

Falls contribute to fractures, and thus fall prevention offers another opportunity to protect the bones throughout life, particularly in those over age 60. While low bone mass may put an individual at high risk of fracture, it is often a fall that precipitates the injury. Falls are one of the most common problems that threaten the independence of older individuals. About 10–15 percent of falls in the elderly result in fracture (Nevitt et al. 1991), and some may result in death. The risk of falling increases with age and varies according to living status. One study found that between 30–40 percent of those over age 65 who live in the community fall each year (Tinetti et al. 1988). The rate of falls is even greater in long-term care settings, as the general health of these individuals is more fragile (Thapa et al. 1996). An elderly individual's level of social integration—that is, the degree to which he or she has developed and maintained networks of family members and friends, also has an impact on falls. Those with stronger networks have a lower risk of falling (Faulkner 2003). A history of falling is also an important predictor of future falls, as almost 60 percent of those who fell during the previous year will fall again (Nevitt et al. 1991).

Falls in older individuals are rarely due to a single cause. They usually result when a threat to the normal mechanisms that maintain posture occurs in someone who already has problems with balance, mobility, sensory changes and lower extremity weakness, and/or blood pressure or circulation. The new threat may involve an acute illness (e.g., infection, fever, dehydration, arrhythmia), or an environmental stress (e.g., taking a new drug or walking on an unsafe surface). Since they may already have several health problems as a result of aging or chronic disease, many elderly people cannot compensate for the additional burden posed by the new threat.

Some Facts About the Prevalence of Falls

- One third of people over age 65 fall each year, with half of those falls being recurrent (i.e., the individual has fallen before).
- One in 10 falls results in a serious injury, such as a hip fracture. In fact, 90 percent of hip fractures result from falls.
- Falls account for 10 percent of visits to emergency room visits and 6 percent of urgent hospitalizations in the elderly.
- The risk of falling varies tremendously depending upon an individual's risk factors. An elderly person with no risk factors has only a 10 percent chance of falling each year, compared to an 80 percent likelihood of falling for a person with four or more risk factors.

(Tinetti 2003)

Risk Factors for Falls

- Age
- Arthritis
- Depression
- Fall in blood pressure upon standing (i.e., orthostasis)
- Poor cognition
- Poor vision, gait, or balance
- Need for home health care
- Use of four or more medications

(Tinetti 2003)

Falls and Fall Prevention: A Review of the Evidence

Many well-designed studies of risk factors for falls have been published over the several decades (Tinetti et al. 1988, Nevitt et al. 1991). These studies show that the more risk factors an individual has, the more likely he or she is to fall (Tinetti et al. 1988, Nevitt et al. 1991). As noted previously, one of the most important risk factors for falls is a previous history of falls. Other risk factors included age, being female, Alzheimer's disease or other types of cognitive impairment, weakness in the legs and feet, balance problems, use of drugs for depression and psychosis, and arthritis. Being hospitalized also increased risk of falling among those who already had other risk factors. Age-related declines in vision, balance and coordination, inner ear function, muscle amount and responsiveness, blood pressure regulation, and problems with staying hydrated also can lead to falls. Finally, those requiring bi- or tri-focal glasses are also at increased risk of falls and hip fractures (Lord et al. 2002, Felson et al. 1989).

Medication use is one of the most modifiable risk factors for falls. Drugs that affect the central nervous system (CNS) frequently have been linked to risk of falling. Examples of these drugs include neuroleptic drugs (used to treat psychotic behavior), benzodiazepines (used to treat anxiety), and tricyclic or serotonin reuptake inhibitors (used to treat depression) (Ensrud et al. 2002). Drugs to control blood pressure may also increase the risk of falling (Mukai and Lipsitz 2002). In addition to these specific drug classes, recent changes in the dose of a medication and the total number of prescriptions appear to be associated with an increased risk of falling (Cumming et al. 1991). Attention by physicians to the potential effects of medications on falls in the elderly may lead to some modification of therapy (e.g., changes in dose or timing of use) and/or to enhanced fall prevention activities.

Environmental factors, such as poor lighting or loose rugs, may also increase the risk of falling. Most well-designed studies on methods to prevent falls combine efforts to improve the individual's health-related risks with efforts to remove environmental hazards, making it difficult to separate out the unique contribution of either set of factors (Tinetti et al. 1994). One study, for example, investigated the usefulness of having an experienced occupational therapist visit the home to assess and help modify potential environmental hazards (Cumming et al. 1999). The visits reduced the risk of falling by 36 percent in high-risk patients (e.g., those who fell one or more times in the previous year). However, the therapist's visit may have also prompted behavior changes in these patients that lowered their falling risk.

A different study examined the role of hazard reduction more directly. In that study, people age 70 and older were randomly assigned either to a group that received a home hazard assessment, information on hazard reduction, and installation of safety devices, or to a control group that did not receive these things (Stevens et al. 2001a and b). A research nurse visited the homes of people in both groups once. At the end of the study, there were fewer hazards in the homes of the group that received the information and safety devices than in the control group, but the number of falls did not differ between the two groups (Stevens et al. 2001a and b).

Fall prevention in the hospital and nursing home settings are also important. In hospital settings, bed rails do not appear to change the total number of falls, although they can decrease the number of serious falls (Hanger et al. 1999).

Several studies to identify effective ways to reduce falling risk have been conducted over the past decade. The approaches studied include programs to improve strength or balance, educational programs, optimization of medications, and environmental modifications.

Figure 6–8. Rationale for the Use of Hip Protectors to Prevent Fractures

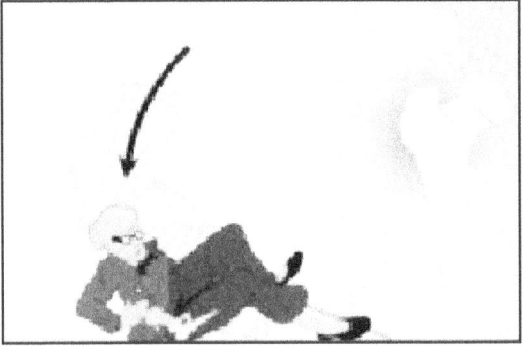
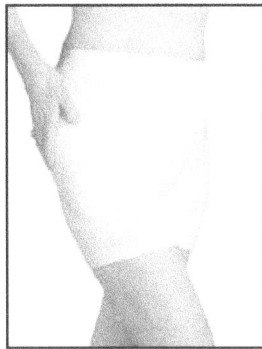

Note: Falls to the side are associated with the majority of hip fractures. Energy absorption in soft tissue may account for up to 75% of the energy in a fall. Hip protector systems can be designed to be energy absorbing or energy shunting. The protective effect of this intervention is immediate, as opposed to the typical 1-2 years required for pharmacologic therapies.

Source: Kiel 2002.

Some approaches have targeted a single risk factor, while others have focused on modifying several factors simultaneously. The latter have been more successful, since falls are generally caused by more than one risk factor (Gillespie et al. 2001). Specific approaches that have demonstrated benefit included: a) muscle strengthening and balance retraining; b) professional home hazard assessment and modification; and c) stopping or reducing psychotropic medication (Tinetti et al. 1994, Tinetti 2003). The optimal duration or intensity of these approaches has not been defined. As noted earlier in this chapter, vitamin D deficiency is associated with an increased risk of falls and hence the use of vitamin D supplementation to reduce falls may be promising (Bischoff et al. 2003, Bischoff-Ferrari et al. 2004, Dukas 2004).

Finally, a complementary approach to reducing fractures due to falls is to attempt to minimize the impact of those falls that do occur through use of a hip protector or hip pad that helps to "cushion the blow" from a fall, as shown in Figure 6-8. A recently updated systematic review of the efficacy of hip protectors concluded that hip protectors reduce the risk of hip fracture for elderly individuals who live in nursing homes and residential care facilities, as well as those in supported living at home; the generalization of the results beyond this high risk population is unknown (Parker 2003). One of the larger studies (Kannus 2000) included in this systematic review found that 41 patients would need to be offered treatment with a hip protector to prevent one hip fracture over the course of one year, a finding that suggests that hip protectors may be a reasonable and cost-effective option for patients at high risk of falls.

While hip protectors appear to be effective when used, the biggest problem may relate to getting people to wear them. A recent randomized controlled trial among women over age 70 living in the community found that hip protectors offered no significant reduction in the risk of hip fracture (Birks et al. 2004). But compliance rates were quite low (roughly 30 percent). This study, the Kannus study described above, and others have documented low rates of compliance (i.e., those who have hip protectors do not wear them), suggesting the need to develop more acceptable, easy-to-use devices that can protect fragile bones by absorbing some of the energy of falls. The policies of nursing homes and other residential care facilities might also influence usage rates. While hip protectors may be relatively inexpensive, the decision to use them for residents of these facilities may be influenced by the cost and how much staff time is required in helping residents to put them on and take them off. But a recent economic analysis of ambulatory nursing facility residents demonstrated that hip protectors save money and are economically attractive over a wide range of cost and utility assumptions (Colon-Emeric 2003).

The Bottom Line on Fall Prevention

The approaches summarized above have modestly reduced the frequency and/or impact of falling. When combined with strategies to improve underlying bone strength, they can likely decrease fracture risk. In fact, based on a review of the evidence, the USPSTF recommends counseling elderly patients on specific measures to prevent falls. The USPSTF also recommends that more intensive individualized multi-factorial interventions be implemented for high-risk elderly patients in settings where adequate resources to deliver such services are available (USPSTF 1996).

Reproductive Factors

Reproductive Factors and Bone Health: What the Evidence Tells Us
- Pregnancy and lactation generally do not harm the skeleton of healthy adult women.
- Amenorrhea (cessation of menstrual periods) is linked to low bone mass.
- Bilateral oophorectomy (removal of both ovaries) is linked to increased bone loss and fracture risk.
- The effects of oral contraceptives on bone health may differ depending on type, and have not been clearly established.

Reproductive hormones play a central role in BMD levels among both women and men, but these hormones have been most widely evaluated in young to middle-aged women, particularly with respect to pregnancy, lactation, and contraception.

Pregnancy and Lactation

Several changes occur during pregnancy and lactation that can affect bone mass, including changes in reproductive hormones and in hormones that affect calcium metabolism. Since fetal and infant bone growth during pregnancy and lactation depends on calcium transfer from the mother, the possibility that pregnancy and lactation affect risk for osteoporosis later in life has been investigated. Intestinal calcium absorption increases during pregnancy to meet much of the fetal calcium needs, but maternal bone loss may occur in the last months of pregnancy (Reed et al. 2003). The mother's skeleton also loses bone during breastfeeding, but this loss is largely restored during weaning, as ovulation and menses is re-established. This bone loss and its subsequent restoration appear to be independent of lifestyle behaviors, including dietary calcium intake and physical activity patterns (Kalkwarf and Specker 2002).

Epidemiologic studies indicate that neither extended lactation nor multiple pregnancies are associated with subsequent osteoporosis, whether measured by BMD levels (Karlsson et al. 2001, Paton et al. 2003) or by assessment of fracture risk. In fact, the risk of hip fracture in women has been found to decrease by 5–10 percent with each additional child, and there is no apparent association between the duration of lactation and fracture risk (Michaelsson et al. 2001). Thus, in general, pregnancy and lactation in healthy adult women do not appear to cause lasting harm to the skeleton. For example, in one recent study, women with more than 10 pregnancies and extended lactation had BMD levels similar to those in women who have not been pregnant (Henderson et al. 2000). Having more children also does not appear to increase fracture risk (Cumming and Klineberg 1993). For pregnant teens who have not yet reached peak bone mass, the 30 g of calcium required for the fetal skeleton competes with the demands of calcium for the teen's mineral accrual. Whether peak bone mass is compromised in women who experience teen pregnancies remains controversial (Lloyd et al. 2002).

Menstrual Cycling

Regular menstrual cycles are the outward vital sign of a normally functioning reproductive system in the premenopausal female. The impact on bone health of irregular cycles or subtle hormonal changes during the menstrual cycle has not been clearly established. However, amenorrhea, or the cessation of menstrual periods, should be viewed with concern, and its cause should be investigated. Primary amenorrhea may be due to a variety of endocrine abnormalities, but the cessation of regular cycling can also be due to an imbalance of energy intake (nutrition) and energy expenditure (exercise). Anorexia nervosa is the most serious cause of secondary amenorrhea and the most difficult to treat. The onset of anorexia nervosa frequently occurs during adolescence when maximal bone mineral accrual takes place, thereby making adolescent girls with anorexia nervosa at high risk for reduced peak bone mass (Soyka et al. 2002).

Female athletes may also experience amenorrhea, especially those participating in sports where leanness is an advantage and very strenuous training is the norm (e.g., cross country running, ballet). While some athletes experience amenorrhea due to disordered eating patterns, others experience it because of chronically inadequate caloric intake that does not compensate for the energy expended. Complications associated with amenorrhea include compromised bone density, failure to attain peak bone mass in adolescence, and increased risk of stress fractures. The most effective treatment is to decrease the intensity of the exercise and increase the nutritional intake (Warren 2003). Adolescent and young adult women who experience amenorrhea lasting for more than 3 months (regardless of the cause) should consult their health care provider.

Contraceptive Practices

Oral contraceptives were first marketed in the United States in 1960, gaining immediate and widespread use. It is estimated that 80 percent of American women born since 1945 have used birth control pills at some point in their lives. About 45 percent of the estimated 24 million women who report using reversible methods of birth control use oral contraceptives (Piccinino et al. 1998). Use is highest in women under age 30, who are also completing bone mass accrual.

Oral contraceptives contain variable amounts of the hormones estrogen and progesterone. Given the known impact of these hormones on bone, it is natural to ask what effect oral contraceptives have on bone mass and density. The factors that determine the effect of an oral contraceptive on bone health are the dose of estrogen and the age of the woman. The formulations of oral contraceptives have changed dramatically over the years, with older types having higher estrogen levels than do newer ones. These different formulations have a different overall impact on total estrogen exposure and ultimately on fracture risk. Both the short- and long-term effects of oral contraceptives on bone health are unclear at this time (Reed et al. 2003). There may be may relatively little impact on bone health from oral contraceptives in women who have already achieved peak bone mass, but low-dose oral contraceptives could potentially compromise the acquisition of bone in younger women (Cromer 2003).

Hysterectomy and Oophorectomy

Roughly 600,000 hysterectomies are performed annually in the United States, and 55 percent of women undergoing this procedure also have both ovaries removed (Keshavarz et al. 2002). Removing the ovaries (oophorectomy) affects calcium metabolism, fracture risk, and bone mineral content because it results in estrogen deficiency.

Bilateral oophorectomy in postmenopausal women results in a 54 percent increase in fractures of the hip, spine, and wrist, and a 35 percent increase in fractures at other sites. The increase in fracture risk among women who underwent bilateral oophorectomy after natural menopause is consistent with the hypothesis that androgens produced by the postmenopausal ovary may be important for endogenous estrogen production that protects against fractures (Melton et al. 2003).

Medical Conditions and Drugs

Medical Conditions and Drugs: What the Evidence Tells Us

- Several medical conditions and prescription medications can affect bone health through various mechanisms. A detailed list of conditions and medications is shown in Chapter 3 and further described below.

Many individuals have medical conditions or take medications that can affect bone health. Chapter 3 contains two tables with a reasonably complete list of these drugs and diseases. This section will discuss the more common prescription drugs and medical conditions that affect bone health. These medical situations, which are known as secondary causes of osteoporosis (Schneider and Shane 2001), should act as a "red flag" to individuals and health care professionals about bone health. A person who has one of these conditions or takes one of these drugs should speak to his or her health care provider about safeguarding bone health. Children who must take one or more of these prescription drugs or who have one of these medical conditions may not accumulate as much bone as they should during adolescence and thus may enter adulthood with abnormally low BMD. Adults who develop one of these diseases or begin taking one or more of these prescription drugs may experience even larger or more rapid bone loss than they would normally have during menopause and aging. In most cases, therefore, measurement of bone density will be necessary to determine whether there has been excessive bone loss.

Medications that can affect skeletal health include the following:

Corticosteroids are a class of drugs that reduce inflammation and suppress the body's immune response. They are called by a number of different names, including cortisone, glucocorticoids, prednisone, prednisolone, steroids, and ACTH. Corticosteroids may be inhaled, taken by mouth, given through the veins, or rubbed on the skin. They are used most commonly to treat lung diseases (emphysema, asthma, cystic fibrosis, sarcoidosis), diseases of the joints (lupus, rheumatoid arthritis, polymyalgia rheumatica), gastrointestinal tract diseases (ulcerative colitis, Crohn's disease), kidney diseases (glomerulonephritis), and certain skin diseases (psoriasis, eczema). Corticosteroids are the most common cause of secondary osteoporosis. They have powerful effects on bone (Saag 2002). For example, doses of prednisone (a corticosteroid) above 7.5 mg per day have been shown to completely shut off formation of new bone, while the loss of older bone continues at a faster rate than normal. As a result, bone is lost very rapidly, particularly during the first year or so after beginning corticosteroids. As shown in Figure 3-4 in Chapter 3, even very small doses may increase risk of spine fractures (van Staa et al. 2000, Kanis et al. 2004a). The risk of fracture increases rapidly after the start of oral corticosteroid therapy (within 3 to 6 months) and decreases after stopping therapy. This increase in risk is independent of underlying disease, age, and gender (van Staa et al. 2002).

Elevated thyroid hormone is associated with secondary osteoporosis (Ross 1994). High levels of thyroid hormone can be the consequence of endogenous conditions such as Grave's disease or thyrotoxicosis (an overly active thyroid gland that produces too much of this hormone). However, prolonged, elevated levels are much more likely to be the result of prescribing thyroid hormone as a drug to treat an underactive or enlarged thyroid gland or to control growth of nodules in the thyroid gland. Too much thyroid hormone, no matter what the source, increases

both the breakdown of old bone and the formation of new bone to take its place. However, more bone is lost than is formed. People with abnormally high levels of thyroid hormone are at increased risk for fracture, and the fractures often occur at younger ages. Postmenopausal women are probably at greater risk than premenopausal women or men, but all patients with a history of an overactive thyroid gland or those who must take thyroid hormone for any reason should have bone density testing. The lowest possible dose of thyroid hormone that corrects the medical problem being addressed should be used, since the effects on bone are related to the dose.

Gonadotrophin-releasing hormone agonists are drugs that lower the blood levels of male and female sex hormones (testosterone, estrogen). They may be referred to as GnRH agonists or hormone deprivation therapy. In men, these drugs are used to treat prostate cancer. In premenopausal women, they may be used to treat endometriosis or as a form of contraception. Hormone deprivation therapy causes levels of bone loss that are similar to that seen in women after menopause. Both men and premenopausal women undergoing this therapy have lower-than-expected BMD, while fracture rates are higher in men with prostate cancer who have undergone this treatment (Smith 2003).

Antiseizure or anticonvulsant medications, particularly diphenylhydantoin, phenobarbital, carbamazepine, and sodium valproate, can cause bone loss (Schneider and Shane 2001, Ensrud et al. 2004). The effect on bone health differs depending on the specific drug prescribed, and the mechanisms by which the drug affects bone are not fully understood. Effects on vitamin D metabolism and on bone or the parathyroid glands have been implicated (Fitzpatrick 2004). Individuals who take these drugs are more likely to have bone disease if they: a) have been on the drugs for years; b) require high doses and/or more than one anticonvulsant; c) avoid dairy products and do not take multivitamins and thus have low dietary intake of vitamin D; d) have chronic illnesses; and e) are institutionalized and thus get little sunlight. However, all patients taking these drugs should be evaluated for osteoporosis and vitamin D deficiency.

Medical conditions or events that should prompt a discussion of bone health fall into three major categories:

1. Warning signs that osteoporosis may already be present include any fracture that occurs during adulthood, loss of height, and the development of osteoporosis in another family member, such as a parent, sibling, or child.

2. The development of any disorder that increases the risk of falling is an important risk factor to consider. For example, an individual who has had a stroke that affects the ability to walk or causes difficulty with balance might be expected to fall more often and thus be at increased risk of fracture. Other diseases that fall into this category include Parkinson's disease, spinal cord injuries, any disorder that causes muscle weakness, and the onset of frailty in the elderly. Similarly, it is important for individuals who are beginning to take medications that increase the risk of falling (tranquilizers, sleeping pills, diuretics, and certain blood pressure pills) to discuss this risk with their health care providers.

3. Many medical conditions can result in low bone mass. The most common are genetic diseases (cystic fibrosis, muscular dystrophy), diseases that lower estrogen levels before menopause (eating disorders, excessive physical activity, ovarian failure of any cause), endocrine disorders (diabetes, hyperparathyroidism, Cushing's syndrome), gastrointestinal diseases (celiac disease, intestinal malabsorption, primary biliary cirrhosis, Crohn's disease), blood disorders (hereditary anemias, multiple myeloma, leukemia), rheumatoid arthritis, lupus, and depression. Anyone with these conditions should consult with a physician about bone health and potential preventive measures.

Smoking, Alcohol, and Environmental Threats to Bone Health

Smoking, Alcohol, and Environmental Threats: What the Evidence Tells Us

- Smoking is associated with reduced bone mass and increased fracture risk.
- Alcohol may have both harmful and beneficial effects on bone.
  - ~ Heavy alcohol consumption is associated with reduced bone mass and increased fracture risk
  - ~ Moderate alcohol use has been associated with higher bone density in some studies.
- Lead is among the most significant environmental threats to bone health in the United States.

Smoking

Smoking may harm the skeleton both directly and indirectly (USDHHS 2004). The nicotine and cadmium found in cigarettes can have a direct toxic effect on bone cells (Riebel et al. 1995, Fang et al. 1991). Smoking may also harm bone indirectly by lowering the amount of calcium absorbed from the intestine, altering the body's handling of vitamin D and various hormones needed for bone health, or lowering body weight (Michnovicz et al. 1986, Baron et al. 1995, Krall and Dawson-Hughes 1999, Brot et al. 1999). Smokers may also be less physically active. Smoking influences estrogen metabolism and the risk for multiple estrogen-sensitive outcomes. Smokers are likely to require higher doses of hormone therapy to achieve clinical effects on bone density that are comparable to those observed in nonsmokers (Tansavatdi et al. 2004). All of these factors can lead to lower bone density and higher risk of fracture (Cummings et al. 1995, Baron et al. 2001).

Several studies have linked smoking to higher fracture risk. A meta-analysis of data from postmenopausal women (Law and Hackshaw 1997) demonstrates that smoking increases the risk of hip fracture. More recent data on the association between smoking and fractures at other skeletal sites, while more limited, also support a relationship between smoking and fracture risk (Honkanen et al. 1998, Jacqmin et al. 1998). A recent meta-analysis, using data from 10 different observational studies from around the world, found that smoking was associated with an increased risk of hip and other fractures in both men and women (Kanis et al. 2004b). Although the lower BMD and BMI of smokers were found to contribute to the increased risk of fracture, these factors did not completely explain the increased risk. After adjustment for BMD, BMI, and age, the risk of hip fracture was 55 percent higher in smokers than in non-smokers. In addition to current smoking, a history of smoking was also associated with a higher risk of fracture, although the risk for former smokers was not as high as for current smokers.

Alcohol

Alcoholism is known to have negative effects on bone (Scharpira 1990), but moderate alcohol use in women has been associated with higher bone density in some studies (Felson et al. 1995,

Sampson 2002). This apparent beneficial effect of moderate alcohol intake may be seen in women and not men because of the effect of alcohol on adrenal androgens or estrogen (Wild et al. 1987). Alcohol inhibits bone remodeling, possibly by affecting vitamin D or by reducing bone formation (Laitinen et al. 1991). It may also increase calcium and magnesium losses from the body. Although some studies suggest moderate alcohol intake increases bone density, it does not seem to lower fracture risk (Cummings et al. 1995, Hoidrup et al. 1999), and high alcohol intake may increase likelihood of fracture (Grisso et al. 1994). It is conceivable that the higher fracture risk is caused by an increased risk of falling or other types of trauma.

Environmental Threats to Bone

While a number of heavy metals can be detrimental to bone health, lead is among the most significant environmental threats to bone health in the United States Lead may accumulate in bone due to environmental or dietary exposures. Periods of high remodeling (pregnancy, lactation, postmenopausal period) are particularly critical since lead can have both a direct effect on bone and a latent effect on other organ systems through release from bone long after the initial exposure (Silbergeld and Flaws 2002, Gulson et al. 2003). High calcium intake may actually blunt the effect of stored lead release from bone in pregnant women (Hernandez-Avila et al. 2003). One potential dietary source of lead is calcium supplements. Certain preparations of calcium (e.g., bone meal and dolomite) can have significant contamination with lead and other heavy metals. However, most commercial calcium preparations are tested to ensure that they do not contain significant contamination of heavy metals (Optimal 1994).

Key Questions for Future Research

Much remains to be learned about the genetic and environmental factors that affect bone health, and, as discussed in Chapter 7, the behavior changes that are necessary to promote bone health throughout life. Some of the most important research questions for Chapters 6 and 7 are listed below:

- What are the genetic factors involved in regulating bone mass acquisition, bone loss, and the response of bone to environmental factors such as nutrients and loading?
- What are the optimal physical activity programs to maximize peak bone mass in children and adolescence and to minimize bone loss in adults?
- What is the potential for changes in the acid/base balance in blood and extra-cellular fluid—either through dietary manipulation or potassium supplementation—to influence bone and muscle health? Over a long period of time, a more acidic balance may create an environment in which the breakdown of existing bone is favored over the formation of new bone.

- What are the optimal muscle loading regimens to prevent sarcopenia and bone loss in the frail elderly?
- What can be done to imitate the effects of exercise (i.e., "exercise mimetics") in individuals who are paralyzed, chronically immobile, traveling in space, or otherwise not capable of engaging in loading activities that benefit bone health?
- What mechanisms and interventions can preserve bone mass during weight loss?
- What is the relationship between weight and weight loss, bone density, and fracture risk in men?
- What are the best ways to promote the adoption of bone-healthy practices by individuals?
- What are the best comprehensive fall prevention programs that can be easily adopted by communities and individuals?
- What impact do different oral and injectable contraceptives have on bone health? How does this impact vary by age?
- What interventions optimize bone health in children and adolescents who need to take glucocorticoids or other drugs that can be harmful to bone?

References

Antoniades L, MacGregor AJ, Andrew T, Spector TD. Association of birth weight with osteoporosis and osteoarthritis in adult twins. Rheumatology (Oxford) 2003 Jun;42(6):791-6.

Avenell A, Handoll H. Nutritional supplementation for hip fracture aftercare in the elderly. Cochrane Database Syst Rev 2004;1:CD001880.

Bachrach LK, Guido D, Katzman D, Litt IF, Marcus R. Decreased bone density in adolescent girls with anorexia nervosa. Pediatrics. 1990 Sep;86(3):440-7.

Bachrach LK. Acquisition of optimal bone mass in childhood and adolescence. Trends Endocrinol Metab 2001 Jan-Feb;12(1):22-8.

Bailey DA, Martin AD, McKay HA, Whiting S, Mirwald R. Calcium accretion in girls and boys during puberty: A longitudinal analysis. J Bone Miner Res 2000 Nov;15(11):2245-50.

Baron JA, Comi RJ, Cryns V, Brinck-Johnsen T, Mercer NG. The effect of cigarette smoking on adrenal cortical hormones. J Pharmacol Exp Ther 1995; 272(1):151-5.

Baron JA, Farahmand BY, Weiderpass E, Michaelsson K, Alberts A, Persson I, Ljunghall S. Cigarette smoking, alcohol consumption, and risk of hip fracture in women. Arch Intern Med 2001 Apr 9;161(7):983–8.

Barzel US. The skeleton as an ion exchange system: Implications for the role of acid-base imbalance in the genesis of osteoporosis. J Bone Miner Res 1995 Oct;10(10):1431-6.

Bass S, Pearce G, Hendrich E, Delmas P, Bradney M, Harding A, Seeman E. Exercise before puberty may confer residual benefits in bone density in adulthood: Studies in active prepubertal and retired female gymnasts. J Bone Miner Res. 1998 Mar;13(3):500–7.

Bass SL, Saxon L, Daly RM, Turner CH, Robling AG, Seeman E, Stuckey S. The effect of mechanical loading on the size and shape of bone in pre-, peri-, and postpubertal girls: A study in tennis players. J Bone Miner Res 2002 Dec;17(12):2274-80.

Bassey E, Ramsdale S. Increase in femoral bone density in young women following high-impact exercise. Osteoporos Int 1994;4(2):72-5.

Beck TJ, Looker AC, Ruff CB, Sievanen H, Wahner HW. Structural trends in the aging femoral neck and proximal shaft: Analysis of the Third National Health and Nutrition Examination Survey dual-energy X-ray absorptiometry data. J Bone Miner Res 2000 Dec;15(12):2297-304.

Biller BM, Saxe V, Herzog DB, Rosenthal DI, Holzman S, Klibanski A. Mechanisms of osteoporosis in adult and adolescent women with anorexia nervosa. J Clin Endocrinol Metab 1989 Mar;68(3):548-54.

Birks YF, Porthouse J, Addie C, Loughney K, Saxon L, Baverstock M, Francis RM, Reid DM, Watt I, Torgerson DJ. Randomized controlled trial of hip protectors among women living in the community. Osteoporos Int. 2004 Mar 3.

Bischoff HA, Stahelin HB, Dick W, Akos R, Knecht M, Salis C, Nebiker M, Theiler R, Pfeifer M, Begerow B, et al. Effects of vitamin D and calcium supplementation on falls: A randomized controlled trial. J Bone Miner Res 2003;18(2):343-51.

Bischoff HA, Borchers M, Gudat F, Duermueller U, Theiler R, Stahelin HB, Dick W. In situ detection of 1,25-

dihydroxyvitamin D3 receptor in human skeletal muscle tissue. Histochem J. 2001 Jan;33(1):19-24

Bischoff-Ferrari HA, Dawson-Hughes B, Willett WC, Staehelin HB, Bazemore MG, Zee RY, Wong JB. Effect of Vitamin D on falls: A meta-analysis. JAMA. 2004 Apr 28;291(16):1999-2006.

Blumenthal JA, Emery CF, Madden DJ, Schniebolk S, Riddle MW, Cobb FR, Higginbotham M, Coleman RE. Effects of exercise training on bone density in older men and women. JAm Geriatr Soc 1991;39(11): 1065-70.

Bonaiuti D, Shea B, Iovine R, Negrini S, Robinson V, Kemper HC, Wells G, Tugwell P, Cranney A. Exercise for preventing and treating osteoporosis in postmenopausal women. Cochrane Database Syst Rev. 2002;(3):CD000333.

Bonjour JP, Chevalley T, Ammann P, Slosman D, Rizzoli R. Gain in bone mineral mass in prepubertal girls 3.5 years after discontinuation of calcium supple-mentation: A follow-up study. Lancet 2001;358(9289):1208-12.

Bowden LS, Jones CJ, Ryan SW. Bone mineralisation in ex-preterm infants aged 8 years. Eur J Pediatr 1999 Aug;158(8):658-61.

Brot C, Jorgensen NR, Sorensen OH. The influence of smoking on vitamin D status and calcium metabolism. Eur J Clin Nutr 1999 Dec; 53(12):920-6.

Cadogan J, Eastell R, Jones N, Barker ME. Milk intake and bone mineral acquisition in adolescent girls: Randomised, controlled intervention trial. BMJ 1997;315(7118):1255-60.

Chan GM, Hoffman K, McMurry M. Effects of dairy products on bone and body composition in pubertal girls. J Pediatr 1995 Apr;126(4):551-6.

Chapuy MC, Arlot ME, Duboeuf F, Brun J, Crouzet B, Arnaud S, Delmas PD, Meunier PJ. Vitamin D3 and calcium to prevent hip fractures in the elderly women. N Engl J Med 1992 Dec 3;327(23):1637-42.

Colon-Emeric CS, Datta SK, Matchar DB. An economic analysis of external hip protector use in ambulatory nursing facility residents. Age Ageing 2003 Jan;32(1):47-52.

Cooper C, Eriksson JG, Forsen T, Osmond C, Tuomilehto J, Barker DJP. Maternal height, childhood growth and risk of hip fracture in later life: A longitudinal study. Osteoporos Int 2001:12(8):623-9.

Cromer BA. Bone mineral density in adolescent and young adult women on injectable or oral contraception. Curr Opin Obstet Gynecol. 2003 Oct;15(5):353-7.

Cumming RG, Miller JP, Kelsey JL, Davis P, Arfken CL, Birge SJ, Peck WA. Medications and multiple falls in elderly people: The St. Louis OASIS study. Age Ageing 1991Nov; 20(6):455-61.

Cumming RG, Klineberg RJ. Breastfeeding and other reproductive factors and the risk of hip fractures in elderly women. Int J Epidemiol 1993 Aug;22(4):684-91.

Cumming RG, Thomas M, Szonyi G, Salkeld G, O'Neill E, Westbury C, Frampton G. Home visits by an occupational therapist for assessment and modification of environmental hazards: A randomized trial of falls prevention. J Am Geriatr Soc 1999; 47 (12):1397-402.

Cummings SR, Black DM, Nevitt MC, Browner W, Cauley J, Ensrud K, Genant HK, Palermo L, Scott J, Vogt TM; Study for Osteoporotic Fractures Research Group. Bone density at various sites for prediction of hip fractures. Lancet. 1993 Jan 9;341(8837):72-5.

Cummings SR, Nevitt MC, Browner WS, Stone K, Fox KM, Ensrud KE, Cauley J, Black D, Vogt TM; Study of Osteoporotic Fractures Research Group. Risk factors for hip fracture in white women. N Engl J Med 1995 Mar 23;332(12):767-73.

Dawson-Hughes B, Harris SS, Krall EA, Dallal GE. Effect of calcium and vitamin D supplementation on bone density in men and women 65 years of age or older. N Engl J Med 1997 Sep 4;337(10):670-6.

Dawson-Hughes B. Calcium and protein in bone health. Proc Nutr Soc. 2003 May;62(2):505-9.

Dawson-Hughes B, Harris SS, Rasmussen H, Song L, Dallap GE. Effect of dietary protein supplements on calcium excretion in healthy older men and women. J Clin Endocrinol Metab 2004 Mar;89(3): 1169-73.

Devine A, Criddle RA, Dick IM, Kerr DA, Prince RL. A longitudinal study of the effect of sodium and calcium intakes on regional bone density of postmenopausal women. Am J Clin Nutr 1995 Oct;62(4):740-5.

Dibba B, Prentice A, Ceesay M, Stirling DM, Cole TJ, Poskitt EM. Effect of calcium supplementation on bone mineral accretion in Gambian children accustomed to a low calcium diet. Am J Clin Nutr 2000 Feb;71(2):544-9.

Doherty TJ. Invited review: Aging and sacropenia. J Appl Physiol 2003 Oct; 95(4):1717-27.

Dukas LH, Bischoff A, Lindpaintner LS, Schacht E, Birkner-Bidner D, Damm TN, Thalmann B, Stahelin HB. Alfacalcidol reduces the number of fallers in a community-dwelling elderly population with a minimum calcium intake of more than 500 mg daily. J Am Geriatr Soc 2004 Feb;52(2):230-6.

Ensrud KE, Cauley J, Lipschutz R, Cummings SR. Weight change and fractures in older women. Arch Intern Med 1997;157(8):857-863.

Ensrud KE, Blackwell TL, Mangione CM, Bowman PJ, Whooley MA, Bauer DC, Schwartz AV, Hanlon JT, Nevitt MC; Study of Osteoporotic Fractures Research Group. Central nervous system-active medications and risk for falls in older women. J Am Geriatr Soc 2002 Oct; 50(10):1629-37.

Ensrud KE, Ewing SK, Stone KL, Cauley JA, Bowman PJ, Cummings SR; Study of Osteoporotic Fractures Research Group. Intentional and unintentional weight loss increase bone loss and hip fracture risk in older women. J Am Geriatr Soc 2003 Dec; 51(12): 1740-7.moved

Ensrud KE, Walczak TS, Blackwell T, Ensrud ER, Bowman PJ, Stone KL. Antiepileptic drug use increases rates of bone loss in older women: A prospective study. Neurology 2004 Jun 8;62(11):2051-7.

Fang MA, Frost PJ, Iida-Klein A, Hahn TJ. Effects of nicotine on cellular function in UMR 106-01 osteoblast-like cells. Bone 1991; 12(4):283-6

Farmer ME, Harris T, Madans JH, Wallace RB, Cornoni-Huntley J, White LR. Anthropometric indicators and hip fracture. The

NHANES I epidemiologic follow-up study. J Am Geriatr Soc 1989. Jan;37(1):9-16.

Faulkner KA, Cauley JA, Zmuda JM, Griffin JM, Nevitt, MC. Is social integration associated with the risk of falling in older community-dwelling women? J Gerontol A Biol Sci Med Sci 2003 Oct;58(10): M954-9.

Feldman D. Vitamin D, parathyroid hormone, and calcium: A complex regulatory network. Am J Med 1999 Dec;107(6):637-9.

Felson DT, Anderson JJ, Hannan MT, Milton R, Wilson PW, Kiel DP. Impaired vision and hip fracture: The Framingham Study. J Am Geriatr Soc 1989 Jun; 37(6):495-500.

Felson DT, Zhang Y, Hannan MT, Kannel WB, Kiel DP. Alcohol intake and bone mineral density in elderly men and women: The Framingham Study. Am J Epidemiol 1995 Sep 1;142(5):485-92.

Feskanich D, Willett W, Colditz G. Walking and leisure-time activity and risk of hip fracture in postmenopausal women. JAMA 2002 Nov 13;288(18):2300-6.

Fewtrell MS, Prentice A, Jones SC, Bishop NJ, Stirling D, Buffenstein R, Lunt M, Cole TJ, Lucas A. Bone mineralisation and turnover in preterm infants at 8-12 years of age: The effect of early diet. J Bone Miner Res 1999 May;14(5):810-20.

Fiatarone MA, Marks EC, Ryan ND, Meredith CN, Lipsitz LA, Evans WJ. High-intensity strength training in nonagenarians. Effects on skeletal muscle. JAMA 1990 Jun 13;263(22):3029-34.

Fitzpatrick L, Heaney RP. Got soda? J Bone Miner Res 2003 Sep;18(9):1570-2.

Fitzpatrick LA. Pathophysiology of bone loss in patients receiving anticonvulsant therapy. Epilepsy Behav. 2004 Feb;5 Suppl 2:S3-15.

Flegal KM, Carroll MD, Ogden CL, Johnson CL. Prevalence and trends in obesity among US adults, 1999 – 2000. JAMA 2002 Oct 9;288(14):1723-7.

Flicker L, Mead K, MacInnis RJ, Nowson C, Scherer S, Stein MS, Thomasz J, Hopper JL, Walker JD. Serum vitamin D and falls in older women in residential care in Australia. J Am Geriatr Soc 2003 Nov;51(11):1533-8.

Fuchs RK, Bauer JJ, Snow CM. Jumping improves hip and lumbar spine bone mass in prepubescent children: A randomized controlled trial. J Bone Miner Res. 2001 Jan;16(1):148-56.

Fuchs RK, Snow CM. Gains in hip bone mass from high-impact training are maintained: A randomized controlled trial in children. J Pediatr 2002 Sep;141(3):357-62.

Gartner LM, Greer FR; Section on Breastfeeding and Committee on Nutrition. Prevention of rickets and vitamin D deficiency: New guidelines for vitamin D intake. Pediatrics 2003 Apr;111(4 Pt 1):908-10.

Gillespie LD, Gillespie WJ, Robertson MC, Lamb SE, Cumming RG, Rowe BH. Interventions for preventing falls in elderly people. Cochrane Database Syst Rev 2001;(3):CD000340.

Going S, Lohman T, Houtkooper L, Metcalfe L, Flint-Wagner H, Blew R, Stanford V, Cussler E, Martin J, Teixeira P, et al. Effects of exercise on bone mineral density in calcium-replete postmenopausal women with and without hormone replacement therapy. Osteoporos Int. 2003 Aug;14(8):637-43.

Goldring SR, Krane SM, Aviolo LV. Disorders of calcification: Osteomalacia and rickets. In: LJD, ed.. Endocrinology 3rd ed. Philadelphia (PA): WB Saunders 1995:1204-27.

Gordon-Larsen P, McMurray RG, Popkin BM. Adolescent physical activity and inactivity vary by ethnicity: The National Longitudinal Study of Adolescent Health. J Pediatr 1999 Sep; 135(3): 301-6.

Greenlund LJ, Nair KS. Sarcopenia-consequences, mechanisms, and potential therapies. Mech Ageing Dev 2003 Mar; 124(3):287-99.

Gregg EW, Cauley JA, Seeley DG, Ensrud KE, Bauer DC; Study of Osteoporotic Fractures Research Group. Physical activity and osteoporotic fracture risk in older women. Ann Intern Med 1998 Jul 15;129(2):81-8.

Gregg EW, Pereira MA, Caspersen CJ. Physical activity, falls and fractures among older adults: A review of the epidemiologic evidence. J Am Geriatr Soc 2000;48(8):883-93.

Grisso JA, Kelsey JL, Strom BL, O'Brien LA, Maislin G, LaPann K, Samelson L, Hoffman S; The Northeast Hip Fracture Study Group. Risk factors for hip fracture in black women. N Engl J Med 1994 Jun 2; 330(22):1555-9.

Gulson BL, Mizon KJ, Korsch MJ, Palmer JM, Donnelly JB. Mobilization of lead from human bone tissue during pregnancy and lactation—a summary of long-term research. Sci Total Environ. 2003 Feb 15;303(1-2):79-104.

Hanger HC, Ball MC, Wood LA. An analysis of falls in the hospital: Can we do without bedrails? J Am Geriatr Soc 1999 May; 47(5):529-31.

Harwood RH, Sahota O, Gaynor K, Masud T, Hosking DJ; The Nottingham Neck of Femur (NONOF) Study. A randomised, controlled comparison of different calcium and vitamin D supplementation regimens in elderly women after hip fracture: The Nottingham Neck of Femur (NONOF) Study. Age Ageing 2004 Jan;33(1): 45-51.

Heaney RP, Recker RR, Stegman MR, Moy AJ. Calcium absorption in women: Relationships to calcium intake, estrogen status, and age. J Bone Miner Res. 1989 Aug;4(4):469-75.

Heaney RP, Abrams S, Dawson-Hughes B, Looker A, Marcus R, Matkovic V, Weaver C. Peak bone mass. Osteoporosis Int 2000;11(12): 985-1009.

Heaney RP. Constructive interactions among nutrients and bone-active pharmacologic agents with principal emphasis on calcium, phosphorus, vitamin D and protein. J Am Coll Nutr 2001 Oct;20(5 Suppl):403S-9S;discussion 417S-20S.

Heaney RP. Is the paradigm shifting? Bone 2003 Oct;33(4):457-65.

Heaney RP. Phosphorus nutrition and the treatment of osteoporosis. Mayo Clin Proc 2004 Jan;79(1): 91-7.

Heaney RP, Abrams SA. Improved estimation of the calcium content of total digestive secretions. J Clin Endocrinol Metab 2004;Mar;89(3):1193-5.

Heikinheimo JR, Inkovaara JA, Harju EJ, Haavisto MV, Kaarela RH, Kataja JM, Kokko AM, Kolho LA, Rajala SA. Annual injection of vitamin D and fractures of aged bones. Calcif. Tissue Int 1992 Aug;51(2):105-10.

Henderson PH 3rd, Sowers M, Kutzko KE, Jannausch ML. Bone mineral density in grand multiparous women with extended lactation. Am J Obstet Gynecol 2000 Jun; 182(6):1371-7.

Hernandez-Avila M, Gonzalez-Cossio T, Hernandez-Avila JE, Romieu I, Peterson KE, Aro A, Palazuelos E, Hu H. Dietary calcium supplements to lower blood lead levels in lactating women: A randomized placebo-controlled trial. Epidemiology. 2003 Mar;14(2):206-12.

Higgs G and American Academy of Orthopaedic Surgeons. The progression of osteoporosis: An orthopedist's challenge (photo). Rosemont (IL): 2001.

Hoidrup S, Gronbaek M, Gottschau A, Lauritzen JB, Schroll M; Copenhagen Centre for Prospective Population Studies. Alcohol intake, beverage preference, and risk of hip fracture in men and women. Am J Epidemiol 1999 Nov 15; 150(10):1085-93.

Honkanen R, Tuppurainen M, Kroger H, Alhava E, Saarikoski S. Relationships between risk factors and fractures differ by type of fracture: a population-based study of 12,192 perimenopausal women. Osteoporosis Int1998;8(1):25-31.

Institute of Medicine. Dietary reference intakes for calcium, phosphorus, magnesium, vitamin D, and fluoride. Washington, DC: National Academy of Sciences; 1997. 432p.

Jackson KA, Savaiano DA. Lactose maldigestion, calcium intake and osteoporosis in African-, Asian-, and Hispanic-Americans. J Amer Coll Nutr. 2001 April;20(2 Suppl):198S-207S.

Jackson RD, LaCroix AZ, Cauley JA, McGowan J. The Women's Health Initiative calcium-vitamin D trial: Overview and baseline characteristics of participants. Ann Epidemiol. 2003 Oct;13(9 Suppl):S98-106.

Jacqmin-Gadda H, Fourrier A, Commenges D, Dartigues JF. Risk factors for fractures in the elderly. Epidemiology 1998 Jul; 9(4):417-23.

Jarvinen TL, Kannus P, Sievanen H. Have the DXA-based exercise studies seriously underestimated the effects of mechanical loading on bone? J Bone Miner Res 1999 Sep;14(9):1634-5.

Johnston CC Jr, Miller JZ, Slemenda CW, Reister TK, Hui S, Christian JC, Peacock M. Calcium supplementation and increases in bone mineral density in children N Eng J Med 1992 Jul 9;327(2):82-7.

Kalkwarf HJ, Specker BL. Bone mineral changes during pregnancy and lactation. Endocrine. 2002 Feb;17(1):49-53.

Karlsson C, Obrant KJ, Karlsson M. Pregnancy and lactation confer reversible bone loss in humans. Osteoporos Int. 2001;12(10):828-34.

[a]Kanis JA, Johansson H, Oden A, Johnell O, De Laet C, Melton III LJ, Tenenhouse A, Reeve J, Silman AJ, Pols HA, et al. A meta-analysis of prior corticosteroid use and fracture risk. J Bone Miner Res. 2004 Jun;19 (6):893-899.

[b]Kanis JA, Johnell O, Oden A, Johansson H, De Laet C, Eisman JA, Fujiwara S, Kroger H, McCloskey EV, Mellstrom D, et al. Smoking and fracture risk: A meta-analysis. Osteoporos Int. 2004 Jun 3 [Epub ahead of print].

Kannus P, Haapasalo H, Sankelo M, Sievanen H, Pasanen M, Heinonen A, Oja P, Vuori I. Effect of starting age of physical activity on bone mass in the dominant arm of tennis and squash players. Ann Intern Med. 1995 Jul 1;123(1):27-31.

Kannus P, Parkkari J, Niemi S, Pasanen M, Palvanen M, Jarvinen M, Vuori I. Prevention of hip fracture in elderly people with use of a hip protector. N Engl J Med 2000 Nov 23;343(21):1506-13.

Kaptoge S, Dalzell N, Jakes RW, Wareham N, Day NE, Khaw KT, Beck TJ, Loveridge N, Reeve J. Hip section modulus, a measure of bending resistance, is more strongly related to reported physical activity than BMD. Osteoporos Int 2003 Nov;14(11):941-9

Karlsson MK, Linden C, Karlsson C, Johnell O, Obrant K, Seeman E. Exercise during growth and bone mineral density and fractures in old age. Lancet 2000 Feb 5;355(9202):469-70.

Karlsson M. Does exercise reduce the burden of fractures? A review. Acta Orthop Scand 2002 Dec;73(6):691-705.

Katzman DK, Bachrach LK, Carter DR, Marcus R. Clinical and anthropometric correlates of bone mineral acquisition in healthy adolescent girls. J Clin Endocrinol Metab 1991 Dec;73(6):1332-9.

Kelley GA, Kelley KS, Tran ZV. Exercise and bone mineral density in men: A meta-analysis. J Appl Physiol. 2000 May; 88(5):1730-6.

Kelley GA, Kelley KS, Tran ZV. Resistance training and bone mineral density in women: A meta-analysis of controlled trials. Am J PhysMed Rehabil 2001 Jan;80(1):65-77.

Kemmler W, Lauber D, Weineck J, Hensen J, Kalender W, Engelke K. Benefits of 2 years of intense exercise on bone density, physical fitness, and blood lipids in early postmenopausal osteopenic women: Results of the Erlangen Fitness Osteoporosis Prevention Study (EFOPS). Arch Intern

Med. 2004 May 24;164(10):1084-91.

Kerstetter J, O'Brien KO, Insogna KL. Low protein intake: The impact on calcium and bone homeostasis in humans. J Nutr 2003 Mar;133(3):855S-61S.

Keshavarz H, Jikis SD, Kicke BA, Marchbanks PA; Centers for Disease Control and Prevention. Hysterectomy surveillance – United States, 1994-1999. MMWR Morb Mortal Wkly Rep 2002 Jul;51(SS05); 1-8.

Kiel DP, Felson DT, Anderson JJ, Wilson PW, Moskowitz MA. Hip fracture and the use of estrogens in postmenopausal women. The Framingham Study. N Engl J Med. 1987 Nov 5;317(19):1169–74.

Khan K, McKay HA, Haapasalo H, Bennell KL, Forwood MR, Kannus P, Wark JD. Does childhood and adolescence provide a unique opportunity for exercise to strengthen the skeleton? J Sci Med Sport 2000 Jun;3(2):150-64. Review.

Khosla S, Melton LJ 3rd, Dekutoski MB, Achenbach SJ, Oberg AL, Riggs BL. Incidence of childhood distal forearm fractures over 30 years: A population-based study. JAMA 2003 Sep 17;290(11):1479-85.

Kiel D. Hip protectors. Slide presentation at the Surgeon General's Workshop on Osteoporosis and Bone Health; 2002 Dec 12-13; Washington, DC.

Kohrt WM, Snead DB, Slatopolsky E, Birge SJ Jr. Additive effects of weight-bearing exercise and estrogen on bone mineral density in older women. J Bone Miner Res 1995 Sep;10(9):1303-11.

Kontulainen S, Kannus P, Haapasalo H, Sievanen H, Pasanen M, Heinonen A, Oja

P, Vuori I. Good maintenance of exercise-induced bone gain with decreased training of female tennis and squash players: A prospective 5 year follow-up study of young and old starters and controls. J Bone Miner Res. 2001 Feb;16(2):195–201.

Krall EA, Dawson-Hughes B. Smoking increases bone loss and decreases intestinal calcium absorption. J Bone Miner Res 1999 Feb;14(2):215-20.

Kruger J, Brown DR, Galuska DA, Buchner D; Centers for Disease Control and Prevention. Strength training among adults aged >/=65 years—United States, 2001. MMWR Morb Mortal Wkly Rep 2004 Jan 23;53(2):25-8.

Kujala UM, Kaprio J, Kannus P, Sarna S, Koskenvuo M. (2000) Physical activity and osteoporotic hip fracture risk in men. Arch Intern Med 2000 Mar 13;160(5):705-8.

Laitinen K, Lamberg-Allardt C, Tunninen R, Karonen SL, Ylikahri R, Valimaki M. Effects of 3 weeks' moderate alcohol intake on bone and mineral metabolism in normal men. Bone Miner 1991 May;13(2):139-51.

Langlois JA, Mussolino ME, Visser M, Looker AC, Harris T, Madans J Weight loss from maximum body weight among middle-aged and older white women and the risk of hip fracture: The NHANES I epidemiologic follow-up study. Osteoporos Int. 2001;12 (9):763-8.

Latham NK, Anderson CS, Reid IR. Effects of vitamin D supplementation on strength, physical performance, and falls in older persons: A systematic review. J Am Geriatr Soc 2003 Sep;51(9):1219-26.

Law MR, Hackshaw AK. A meta-analysis of cigarette smoking, bone mineral density and risk of hip fracture: Recognition of a major effect. BMJ 1997 Oct 18;315(7114):973-80.

LeBoff MS, Kohlmeier L, Hurwitz S Franklin J, Wright J, Glowacki J. Occult vitamin D deficiency in postmenopausal US women with acute hip fracture. JAMA 1999 Apr 28;281(16):1505-11.

Lee WT, Leung SS, Wang SH, Xu YC, Zeng WP, Lau J, Oppenheimer SJ, Cheng JC. Double blind controlled calcium supplementation and bone mineral accretion in children accustomed to a low calcium diet. Am J Clin Nutr 1994 Nov,60(5):744-50.

Lee WT, Leung SS, Leung DM, Tsang HS, Lau J, Cheng JC. A randomized double blind controlled calcium supplementation trial and bone and height acquisition in children. Br J Nutr 1995 Jul;74(1):125-39.

Lee WT, Leung SS, Leung DM, Cheng JC. A follow-up study on the effects of calcium-supplement withdrawal and puberty on bone acquisition of children. Am J Clin Nutr 1996 Jul;64(1):71-7.

Lin PH, Ginty F, Appel LJ, Aickin M, Bohannon A, Garnero P, Barclay D, Svetkey LP. The DASH diet and sodium reduction improve markers of bone turnover and calcium metabolism in adults. J Nutr 2003 Oct;133(10):3130-6.

Lin YC, Lyle RM, Weaver CM, McCabe LD, McCabe GP, Johnston CC, Teegarden D. Peak spine and femoral neck bone mass in young women. Bone 2003 May;32(5):546-53.

Lloyd T, Andon MB, Rollings N, Martel JK, Landis JR, Demers LM, Eggli DF, Kieselhorst K, Kulin HE. Calcium supplementation and bone mineral density in adolescent girls. JAMA 1993 Aug 18;270(7):841-4.

Lloyd T, Lin HM, Eggli DF, Dodson WC, Demers LM, Legro RS. Adolescent Caucasian mothers have reduced adult hip bone density. FertilSteril 2002 Jan; 77(1):136-40.

Looker AC. Interaction of science, consumer practices and policy: Calcium and bone health as a case study. J Nutri. 2003 Jun;133(6):1987S-1991S.

Lord SR, Dayhew J, Howland A. Multifocal glasses impair edge-contrast sensitivity and depth perception and increase the risk of falls in older people. J Am Geriatr Soc 2002 Nov; 50(11):1760-6.

MacKelvie KJ, McKay HA, Khan KM, Crocker PR. A school-based exercise intervention augments bone mineral accrual in early pubertal girls. J Pediatr. 2001 Oct; 139(4):501-8.

MacKelvie KJ, Khan KM, McKay HA. Is there a critical period for bone response to weight-bearing exercise in children and adolescents? A systematic review. Br J Sports Med 2002 Aug;36(4):250-7.

MacKelvie KJ, Khan KM, Petit MA, Janssen PA, McKay HA. A school-based exercise intervention elicits substantial bone health benefits: A 2-year randomized controlled trial in girls. Pediatrics 2003 Dec;112(6 Pt 1):e447.

Matkovic V, Kostial K, Simonovic I, Buzina R, Brodarec A, Nordin BE. Bone status and fracture rates in two regions of Yugoslavia. Am J Clin Nutr 1979 Mar;32(3):540-9.

Melton LJ 3rd, Khosla S, Malkasian GD, Achenbach SJ, Oberg AL, Riggs BL. Fracture risk after bilateral oophorectomy in elderly women. J Bone Miner Res 2003 May;18(5):900-5.

Merrilees MJ, Smart EJ, Gilchrist NL, Frampton C, Turner JG, Hooke E, March RL, Maguire P. Effects of dairy food supplements on bone mineral density in teenage girls. Eur J Nutr 2000 Dec; 39(6):256-62.

Michaelsson K, Baron JA, Farahmand BY, Ljunghall S. Influence of parity and lactation on hip fracture risk. Am J Epidemiol. 2001 Jun 15;153(12):1166-72.

Michnovicz JJ, Hershcopf RJ, Naganuma H, Bradlow HL, Fishman J. Increased 2-hydroxylation of estradiol as a possible mechanism for the anti-estrogenic effect of cigarette smoking. New Engl J Med 1986 Nov 20; 315(21):1305-9.

Morris FL, Naughton GA, Gibbs JL, Carlson JS, Wark JD. Prospective ten-month exercise intervention in premenarcheal girls: Positive effects on bone and lean mass. J Bone Miner Res 1997 Sep;12(9):1453-62.

Morris JN, Fiatarone M, Kiely DK, Belleville-Taylor P, Murphy K, Littlehale S, Ooi WL, O'Neill E, Doyle N. Nursing rehabilitation and exercise strategies in the nursing home. J Gerontol A Biol Sci Med Sci 1999 Oct; 54(10): M494-500.

Mukai S, Lipsitz LA. Orthostatic hypotension. Clin Geriatr Med. 2002 May;18(2):253-68.

National Institutes of Health. Osteoporosis prevention, diagnosis and therapy. NIH Consensus Statement 2000 Mar 27-29;17(1):1-52.

National Women's Health Information Center [homepage on the Internet]. Washington

(DC): A project of the U.S. Department of Health and Human Services, Office of Women's Health; April 2002 [cited 2004 June 25]. Lactose intolerance. Available from: http://www.4woman.gov/faq/lactose.htm#3.

Nelson HD, Morris CD, Kraemer DF, Mahon S, Carney N, Nygren PM, Helfand MH (Oregon Health & Science University Evidence-based Practice Center, Portland, OR). Osteoporosis in postmenopausal women: Diagnosis and monitoring Evidence Report/Technology Assessment No. 28. Rockville (MD): Agency for Healthcare Research and Quality; 2001 Nov. Publication No.: 01-E032. Contract No.:290-97-0018.

Nevitt MC, Cummings SR, Hudes ES. Risk factors for injurious falls: A prospective study. J Gerontol 1991 Sep; 46(5):M164-70.

New SA, Robins SP, Campbell MK, Martin JC, Garton MJ, Bolton-Smith C, Grubb DA, Lee SJ, Reid DM. Dietary influences on bone mass and bone metabolism: Further evidence of a positive link between fruit and vegetable consumption and bone health? Am J Clin Nutr 2000 Jan;71(1):142-51.

New SA, MacDonald HM, Campbell MK, Martin JC, Garton MJ, Robins SP, Reid DM. Lower estimates of net endogenous non-carbonic acid production are positively associated with indexes of bone health in premenopausal and perimenopausal women. Am J Clin Nutr 2004 Jan;79(1):131-8.

Nowson CA, Green RM, Hopper JL, Sherwin AJ, Young D, Kaymakci B, Guest CS, Smid M, Larkins RG, Wark JD. A co-twin study of the effect of calcium supplementation on bone density during adolescence. Osteoporos Int 1997;7(3):219-25.

Obermayer-Pietsch BM, Bonelli CM, Walter DE, Kuhn RJ, Fahrleitner-Pammer A, Berghold A, Goessler W, Stepan V, Dobnig H, Leb G, Renner W. Genetic predisposition for adult lactose intolerance and relation to diet, bone density, and bone fractures. J Bone Miner Res 2004 Jan;19(1): 42-7.

Ooms ME, Roos JC, Bezemer PD, van Der Vijgh WJ, Bouter LM, Lips P. Prevention of bone loss by vitamin D supplementation in elderly women: A randomized double-blind trial. J Clin Endocrinol Metab 1995 Apr;80(4):1052-8.

Optimal Calcium Intake. NIH Consens Statement Online 1994 June 6-8;12(4):1-31. Available from: http://consensus.nih.gov/cons/097/097_intro.htm.

Paganini-Hill A, Chao A, Ross RK, Henderson BE. Exercise and other factors in the prevention of hip fracture: The Leisure World study. Epidemiology. 1991 Jan;2(1):16-25.

Papadimitropoulos E, Wells G, Shea B, Gillespie W, Weaver B, Zytaruk N, Cranney A, Adachi J, Tugwell P, Josse R, Greenwood C, Guyatt G; Osteoporosis Methodology Group and The Osteoporosis Research Advisory Group. Meta-analyses of therapies for postmenopausal osteoporosis. VIII: Meta-analysis of the efficacy of vitamin D treatment in preventing osteoporosis in postmenopausal women. Endocr Rev 2002 Aug;23(4):560-9.

Parfitt AM, Gallagher JC, Heaney RP, Johnston CC, Neer R, Whedon GD. Vitamin D and bone health in the elderly. Am J Clin Nutr 1982 Nov;36(5 Suppl):1014-31.

Parker MJ, Gillespie LD, Gillespie WJ. Hip protectors for preventing hip fractures in the elderly. Cochrane Database Syst Rev. 2003;(3):CD001255.

Paton LM, Alexander JL, Nowson CA, Margerison C, Frame MG, Kaymakci B, Wark JD. Pregnancy and lactation have no long-term deleterious effect on measures of bone mineral in healthy women: A twin study. Am J Clin Nutr. 2003 Mar;77(3):707-14.

Peacock M, Liu G, Cary M, McClintock R, Ambrosius W, Hui S, Johnston CC. Effect of calcium or 25 OH vitamin D3 dietary supplementation as bone loss at the hip in men and women over the age of 60. J Clin Endocrinol Metab 2000 Sep; 85(9):3011-9.

Piccinino LJ, Mosher WD. Trends in contraceptive use in the United States: 1982-1995. Fam Plann Perspect 1998 Jan-Feb;30(1):4-10, 46.

Province MA, Hadley EC, Hornbrook MC, Lipsitz LA, Miller JP, Mulrow CD, Ory MG, Sattin RW, Tinetti ME, Wolf SL. The effects of exercise on falls in elderly patients: A preplanned meta-analysis of the FICSIT trials. Frailty and Injuries: Cooperative Studies of Intervention Techniques. JAMA 1995 May 3; 273(17):1341-7.

Recker RR, Deng HW. Role of genetics in osteoporosis. Endocrine 2002 Feb;17(1):55-66.

Reed SD, Scholes D, LaCroix AZ, Ichikawa LE, Barlow WE, Ott SM. Longitudinal changes in bone density in relation to oral contraceptive use. Contraception 2003 Sep;68(3):177-82.

Reid IR. Relationships among body mass, its components, and bone. Bone 2002 Nov;31(5):547-55.

Ricci TA, Chowdhury HA, Heymsfield SB, Stahl T, Pierson RN Jr, Shapses SA. Calcium supplementation suppresses bone turnover during weight reduction in postmenopausal women. J Bone Miner Res 1998 Jun;13(6):1045-50.

Riebel GD, Boden SD, Whitesides TE, Hutton WC. The effect of nicotine on incorporation of cancellous bone graft in an animal model. Spine 1995 Oct 15; 20(20):2198-202.

Riggs BL, Khosla S, Melton LJ 3rd. Sex steroids and the construction and conservation of the adult skeleton. Endocr Rev 2002 June;23(3):279-302.

Rizzoli R, Bonjour JP. Dietary protein and bone health. J Bone Miner Res 2004;19(4): 527-31.

Robertson MA, Campbell AJ, Gardner MM, Devlin N. Preventing injuries in older people by preventing falls: A meta-analysis of individual-level data. JAmGeriatr Soc 2002;50:905-11.

Ross DS. Hyperthyroidism, thyroid hormone therapy, and bone. Thyroid 1994 Fall;4(3):319-26.

Ryan AS, Treuth MS, Rubin MA, Miller JP, Nicklas BJ, Landis DM, Pratley RE, Libanati CR, Gundberg CM, Hurley BF. Effects of strength training on bone mineral density: Hormonal and bone turnover relationships. J Appl Physiol 1994 Oct;77(4):1678-84.

Saag KG. Glucocorticoid use in rheumatoid arthritis. Curr Rheumatol Rep. 2002 Jun;4(3):218-25.

Salamone LM, Cauley JA, Black DM, Simkin-Silverman L, Lang W, Gregg E, Palermo L, Epstein RS, Kuller LH, Wing R. Effect of a lifestyle intervention on bone mineral density in premenopausal women: A randomized trial. Am J Clin Nutr 1999 Jul;70(1):97-103.

Sampson HW. Alcohol and other factors affecting osteoporosis risk in women. Alcohol Res Health 2002;26(4):292-8.

Schapira D. Alcohol abuse and osteoporosis. Semin Arthritis Rheum 1990 Jun;19(6):371–6.

Schiller JS, Coriaty-Nelson Z, Barnes P. Early release of selected estimates based on data from the 2003 National Health Interview Survey. National Center for Health Statistics. c2004 [cited 2004 July 9]. Available from: http://www.cdc.gov/nchs/about/major/nhis/released200406.htm.

Schneider A, Shane E. Osteoporosis secondary to illnesses and medications. In: Osteoporosis. 2nd ed. San Diego (CA): Academic Press; 2001. p. 303-27. 2 vols. (Marcus R, Feldman D, Kelsey J editors).

School Health Policies and Programs Study 2000 (SHPPS): A summary report. Journal of School Health 2001 Sep;71(7): 251-350.

Schurch MA, Rizzoli R, Slosman D, Vadas L, Vergnaud P, Bonjour JP. Protein supplements increase serum insulin-like growth factor I levels and attenuate proximal femur bone loss in patients with recent hip fracture. A randomized, double-blind, placebo-controlled trial. Ann Intern Med 1998 May 15;128(1):801-9.

Sebastian A, Harris ST, Ottaway JH, Todd KM, Morris RC Jr. Improved mineral balance and skeletal metabolism in postmenopausal women treated with potassium bicarbonate. N Engl J Med. 1994 Jun 23;330(25):1776-81.

Seeman E. The Achilles' heel of exercise-induced bone mass increments: Cessation of exercise. J Bone Miner Res. 2001 Jul; 16(7):1370-3.

Sellmeyer DE, Schloetter M, Sebastian A. Potassium citrate prevents increased urine calcium excretion and bone resorption induced by a high sodium chloride diet. J Clin Endocrinol Metab 2002 May;87(5):2008-12.

Shea, Beverley, George Wells, Ann Cranney, Nicole Zytaruk, Vivian Robinson, Lauren Griffith, Zulma Ortiz, Joan Peterson, Jonathan Adachi, Peter Tugwell, and Gordon Guyatt VII. Meta-Analysis of Calcium Supplementation for the Prevention of Postmenopausal Osteoporosis Endocr Rev 2002 23: 552-559.

Sheven BA, Hamilton NJ. Retinoic acid and 1,25-dihydroxyvitamin D3 stimulate osteoclast formation by different mechanisms. Bone 1990;11:53-9.

Shortt KC, Madden A, Flynn A, Morrissey PA. Influence of dietary sodium intake on urinary calcium excretion in selected Irish individuals. Eur J Clin Nutr 1988 Jul;42(7):595-603.

Silbergeld EK, Flaws JA. Environmental exposures and women's health. Clin Obstet Gynecol. 2002 Dec;45(4):1119-28.

Singh MA. Exercise comes of age: Rationale and recommendations for a geriatric exercise prescription. J Gerontol A Biol Sci Med Sci 2002 May;57(5):M262-82.

Slemenda CW, Peacock M, Hui S, Zhou L, Johnston CC. Reduced rates of skeletal remodeling are associated with increased bone mineral density during the development of peak skeletal mass. J Bone Miner Res 1997 Apr;12(4):676-82.

Smith MR. Diagnosis and management of treatment-related osteoporosis in men with prostate carcinoma. Cancer 2003 Feb 1;97(3 Suppl): 789-95.

Snow-Harter C, Bouxsein ML, Lewis BT, Carter DR, Marcus R. Effects of resistance and endurance exercise on bone mineral status of young women: A randomized exercise intervention trial. J Bone Miner Res 1992 Jul;7(7):761-9.

Sowers MF, Shapiro B, Gilbraith MA, Jannausch M. Health and hormonal characteristics of premenopausal women with lower bone mass. Calcif Tissue Int 1990 Sep; 47(3):130-5.

Soyka LA, Misra M, Frenchman A, Miller KK, Grinspoon S, Schoenfeld DA, Klibanski A. Abnormal bone mineral accrual in adolescent girls with anorexia nervosa. J Clin Endocrinol Metab. 2002 Sep;87(9):4177-85.

Specker BL. Evidence for an interaction between calcium intake and physical activity on changes in bone mineral density. J Bone Miner Res 1996 Oct;11(10): 1539-44.

Specker BL, Mulligan L, Ho ML. Longitudinal study of calcium intake, physical activity, and bone mineral content in infants 6-18 months of age. J Bone Miner Res 1999 Apr;14(4):569-76.

Specker B, Binkley T. Randomized trial of physical activity and calcium supplementation on bone mineral content in 3- to 5-year-old children. J Bone Miner Res 2003 May;18(5):885-92.

[a]Stevens M, Holman CD, Bennett N, de Klerk N. Preventing falls in older people: Outcome evaluation of a randomized controlled trial. J Am Geriatr Soc 2001 Nov; 49(11):1448-55.

[b]Stevens M, Holman CD, Bennett N. Preventing falls in older people: Impact of an intervention to reduce environmental hazards in the home. J Am Geriatr Soc 2001; 49(11):1442-7.

Suarez F, Levitt MD. Abdominal symptoms and lactose: The discrepancy between patients'

claims and the results of blinded trials. Am J Clin Nutr 1996 Aug;64(2):251-2.

Taaffe DR, Snow-Harter C, Connolly DA, Robinson TL, Brown MD, Marcus R. Differential effects of swimming versus weight-bearing activity on bone mineral status of eumenorrheic athletes. J Bone Miner Res 1995 Apr;10(4):586-93.

Tansavatdi K, McClain B, Herrington DM. The effects of smoking on estradiol metabolism. Minerva Ginecol. 2004 Feb;56(1):105-14.

Thapa PB, Brockman KG, Gideon P, Fought RL, Ray WA. Injurious falls in nonambulatory nursing home residents: A comparative study of circumstances, incidence, and risk factors. J Am Geriatr Soc 1996 Mar;44(3):273-8.

Thomas MK, Lloyd-Jones DM, Thadhani R, Shaw AC, Deraska DJ, Kitch BT, Vamvakas E, Dick IM, Prince RL, Finkelstein JS. Hypovitaminosis D in medical inpatients. N Engl J Med 1998 Mar 19;338(12):777-83.

Tinetti ME, Speechley M, Ginter SF. Risk factors for falls among elderly persons living in the community. N Engl J Med 1988 Dec 29; 319(26):1701-7.

Tinetti ME, Baker DI, McAvay G, Claus EB, Garrett P, Gottschalk M, Koch ML, Trainor K, Horowitz RI. A multifactorial intervention to reduce the risk of falling among elderly people living in the community. N Engl J Med 1994 Sep 29; 331(13):821-7.

Tinetti ME. Clinical practice. Preventing falls in elderly persons. N Engl J Med. 2003 Jan 2;348(1):42-9.

Tucker KL, Hannan MT, Chen H, Cupples LA, Wilson PW, Kiel DP. Potassium, magnesium, and fruit and vegetable intakes are associated with greater bone mineral density in elderly men and women. Am J Clin Nutr 1999 Apr;69(4):727-36.

Tylavsky FA, Holliday K, Danish R, Womack C, Norwood J, Carbone L. Fruit and vegetable intakes are an independent pre-dictor of bone size in early pubertal children. Am J Clin Nutr 2004 Feb;79(2):311-7.

U.S. Department of Agriculture; U.S. Department of Health and Human Services. Nutrition and your health: Dietary guidelines for Americans. 5th ed. Washington, DC: The Departments; 2000. 44p. (Home and Garden Bulletin No. 232).

U.S. Department of Health and Human Services. Physical activity and health: A report of the Surgeon General. Atlanta (GA): U.S. Department of Health and Human Services, Centers for Disease Control and Prevention, National Center for Chronic Disease Prevention and Health Promotion, President's Council on Physical Fitness and Sports, 1996. 300p.

U.S. Department of Health and Human Services. Healthy People 2010 2nd ed. With understanding and improving health and objectives for improving health. 2 vols. Washington (DC): U.S. Government Printing Office, November 2000.

U.S. Department of Health and Human Services. The health consequences of smoking: A report of the Surgeon General. Atlanta (GA): U.S. Department of Health and Human Services, Centers for Disease Control and Prevention, National Center for Chronic Disease Prevention and Health Promotion, Office on Smoking and Health, 2004.

U.S. Preventive Services Task Force. Guide to clinical preventive services. 2nd ed. [report on the Internet] Washington (DC): U.S. Department of Health and Human Services, Agency for Healthcare Research and Quality; 1996. Counseling: household and recreational injuries; c2004 [cited 2004 Jun 28]. Available from: http://www.ahrq.gov/clinic/uspstf/uspshrin.htm.

Valimaki VV, Alfthan H, Lehmuskallio E, Loyttyniemi E, Sahi T, Stenman UH, Suominen H, Valiamki MJ. Vitamin D status as a determinant of peak bone mass in young Finnish men. J Clin Endocrinol Metab 2004 Jan;89(1):76-80.

Van Loan MD, Keim NL Influence of cognitive eating restraint on total-body measurements of bone mineral density and bone mineral content in premenopausal women aged 18-45 y: A cross-sectional study. Am J Clin Nutr 2000 Sep;72(3):837-43.

van Staa T, Leufkens H, Abenhaim L, Zhang B, Cooper C. Use of oral corticosteroids and risk of fractures. J Bone Miner Res 2000;15(6): 993-1000.

van Staa TP, Leufkens HG, Cooper C. The epidemiology of corticosteroid-induced osteoporosis: A meta-analysis. Osteoporos Int. 2002 Oct;13(10):777-87.

Wallace BA, Cumming RG. Systematic review of randomized trials of the effect of exercise on bone mass in pre- and postmenopausal women. Calcif Tissue Int. 2000 Jul;67(1):10-8.

Warren MP. Health issues for women athletes: Exercise-induced amenorrhea. J Clin Endocrinol Metab 1999 Jun;84(6):1892-6. Commentary.

Warren MP, Goodman LR. Exercise-induced endocrine pathologies. J Endocrinol Invest 2003 Sep;26(9):873-8.

Webb AR, Kline L, Holick MF. Influence of season and latitude on the cutaneous synthesis of vitamin D3: Exposure to winter sunlight in Boston and Edmonton will not promote vitamin D3 synthesis in human skin. J Clin Endocrinol Metab. 1988 Aug;67(2):373-8.

Webb AR, Pilbeam C, Hanafin N, Holick MF. An evaluation of the relative contributions of exposure to sunlight and of diet to the circulating concentrations of 25-hydroxyvitamin D in an elderly nursing home population in Boston. Am J Clin Nutr 1990;51(6):1075-81.

Welten DC, Kemper HC, Post GB, van Staveren WA. A meta-analysis of the effect of calcium intake on bone mass in young and middle aged females and males. J Nutr 1995 Nov;125(11):2802-13.

Wild RA, Buchanan JR, Myers C, Demers LM. Declining adrenal androgens: An association with bone loss in aging women. Proc Soc Exp Biol Med 1987 Dec;186(3):355–60.

Wolff I, van Croonenborg JJ, Kemper HC, Kostense PJ, Twisk JW. The effect of exercise training programs on bone mass: A meta-analysis of published controlled trials in pre- and postmenopausal women. Osteoporos Int. 1999;9(1):1-12.

Wosje KS, Specker BL. Role of calcium in bone health during childhood. Nutrition Rev 2000 Sep;58(9):253-68.

Wright JD, Wang CY, Kennedy-Stevenson J, Ervin RB. Dietary intakes of ten key nutrients for public health, United States: 1999-2000. Adv Data 2003 Apr 17;(334):1-4.

Yarbrough DE, Barrett-Connor E, Morton DJ. Birth weight as a predictor of adult bone mass in postmenopausal women: The Rancho Bernardo Study. Osteoporos Int 2000;11(7):626-30.

Zamora SA, Rizzoli R, Belli DC, Slosman DO, Bonjour JP. Vitamin D supplementation during infancy is associated with higher bone mineral mass in prepubertal girls. J Clin Endocrinol Metab 1999 Dec;84(12):4541-4.

Chapter 7: Key Messages

- There is much that individuals can do to promote their own bone health, beginning in childhood and continuing into old age. These activities contribute not only to bone health, but to overall health and vitality.

- Since many nutrients are important for bone health, it is important to eat a well-balanced diet containing a variety of foods, including grains, fruits and vegetables, nonfat or low-fat dairy products or other calcium-rich foods, and meat or beans each day.

- Most Americans do not consume recommended levels of calcium, but reaching these levels is a feasible goal. Approximately three 8-ounce glasses of low-fat milk each day, combined with the calcium from the rest of a normal diet, is enough to meet the recommended daily requirements for most individuals. Foods fortified with calcium and calcium supplements can assist those who do not consume an adequate amount of calcium-rich foods.

- For many, especially elderly individuals, getting enough vitamin D from sunshine is not practical. These individuals should look to boost their vitamin D levels through diet. Vitamin D is also available in supplements for those unable to get enough through sunshine and diet.

- In addition to meeting recommended guidelines for physical activity (at least 30 minutes a day for adults and 60 minutes for children), specific strength- and weight-bearing activities are critical to building and maintaining bone mass throughout life.

- Individuals should see a health care provider if they have a medical condition or use medications that can affect the skeleton. Women should also see their health care provider if menstrual periods stop for 3 months.

Chapter 7

LIFESTYLE APPROACHES TO PROMOTE BONE HEALTH

As the evidence presented in the previous chapter makes clear, there is much that individuals can do to promote their own bone health throughout life. This chapter outlines recommendations for diet, physical activity, and other lifestyle practices that can help to achieve that goal. Moreover, the activities and practices suggested in this chapter contribute not only to bone health, but to overall health and vitality. In fact, bone-specific recommendations fit well within an overall program of good nutrition and physical activity that should be followed in order to prevent the onset of many of the major chronic diseases affecting Americans.

Nutrition

Since many nutrients are important for bone health, it is important to eat a well-balanced diet containing a variety of foods. Following the Dietary Guidelines for Americans (USDA 2000, USDHHS 2000) can help, although attention should be paid to serving sizes. These guidelines urge individuals to eat 6–11 servings of grain foods, 3–5 servings of vegetables, 2–4 servings of fruits, 2–3 servings of dairy or other calcium-rich foods, and 2–3 servings of meat or beans each day. The DASH (Dietary Approaches to Stop Hypertension) Eating Plan (USDHHS 2003), which follows these guidelines, is an ex-

ample of a well-balanced diet that can be good for bone and heart health, although bone outcomes from DASH have not been specifically tested. The DASH Eating Plan emphasizes fruits, vegetables, low-fat or fat-free dairy foods, whole grains, fish, poultry, and nuts, making it rich in calcium, magnesium, protein, and potassium while also being low in fat, cholesterol, and sodium. For more information about the Dietary Guidelines and the DASH Eating Plan, refer to Appendix C, Resources and Related Links.

Calcium

The Food and Nutrition Board (FNB) of the Institute of Medicine updated recommended intakes for several nutrients important to the skeleton in 1997, including calcium (IOM 1997). Recommended amounts of calcium, which are shown in Table 7-1, differ by age. These recommendations are meant for healthy people. Those with osteoporosis or other chronic conditions may need more calcium, but unfortunately the calcium requirements for individuals with this disease have not yet been clearly identified (Heaney and Weaver 2003). The highest amount (1,300 mg per day) is recommended for children and adolescents ages 9–18, a period when bones are growing rapidly. Pregnant or lactating women are advised to consume an age-appropriate

Table 7-1. Adequate Intakes (AI) or Recommended Dietary Allowances (RDA) and Tolerable Upper Intake Levels (UL) for Calcium, Vitamin D, Phosphorus, and Magnesium by Life-Stage Group for United States and Canada

Life-stage group	Calcium (mg/day)		Vitamin D (IU/day)		Phosphorus (mg/day)		Magnesium (mg/day)		
							RDA		
	AI	UL	AI	UL	RDA	UL	Male	Female	UL†
0–6 months	210	ND*	200	1000	100	ND*	30	30	ND*
7–12 months	270	ND*	200	1000	275	ND*	75	75	ND*
1–3 years	500	2500	200	2000	460	3000	80	80	65
4–8 years	800	2500	200	2000	500	3000	130	130	110
9–13 years	1300	2500	200	2000	1250	4000	240	240	350
14–18 years	1300	2500	200	2000	1250	4000	410	360	350
19–30 years	1000	2500	200	2000	700	4000	400	310	350
31–50 years	1000	2500	200	2000	700	4000	420	320	350
51–70 years	1200	2500	400	2000	700	4000	420	320	350
>70 years	1200	2500	600	2000	700	3000	420	320	350
Pregnancy:									
<18 years	1300	2500	200	2000	1250	3500		400	350
19–30 years	1000	2500	200	2000	700	3500		350	350
31–50 years	1000	2500	200	2000	700	3500		360	350
Lactation:									
<18 years	1300	2500	200	2000	1250	4000		360	350
19–30 years	1000	2500	200	2000	700	4000		310	350
31–50 years	1000	2500	200	2000	700	4000		320	350

*ND Not determinable
†Represents intake from pharmacological agents only, does not include intake from food and water.

Source: IOM 1997. Reprinted with permission from the National Academy of Sciences courtesy of the National Academies Press, Washington, D.C.

amount of calcium, as shown in Table 7-1. The Institute of Medicine also defined a safe upper limit of 2,500 mg per day for calcium (IOM 1997). Intakes above 2,500 mg per day may increase the risk of adverse effects in susceptible individuals.

Americans obtain most of their calcium from dairy products. In fact, approximately three 8-ounce glasses of milk each day, combined with the calcium from the rest of a normal diet, is enough to meet the recommended daily requirements for most adults. Lowfat or nonfat versions of dairy products are good choices because they have the full amount of calcium, but help to avoid eating too much fat. Foods that have been fortified with calcium are also good sources of the nutrient. There are many foods that serve as

Table 7–2. Selected Food Sources of Calcium

Food	Calcium (mg)	% DV*
Sardines, canned in oil, with bones, 3 oz.	324	32%
Cheddar cheese, 1½ oz. shredded	306	31%
Milk, nonfat, 8 fl oz.	302	30%
Yogurt, plain, low fat, 8 oz	300	30%
Milk, reduced fat (2% milk fat), no solids, 8 fl oz.	297	30%
Milk, whole (3.25% milk fat), 8 fl oz.	291	29%
Milk, buttermilk, 8 fl oz.	285	29%
Milk, lactose reduced, 8 fl oz. (content varies slightly according to fat content; average=300 mg)	285–302	29–30%
Cottage cheese, 1% milk fat, 2 cups unpacked	276	28%
Mozzarella, part skim 1½ oz.	275	28%
Tofu, firm, w/calcium, ½ cup†	204	20%
Orange juice, calcium fortified, 6 fl oz.	200–260	20–26%
Salmon, pink, canned, solids with bone, 3 oz.	181	18%
Pudding, chocolate, instant, made with w/ 2% milk, ½ cup	153	15%
Tofu, soft, w/calcium, ½ cup†	138	14%
Breakfast drink, orange flavor, powder prepared with water, 8 fl oz.	133	13%
Frozen yogurt, vanilla, soft serve, ½ cup	103	10%
Ready to eat cereal, calcium fortified, 1 cup	100–1000	10%–100%
Turnip greens, boiled, ½ cup	99	10%
Kale, raw, 1 cup	90	9%
Kale, cooked, 1 cup	94	9%
Ice Cream, vanilla, ½ cup	85	8.5%
Soy beverage, calcium fortified, 8 fl oz.	80–500	8–50%
Chinese cabbage, raw, 1 cup	74	7%
Tortilla, corn, ready to bake/fry, 1 medium	42	4%
Tortilla, flour, ready to bake/fry, one 6" diameter	37	4%
Sour cream, reduced fat, cultured, 2 tbsp	32	3%
Bread, white, 1 oz.	31	3%
Broccoli, raw, ½ cup	21	2%
Bread, whole wheat, 1 slice	20	2%
Cheese, cream, regular, 1 Tbsp	12	1%

Source: USDA 2002, Heaney et al. 2000.

*DV=Daily Value
†Calcium values are only for tofu processed with a calcium salt. Tofu processed with a non-calcium salt will not contain significant amounts of calcium.

Note: Daily Values (DV) were developed to help consumers determine if a typical serving of a food contains a lot or a little of a specific nutrient. The DV for calcium is based on 1000 mg. The percent DV (% DV) listed on the nutrition facts panel of food labels tells you what percentages of the DV are provided in one serving. For instance, if you consumed a food that contained 300 mg of calcium, the DV would be 30% for calcium on the food label.

A food providing 5% of the DV or less is a low source while a food that provides 10–19% of the DV is a good source and a food that provides 20% of the DV or more is an excellent source for a nutrient. For foods not listed in this table, see the United States Department of Agriculture's Nutrient Database Web site: www.nal.usda.gov/fnic/cgi-bin/nut_search.pl

Table 7–3. Calcium and Lactose in Common Foods

	Calcium Content	Lactose Content
Vegetables, Fruit, Seafood		
Calcium-fortified orange juice, 1 cup	308–344 mg	0
Sardines, with edible bones, 3 oz.	270 mg	0
Salmon, canned, with edible bones, 3 oz.	205 mg	0
Soymilk, fortified, 1 cup	200 mg	0
Broccoli (raw), 1 cup	90 mg	0
Orange, 1 medium	50 mg	0
Pinto beans, ½ cup	40 mg	0
Tuna, canned, 3 oz.	10 mg	0
Lettuce greens, ½ cup	10 mg	0
Dairy Products		
Yogurt, plain, low-fat, 1 cup	415 mg	5 g
Milk, reduced fat, 1 cup	295 mg	11 g
Swiss cheese, 1 oz.	270 mg	1 g
Ice cream, ½ cup	85 mg	6 g
Cottage cheese, ½ cup	75 mg	2–3 g

Source: NIDDIC 2004.

good sources of calcium, including fortified cereal, nonfat milk, and calcium-fortified orange juice from frozen concentrate (Keller et al. 2002). Vegetables also contain calcium, but the amount of calcium absorbed from these sources varies; some, like broccoli and kale, contain calcium that is well absorbed, while others, such as spinach, do not (Weaver et al. 1999). It would be impractical for most people to eat enough vegetables or other low-calcium foods to meet recommended levels if these were the only sources of calcium in the diet. To assist in planning a diet containing adequate levels of calcium, Table 7-2 provides a list of selected food sources of calcium, along with the percent daily value that they contain. These percentages indicate whether a serving of the food contains a high (20 percent or more of the percent daily value) or a low (5 percent or less) amount of a specific nutrient—in this case, calcium. Most individuals can design a diet that is appealing to them (based on their preferences) while also meeting their nutrient needs.

Many individuals, especially non-Whites, suffer from lactose intolerance. These individuals may avoid dairy products, which can result in a low calcium intake unless other good sources of calcium are consumed. Those with lactose intolerance may develop the capability to digest lactose if they slowly build up milk intake over a period of days or weeks so that they develop an intestinal flora capable of digesting milk's lactose (Suarez et al. 1997). Many lactose-intolerant

A Guide to Calculate Calcium Intake

As shown in Figure 6-4 of Chapter 6, most Americans above age 9 on average do not consume recommended levels of calcium. The following guide allows an adult to compare a rough estimate of his or her intake of calcium to the recommended amounts:

- Start by writing down the following amount:
  - ~ 290 if you are a female, regardless of age, or male age 60 or older
  - ~ 370 if you a male under age 60

This is the average amount of calcium that most people eat from non-calcium rich food sources (Cook and Friday 2003, Wright et al. 2003, Weinberg et al. 2004).

- Add 300 mg for each 8-ounce serving of milk or the equivalent serving of other calcium-rich foods (e.g., yogurt, cheese).
- For those taking a calcium supplement or a multi-vitamin containing calcium, add the amount of calcium from that source:
  - ~ Check the supplement label for the amount of calcium per supplement dose.
  - ~ Multiply the amount per supplement dose times the number of doses taken each day.
  - ~ Add the amount from supplements to the base amount and the amount from calcium-rich foods.
- Compare this rough estimate of total calcium intake to the recommended levels shown in Table 7-1. Individuals should try to meet their recommended level of calcium on most days.
- A useful calcium calculator for children can be found at: http://www.cdc.gov/powerfulbones/parents/toolbox/calculator.html.

Figure 7–1. How To Use the Nutrition Facts Panel on Food Labels for Calcium

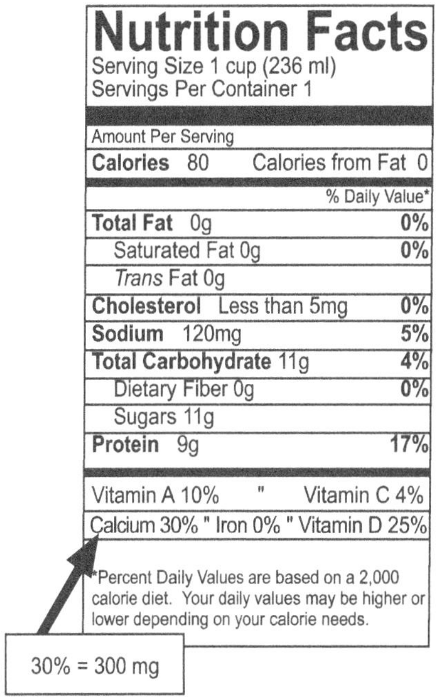

Nutrition Facts

Serving Size 1 cup (236 ml)
Servings Per Container 1

Amount Per Serving	
Calories 80	Calories from Fat 0

	% Daily Value*
Total Fat 0g	0%
Saturated Fat 0g	0%
Trans Fat 0g	
Cholesterol Less than 5mg	0%
Sodium 120mg	5%
Total Carbohydrate 11g	4%
Dietary Fiber 0g	0%
Sugars 11g	
Protein 9g	17%

Vitamin A 10%	"	Vitamin C 4%
Calcium 30% " Iron 0% " Vitamin D 25%		

*Percent Daily Values are based on a 2,000 calorie diet. Your daily values may be higher or lower depending on your calorie needs.

30% = 300 mg

Note: The Nutrition Facts panel on food labels can help individuals choose foods high in calcium. To convert the % Daily Value (DV) for calcium into milligrams (mg) multiply by 10 or add a 0. As an example, a container of yogurt might list 30% DV for calcium. To convert this to milligrams, multiply by 10 or add a 0, which equals 300 mg of calcium for the serving size of 1 cup of yogurt. A food with 20% DV or more contributes a lot of calcium to the daily total, while one with 5% DV or less contributes a little.

Source: FDA 2003.

Tips for Those With Lactose Intolerance

- Choose dairy and other calcium-rich foods with lower amounts of lactose; a list of the amount of calcium and lactose in common foods is shown in Table 7-3:
  - ~ Yogurt with live active cultures (which provide bacterial lactase that digests the lactose).
  - ~ Hard cheeses like cheddar, Colby, Swiss, and Parmesan (the production process for these cheeses breaks down the lactose).
  - ~ Lactose-free or lactose-reduced products, including milk without lactose.
- Gradually increase the amount of lactose-containing foods consumed.
- Consume non-dairy products that contain high levels of calcium, such as fortified soy beverage or fortified cereal or orange juice.

(Jarvis and Miller 2002)

individuals can tolerate up to one cup of milk twice a day if it is consumed with food (McBean and Miller 1998). In addition, some other calcium-rich dairy products such as cheese and yogurt are usually well tolerated by lactose-intolerant people. Finally, there are a number of calcium-rich foods that do not contain lactose, including lactose-free milk, fortified soy beverage, and fortified juice and cereal. Some tips for those with lactose intolerance are shown in the box below.

The Institute of Medicine recommends that nutrients be obtained from food when possible because they provide a package of nutrients that are good for other tissues besides bones. How-ever, fortified foods and supplements can assist those individuals who do not consume an adequate amount of dairy products or other naturally calcium-rich foods to meet recommended levels of calcium intake. Those who take supplements or consume fortified foods should note that: a) all major forms of calcium (e.g., carbonate, citrate) are absorbed well when taken with meals; b) calcium from supplements or fortified foods is best taken in several small doses (no more than 500–600 mg at one time) (Heaney 1975) throughout the day for better absorption; and c) supplements may differ in their absorbability due to manufacturing practices (IOM 1997). One need not choose the most expensive products on the market, as the cost of supplements of comparable quality can vary fivefold (Heaney et al. 2001). In a recent evaluation of calcium sources, calcium carbonate supplements were found to be the least expensive supplemental source of calcium. Since virtually all calcium sources—food or supplement—reduce the absorption of iron, calcium and iron supplements should be taken at different times.

Vitamin D

The current recommended intakes of vitamin D are given in Table 7-1. Most individuals need 200 IU per day, although these recommendations are raised to 400 IU per day in those age 50–70, and to 600 IU per day in those over age 70. There are two sources of vitamin D: sunlight and dietary intake.

As discussed in Chapter 6, vitamin D can be made in the skin by being exposed to sunlight. For some individuals, particularly children and others who get enough exposure during warmer months, the sun can provide adequate levels of vitamin D throughout the entire year. For many, however, it is not practical to get adequate levels of vitamin D from exposure to sunshine. These individuals should instead look to boost their vitamin D levels through diet. This is especially true for elderly individuals who have higher vitamin D needs and who may have difficulty getting outside everyday. People with dark skin and those who live in areas with heavy air pollution may also find it more practical to obtain most or all of their vitamin D from diet, since they need longer periods of sun exposure to get adequate levels of vitamin D. Table 7-4 gives the vitamin D content of several foods, although the most common source is fortified milk. One cup of fortified milk contains 100 IU vitamin D, half of the recommended intake for individuals under age 50. Since vitamin D-fortified milk is not used when making cheese, ice cream, or most yogurts, many other dairy foods are not good sources of vitamin D. Other good dietary sources of vitamin D include fatty fish and vitamin D-fortified orange juice. The best way to know whether a dairy food contains vitamin D is to check the nutrition label.

Vitamin D is also available in dietary supplements. While few supplements contain vitamin D alone, many calcium supplements also contain vitamin D. Multivitamin supplements contain up to 400 IU of vitamin D. The amount of vitamin D in a single dose of many calcium and multivitamin supplements may not be sufficient to meet the recommended levels, especially for people over age 70 who need 600 IU per day. To make sure that the recommended amount of vitamin D is consumed as shown in Table 7-1, check the nutrition label on the supplement for the amount of vitamin D per dose, and, if necessary, supplement vitamin D intake through other sources. However, because vitamin D can have negative effects if taken in very high doses, it is also important to avoid consuming more vitamin D than the tolerable upper level of 2,000 IU per day. Larger doses can initially be given to patients who are deficient as a means of replenishing the stores of vitamin D in the body.

Other Nutrients Important to Bone

As shown in Table 7-1, the Institute of Medicine recently provided recommended intakes for other bone-related nutrients, including phosphorus and magnesium (IOM 1997). Most Americans consume adequate quantities of phospho-

Table 7–4. Dietary Sources of Vitamin D

	Serving Size	Vitamin D (IU)
Milk	1 cup	98
Baked herring	3 oz.	1,775
Baked salmon	3 oz.	238
Canned tuna	3 oz.	136
Sardines	1 oz.	77
Raisin bran cereal	¾ cup	42
Pork sausage	1 oz	31
Egg yolk	1	25

Source: USDA 2002.

Table 7–5.   Other Nutrients and Bone Health at a Glance

Other Nutrients Affecting Bone	What Is the Effect on Bone?	How Much Is Needed?*	What Are the Dietary Sources?	Special Considerations
Potentially Benefical Effects on Bone				
Boron	May enhance calcium absorption and estrogen metabolism.	Not applicable.	Raw avocado, nuts, peanut butter, bottled prune juice.	
Copper	Copper helps certain enzymes and local regulators function properly so that we can form the optimal bone matrix or structure for bone strength.	RDA is 900 µg for men and women over age 30. Daily intakes over 10,000 µg are not recommended.	Organ meats, seafood, nuts, seeds, wheat bran, cereals, whole grain products, cocoa products.	Calcium supplementation may result in lower levels of copper.
Fluoride	Fluoride stimulates the formation of new bone. Necessary for skeletal and dental development.	RDA is 4 mg for men over age 30 and 3 mg for women over age 30. Daily intakes over 10 mg are not recommended.	Fluoridated water, teas, marine fish, fluoridated dental products.	
Iron	Iron helps certain enzymes and local regulators function properly so that we can form the optimal bone matrix or structure for bone strength.	RDA is 8 mg for men over the age of 19. The RDA for women is 18 mg between the ages of 19 and 50 and 8 mg over age 50. Daily intakes over 45 mg are not recommended.	*Non-heme sources* include fruits, vegetables and fortified bread and grain products such as cereal. *Heme sources* include meat and poultry.	
Isoflavones	Isoflavones have been shown to have a protective effect on bone in animal studies. Evidence in humans, however, is conflicting.	Not applicable.	Primarily found in soybeans and soy products, chickpeas and other legumes.	Ipriflavone, a synthetic isoflavone, has been linked to a reduction in lympocytes, a type of white blood cell that fights infection.
Magnesium	60% of the magnesium in our bodies is found in our bones in combination with calcium and phosphorus. Magnesium appears to enhance our bone quality. Studies suggest that it may improve bone mineral density, and not getting enough may interfere with our ability to process calcium.	RDA is 420 mg for men over 30 and 320 mg for women over 30. Daily intakes over 350 mg are not recommended	Good sources include green leafy vegetables such as spinach, potatoes, nuts, seeds, whole grains including bran, wheat, oats, and chocolate. Smaller amounts are found in many foods including bananas, broccoli, raisins and shrimp. Also found in magnesium-containing laxatives and antacids.	Magnesium deficiency is rare in US adults. Magnesium supplements are not recommended for most people.

*Recommended Dietary Allowance (RDA)

Source: NIH ORBD~NRC 2004.

Table 7-5. Other Nutrients and Bone Health at a Glance

Other Nutrients Affecting Bone	What Is the Effect on Bone?	How Much Is Needed?*	What Are the Dietary Sources?	Special Considerations
Potentially Benefical Effects on Bone				
Manganese	Manganese helps certain enzymes and local regulators function properly so that we can form the optimal bone matrix or structure for bone strength.	RDA is 2.3 mg for men over age 30 and 1.8 mg for women over age 30. Daily intakes over 11 mg are not recommended.	Nuts, legumes, tea, whole grains and drinking water.	Manganese supplements may not be a good choice for everyone, including people already consuming high levels of manganese from diets high in plant foods and people with liver disease who are especially susceptible to the adverse effects of excess manganese intake.
Phosphorus	Phosphorus is a component of every cell in our bodies and supports building bone and other tissue during growth. About 85% of the phosphorus in our bodies is found in our bones. In fact, phosphate, a form of phosphorus, makes up more than half of our bone mineral mass.	RDA is 700 mg for men and women over age 30. Daily intakes over 4,000 mg for adults up to age 70 and over 3,000 mg after age 70 are not recommended.	Milk, yogurt, ice cream, cheese, peas, meat, eggs, some cereals, breads, cola soft drinks and many processed foods.	
Potassium		There is no RDA established for potassium. Scientists recommend a daily intake between 1,600 mg and 3,500 mg.	Milk, yogurt, chicken, turkey, fish, many fruits such as bananas, raisins and cantaloupe, and many vegetables such as celery, carrots, potatoes and tomatoes.	
Protein	Proteins are our bodies' building blocks. We use protein to build tissue during growth and to repair and replace tissue throughout life. We also need protein to help heal fractures and to make sure our immune system is functioning properly.	RDA is 56 g for adult men and 46 g for adult women. Nutritionists recommend that 10% to 35% of our calories come from protein. (The rest come primarily from carbohydrates and fats.)	*Complete protein comes from animal sources* including meat, poultry, fish, eggs, milk, cheese, yogurt. *Incomplete protein comes from plant sources* including legumes, grains, nuts, seeds and vegetables.	Getting enough protein is particularly important for elderly people. Studies show that elderly people who have not been getting enough protein and who break their hip are more likely to suffer poor medical outcomes.

*Recommended Dietary Allowance (RDA)

Source: NIH ORBD~NRC 2004.

Table 7–5. Other Nutrients and Bone Health at a Glance

Other Nutrients Affecting Bone	What Is the Effect on Bone?	How Much Is Needed?*	What Are the Dietary Sources?	Special Considerations
Potentially Benefical Effects on Bone				
Vitamin C	Vitamin C helps certain enzymes and local regulators function properly so that we can form the optimal bone matrix or structure for bone strength.	RDA is 90 mg for men over age 30 and 75 mg for women over age 30. Daily intakes over 2,000 mg are not recommended.	Citrus fruits, tomatoes and tomato juice, potatoes, Brussels sprouts, cauliflower, broccoli, strawberries, cabbage and spinach.	People who smoke need 35 mg more vitamin C than the RDA. People who are regularly exposed to second-hand smoke also may need extra vitamin C.
Vitamin K	Vitamin K helps certain enzymes and local regulators function properly so that we can form the optimal bone matrix or structure for bone strength.	RDA is 120 units for men over age 30 and 90 units for women over age 30. No maximum safe intake has been established for vitamin K.	Green vegetables including collards, spinach, salad greens and broccoli, Brussels sprouts, cabbage, plant oils and margarine.	Patients on anticoagulant medication should monitor their vitamin K intake.
Zinc	Zinc helps certain enzymes and local regulators function properly which in turn helps our bodies form the optimal bone matrix or structure for bone strength.	RDA is 11 mg for boys and men over age 19 and 8 mg for girls and women over age 19. Daily intakes over 40 mg are not recommended.	Red meat, poultry, fortified breakfast cereal, some seafood, whole grains, dry beans and nuts.	Nutritionists recommend that vegetarians double the RDA for themselves, because zinc is harder to absorb on a vegetarian diet. Calcium supplementation may reduce the absorption of zinc.

*Recommended Dietary Allowance (RDA)

Table 7–5.   Other Nutrients and Bone Health at a Glance

Other Nutrients Affecting Bone	What Is the Effect on Bone?	How Much Is Needed?*	What Are the Dietary Sources?	Special Considerations
Potentially Adverse Effects on Bone				
Caffeine	Studies suggest that caffeine may interfere with calcium absorption. However, this effect can be neutralized in the presence of adequate dietary calcium.	Not applicable	Coffee, tea, some soft drinks, some over the counter medications.	
Fiber	Fiber has a minor negative impact on calcium absorption.	Men ages 31 to 50 need 38 grams per day and after 50 need 30 grams per day. Women ages 31–50 need 25 gm per day and after 50 need 21 gm per day.	Includes dietary fiber naturally present in grains (oats, wheat or unmilled rice) and functional fiber from plants and animals shown to be of benefit to health.	
Oxalates	When oxalates and calcium are found in the same food, oxalates combine with the calcium, preventing us from absorbing the calcium.	Not applicable	Spinach. Other oxalate-rich foods include rhubarb and sweet potatoes, but since these foods do not contain calcium, the oxalates have no effect on calcium absorption.	Oxalates do not interfere with the absorption of calcium in *other* foods eaten with the oxalate-containing foods.
Phosphorus	Phosphorus is necessary for healthy bones (see above), but some people are concerned that there may be too much in our diet, especially since phosphorus is a component of cola beverages and many processed foods. Some studies suggest that excess amounts of phosphorus may interfere with calcium absorption. The good news is that we can offset the loss by getting adequate amounts of calcium in our diet.	RDA is 700 mg for men and women over age 30. Daily intakes over 4,000 mg for adults up to age 70 and over 3,000 mg after age 70 are not recommended.	Milk, yogurt, ice cream, cheese, peas, meat, eggs, some cereals, breads, cola soft drinks and many processed foods.	Possible negative effects of soft drinks on bone may be due primarily to the replacement of calcium-rich milk with soft drinks, especially by children and teenagers at a time when they need extra calcium to optimize their peak bone mass.

*Recommended Dietary Allowance (RDA)

Source: NIH ORBD~NRC 2004.

Table 7-5.   Other Nutrients and Bone Health at a Glance

Other Nutrients Affecting Bone	What Is the Effect on Bone?	How Much Is Needed?*	What Are the Dietary Sources?	Special Considerations
Potentially Adverse Effects on Bone				
Protein	Protein is essential for good health (see above). However, when we get too much protein, our bodies convert the extra protein into calories for energy, producing a chemical called sulfate in the process. Sulfate causes us to lose some calcium, but these are relatively small losses that we can offset by getting adequate amounts of calcium in our diet.	RDA is 56 g for adult men and 46 g for adult women. It is recommended that 10% to 35% of calories come from protein. (The rest come primarily from carbohydrates and fats.)	*Complete protein comes from animal sources* including meat, poultry, fish, eggs, milk, cheese, yogurt. *Incomplete protein comes from plant sources* including legumes, grains, nuts, seeds and vegetables.	
Sodium	Sodium affects the balance of calcium in our bodies by increasing the amount we excrete in urine and perspiration. The loss of calcium can be significant, but we can replace the lost calcium by making sure we get adequate amounts of calcium in our diet.	The NIH recommends restricting daily sodium intake to less than 2,400 milligrams (equal to about 1 teaspoon of table salt).	Sodium combined with chloride is common table salt. Many processed foods are high in salt.	
Vitamin A	Vitamin A plays an important role in bone growth but excessive amounts of the retinol form of vitamin A may increase the breakdown of our bones and interfere with vitamin D, which we need to help us absorb calcium. The beta carotene form of vitamin A does not appear to cause these problems.	RDAs are 3000 IU for men and 2330 IU for women. Daily intakes over 10,000 IU of the retinol form of vitamin A are not recommended.	*Retinol sources* include animal-source foods such as liver, egg yolks, cheese, milk. Dietary supplements and some acne preparations also contain retinol. *Beta carotene sources* include plant-source foods, such as dark orange and green vegetables including carrots, sweet potatoes, and spinach as well as cantaloupe and kale.	

*Recommended Dietary Allowance (RDA)

Source: NIH ORBD~NRC 2004.

rus through their regular intake of meats, cereals, milk, and processed foods. While some beverages such as soft drinks also contain phosphorus, they are not a preferred source of phosphorus because they may displace calcium-rich beverages like milk (Whiting et al. 2001).

Magnesium intakes may be suboptimal in those who do not eat enough green leafy vegetables, whole grains, nuts, and dairy products. Fortunately, most diets contain adequate levels of other bone-related micronutrients, such as vitamins K and C, copper, manganese, zinc, and iron, to promote bone health.

Some dietary components may potentially have negative effects on bone health, especially if calcium intakes are not adequate. For example, high levels of sodium or caffeine intake can increase calcium excretion in the urine. The effects of these factors can be overcome by increasing the amount of calcium in the diet (Fitzpatrick and Heaney 2003). Studies have linked excessive amounts of phosphorus to altered calcium metabolism, but it appears that the typical level of phosphorus consumed by most individuals in the United States should not negatively affect bone health (IOM 1997). Excessive amounts of preformed vitamin A (e.g., retinol) can also have negative effects on bone, so individuals should not consume more than the recommended dietary allowance for this vitamin (IOM 2000). The vitamin A precursor (beta carotene) found in many fruits and vegetables does not have negative effects on bone, however.

Table 7-5 provides additional information on other nutrients that affect bone, their recommended dietary allowances, and common dietary sources of these nutrients.

Physical Activity

The foundation of a good physical activity regimen involves at least 30 minutes (adults) or 60 minutes (children) of moderate physical activity every day. This regimen can and should involve a variety of activities. Some can be routine activities like walking or gardening. Others may occur more infrequently and differ from day to day and week to week, such as dancing, aerobic classes, biking, swimming, tennis, golf, or hiking. However, it is clear from the evidence presented in Chapter 6 that physical activity to specifically benefit bone health should involve loading (stressing) the skeleton. As a result, weight-bearing activities such as walking should be included in an optimal physical activity regimen to benefit the musculoskeletal system. Moreover, the evidence suggests that the most beneficial physical activity regimens for bone health include strength-training or resistance-training activities. These activities place levels of loading on bone that are beyond those seen in everyday activities; examples include jumping for the lower limbs and weight lifting or resistance training for the lower and upper skeleton. Finally, while a focus on activities that build or maintain bone strength is appropriate and necessary, many older individuals will remain at high risk of fracture. For these individuals, balance training can provide the added benefit of helping to prevent potentially injurious falls.

As noted in Chapter 6, the evidence does not lead to a specific set of exercises or practices but rather a set of principles that can be applied and varied according to the age and current physical condition of an individual. Many of these principles have been reviewed by expert panels of the American College of Sports Medicine (ACSM) (Kraemer et al. 2002, ACSM 1998a, ACSM 1998b) and they lead to the following suggestions for the frequency, intensity, length, and type of physical activity regimens to benefit bone health for individuals of all ages:

- Since continued physical activity provides a positive stimulus for bone, muscle, and other aspects of health, a lifelong commitment to physical activity and exercise is critical.
- Ending a physical activity regimen will result in bone mass returning to the level that existed before the activity began. Since repetitive programs of physical activity may be discontinued due to lack of motivation or interest, variety and creativity are important if physical activity is to be continued over the long term.
- Physical activity will only affect bone at the skeletal sites that are stressed (or loaded) by the activity. In other words, physical activity programs do not necessarily benefit the whole skeleton, although any type of activity provides more benefit to bone than does no activity at all.
- For bone gain to occur, the stimulus must be greater than that which the bone usually experiences. Static loads applied continuously (such as standing) do not promote increased bone mass.
- Complete lack of activity, such as periods of immobility, causes bone loss. When it is not possible to avoid immobility (e.g., bed rest during sickness), even brief daily weight-bearing movements can help to reduce bone loss.
- General physical activity every day and some weight-bearing, strength-building, and balance-enhancing activities 2 or more times a week are generally effective for promoting bone health for most persons.
- Any activity that imparts impact (such as jumping or skipping) may increase bone mass more than will low- and moderate-intensity, endurance-type activities, such as brisk walking. However, endur-

ance activities may still play an important role in skeletal health by increasing muscle mass and strength, balance, and coordination, and they may also help prevent falls in the elderly. Endurance activity is also very important for other aspects of health, such as helping to prevent obesity, diabetes, or cardiovascular disease.
- Load-bearing physical activities such as jumping need not be engaged in for long periods of time to provide benefits to skeletal health. In fact, 5–10 minutes daily may suffice. Most adults should begin with weight-bearing exercise and gradually add some skipping and jumping activity. Longer periods (30–45 minutes) may be needed for weight training or walking/jogging. Those who have been inactive should work up to this amount of time gradually using a progressive program, e.g., start with shorter times and easier activities (light weights or walking) and then increase time or intensity slowly (by no more than 10 percent each week) in order to avoid injury.
- Physical activities that include a variety of loading patterns (such as strength training or aerobic classes) may promote increased bone mass more than do activities that involve normal or regular loading patterns (such as running).

These fundamental principles can be used to develop age-specific regimens, as outlined in the sections that follow.

Physical Activity for Children and Adolescents

For children over age 8 and adolescents, a bone-healthy program of physical activity could include the following:

- At least 60 minutes of moderate intensity, continuous activity on most days, prefer-

Table 7-6. Weight-Bearing Exercise for Kids and Teens

Exercise helps build bone and weight-bearing exercise is particularly helpful in this task. Weight-bearing exercise includes any activity in which your feet and legs carry your own weight. Here are some examples of weight-bearing exercise that can help you build strong bones:

- Walking
- Running
- Jumping
- Jumping rope
- Dancing
- Climbing stairs
- Jogging
- Aerobic dancing
- Hiking
- Inline skating/ice skating
- Racquet sports, such as tennis or racquetball
- Team sports such as soccer, basketball, field hockey, volleyball, and softball or baseball

Source: NICHD 2004.

ably daily. This level of activity can help achieve a healthy body weight and lower the risk of other diseases such as cardiovascular disease and diabetes (USDHHS 1996, USDA 2000, USDHHS 2000, IOM 2002).

- Inclusion of weight-bearing and short, intense impact activities such as basketball, gymnastics, and jumping as part of this regular activity program.
- Performance of weight-bearing activities that increase muscle strength, such as

running, hopping, or skipping. The best activities work all muscle groups. Examples include gymnastics, basketball, volleyball, bicycling, and soccer. Swimming, while highly beneficial to many aspects of health, is not a weight-bearing activity and thus does not contribute to increased bone mass.

Physical Activity for Adults

Adults should strive to get at least 30 minutes of physical activity on most days, preferably daily (USDHHS 1996, USDA 2000, USDHHS 2000, IOM 2002). As part of that regular physical activity program, the following can help enhance bone health:

- For those individuals who can tolerate impact activities, a simple, 10-minute program of physical activity that incorporates 50 3-inch (8-centimeter) jumps per day.
- A progressive program of weight training that uses all muscle groups, with the amount of weight lifted increased gradually over time.
- A jogging or stair-climbing program for those who cannot tolerate higher impact physical activity.
- Active recreational activities such as tennis, hiking, or basketball.

In addition, it is advisable for adults to try to find ways to add extra weight-bearing exercise into everyday activities. For example, consider parking farther away in the parking lot or taking the stairs instead of the elevator.

General recommendations for physical activity in adults are shown in the pyramid in Figure 7-2, with the base of the pyramid being 30 minutes or more of moderate physical activity on most, preferably all, days of the week. It is also recommended that weight-bearing exercises and strength and balance training be added as a

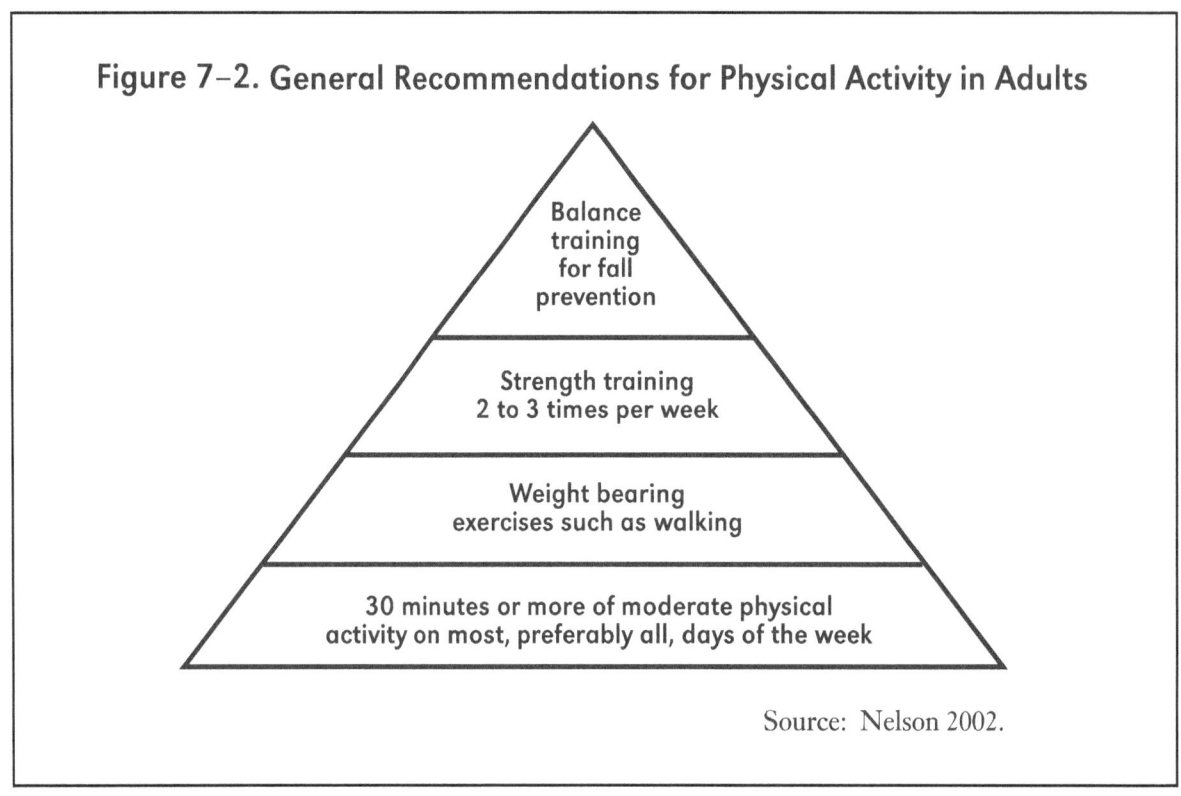

Figure 7–2. General Recommendations for Physical Activity in Adults

Balance training for fall prevention

Strength training 2 to 3 times per week

Weight bearing exercises such as walking

30 minutes or more of moderate physical activity on most, preferably all, days of the week

Source: Nelson 2002.

part of regular physical activity (Nelson 2002, Seguin and Nelson 2003). Lifestyle activities such as walking, gardening, and raking leaves can also be a valuable part of regular physical activity (USDHHS 1996).

It is important to begin any physical activity program slowly and to consider previous activity levels. Those who have been inactive should begin with 5–10 minutes of activity per day and a pre-exercise evaluation by a physician may be advised. Those who are more fit can increase physical activity levels to 20–30 minutes of moderate activity at a higher heart rate (60–85 percent of maximum heart rate). Generally, it is advisable to increase activity levels by no more than 10 percent each week to avoid injury. For example, those who begin with 15 minutes per day can progress to 17 minutes the second week, and so on.

Finally, adults should consult a physician or physical therapist if orthopedic conditions like arthritis, functional limitations, or other medical conditions make these physical activity guidelines difficult or unsafe to follow.

Physical Activity for Older Adults

Most elderly individuals should strongly consider engaging in regular physical activity. Physical activity is the only single therapy that can simultaneously improve muscle mass, muscle strength, balance, and bone strength. As a result, it may decrease the risk of fractures, in part by reducing the risk of falling. In fact, fall-risk reduction may be the biggest benefit of physical activity for the elderly.

The following guidelines should be used to maximize the potential fall prevention benefits of physical activity in the elderly:

Figure 7–3. Examples of Strength Training Exercises

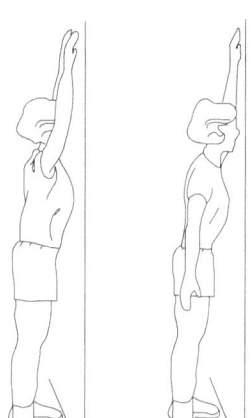

Overhead Press

1. Stand or sit in an armless chair with feet shoulder-width apart. With a dumbbell in each hand, raise your hands, palms facing forward, until the dumbbells are level with your shoulders and parallel to the floor.

2. To a count of two, slowly push the dumbbells up over your head until your arms are fully extended—but don't lock your elbows.

3. Pause. Then, to a count of four, slowly lower the dumbbells back to shoulder level, bringing your elbows down close to your sides.

4. Repeat ten times for one set. Rest for one to two minutes. Then complete a second set of ten repetitions.

Benefit: Strengthens muscles in the arms, upper back, and shoulders.

Wall Arch

1. Face a wall with your feet 6 inches from the wall and 6 inches apart.

2. Stretch your arms up to touch the wall while taking a deep breath in.

3. Concentrate on flattening your stomach.

4. Also, try reaching up with one arm while stretching down with the other.

Benefit: Strengthens stomach and back, stretches shoulders and calves.

Source: CDC 2004, NOF 2003.

- Physical activity needs to be of sufficient intensity to improve muscle strength, since poor muscle strength is a known risk factor for falls. Strength or resistance training is best for building muscle, but even aerobic endurance activity can yield some improvements in muscle strength.

- Improving balance can be an important component of any physical activity program designed to decrease falls. This program may include balance training exercises or a movement activity such as Tai Chi. Any activity that requires weight bearing and challenges the postural system can

Table 7–7. Weight-Bearing Exercise for Adults

Weight-Bearing/High Impact/Resistance Activities:

- Stair-climbing
- Hiking
- Dancing
- Jogging
- Downhill and cross-country skiing
- Aerobic dancing
- Volleyball
- Basketball
- Gymnastics
- Weight lifting or resistance training
- Soccer
- Jumping rope

Weight-Bearing/Low Impact Activities:

- Walking
- Treadmill walking
- Cross-country ski machines
- Stair-step machines
- Rowing machines
- Water aerobics
- Deep-water walking
- Low impact aerobics

Non-Weight-Bearing/Non-Impact Activities:

- Lap swimming
- Indoor cycling
- Stretching or flexibility exercises (avoid forward-bending exercises)
- Yoga
- Pilates

Source: NOF 2003.

Figure 7–4. Resources for Strength Training for Older Adults

"You don't stop exercising because you grow old. You grow old because you stop exercising."
—Anonymous

Growing Stronger: Strength Training for Older Adults
This strength-training program was developed by experts at Tufts University and the Centers for Disease Control and Prevention (CDC). It is based upon sound scientific research involving strengthening exercises—exercises that have been shown to increase the strength of your muscles, maintain the integrity of your bones, and improve your balance, coordination, and mobility. The CDC website features links to the book and animated illustrations of exercises.

Source: CDC 2004.

Exercise: A Guide From the National Institute on Aging
The 48-minute video and 80-page companion booklet were produced by the National Institute on Aging (NIA) to demonstrate how to start and stick with a safe, effective program of stretching, balance, and strength-training exercises. The video features Margaret Richard, star of *Body Electric*, PBS' popular exercise show.

Source: NIA 2004.

Boning Up on Osteoporosis: A Guide to Prevention and Treatment
This 70-page booklet provides information on the prevention, detection, and treatment of osteoporosis. The booklet includes tips on how to begin an exercise program and provides 17 pages of illustrations and instructions on moving safely.

Source: NOF 2003.

improve balance and potentially help reduce falls.

- Physical activity must be performed on average 3 times per week for 30–45 minutes per session for at least three months for strength and balance benefits to be realized, and it must be continued if benefits are to be maintained.

- Those who suffer a fall that requires a visit to a health care provider or an emergency room should ask for a fall risk assessment that includes a program of physical activity. Physical activity is most effective if delivered as a part of a comprehensive fall prevention program (see Chapter 6).

Physical Activity for Those With Fragility Fractures

Individuals who have already experienced osteoporotic fractures should avoid certain types of physical activities and exercises. For example, those who have had vertebral fractures may need to avoid activities that flex the spine. For more information about appropriate physical activity after osteoporotic fracture, see Chapter 9, "Rehabilitation of Osteoporotic Fractures."

Fall Prevention

It is no surprise that falls are often the "precipitating" event that leads to a fracture in individuals with low bone mineral density (BMD), and that therefore preventing these falls can reduce the risk of fracture. Falls are a major contributor to hip fractures and are also associated with a significantly increased risk of many other fractures, including spine, wrist, pelvis, and upper arm. Since falls are usually caused by multiple factors, successful prevention strategies should involve multiple components. The benefit of physical activity in reducing the risk of falls was discussed in the previous section. There is more that can be done to reduce the chances of a fall and to minimize the impact of any fall that does occur. Guidelines issued by the American Geriatrics Society, British Geriatrics Society, and American Academy of Orthopedic Surgeons panel on falls prevention include the following recommendations for older persons (AGS et al. 2001):

- Inform health care providers about any fall, even those that do not result in serious injury. Providers should ask their older patients at least once a year about falls.
- Those who have fallen one or more times should ask their health care providers about the need for a test of their balance and ability to walk.

- Those who need medical attention after a fall or who have fallen several times in the past year should have a fall evaluation. This evaluation should include taking a history related to the circumstances of the fall and performing an examination of vision, balance, walking, muscle strength, heart function, and blood pressure. A specialist, such as a geriatrician, may be needed for this evaluation.
- Health care providers should consider prescribing a program of physical activity and balance training, with an emphasis on those activities that may help reduce risk of falling. Patients can also seek these programs on their own.
- Patients should ask their health care providers to review any medications they are taking (including over-the-counter ones) at least once per year. This step can help to avoid various medication-related problems that commonly lead to falls, such as drug-drug interactions and unnecessarily high doses of certain drugs.
- Vision should be checked annually.
- Individuals should review their homes for possible hazards that could cause a fall, such as loose rugs, poor lighting, electrical cords, or lack of handrails in the tub/shower.
- Individuals should be careful when using step ladders, making sure to use ladders that are stable and have a handrail.

Finally, as discussed in Chapter 6, use of hip protectors or hip pads may help reduce the risk of fractures for persons living in institutionalized care settings.

A good source for tips on how to prevent falls is "The Tool Kit to Prevent Senior Falls," developed by the Injury Center at the Centers for Disease Control and Prevention (CDC). This

Table 7–8.   Preventing Falls Among Seniors

Tips
Falls are not just the result of getting older. Many falls can be prevented. Falls are usually caused by a number of things. By changing some of these things, you can lower your chances of falling. You can reduce your chances of falling by doing these things :
1. Begin a regular exercise program.
Exercise is one of the most important ways to reduce your chances of falling. It makes you stronger and helps you feel better. Exercises that improve balance and coordination (like Tai Chi) are the most helpful. Lack of exercise leads to weakness and increases your chances of falling. Ask your doctor or health care worker about the best type of exercise program for you.
2. Make your home safer.
About half of all falls happen at home. To make your home safer: • Remove things you can trip over (such as papers, books, clothes, and shoes) from stairs and places where you walk. • Remove small throw rugs or use double-sided tape to keep the rugs from slipping. • Keep items you use often in cabinets you can reach easily without using a step stool. • Have grab bars put in next to your toilet and in the tub or shower. • Use non-slip mats in the bathtub and on shower floors. • Improve the lighting in your home. As you get older, you need brighter lights to see well. Lamp shades or frosted bulbs can reduce glare. • Have handrails and lights put in on all staircases. • Wear shoes that give good support and have thin non-slip soles. Avoid wearing slippers and athletic shoes with deep treads.
3. Have your health care provider review your medicines.
Have your doctor or pharmacist look at all the medicines you take (including ones that don't need prescriptions such as cold medicines). As you get older, the way some medicines work in your body can change. Some medicines, or combinations of medicines, can make you drowsy or light-headed which can lead to a fall.
4. Have your vision checked.
Have your eyes checked by an eye doctor. You may be wearing the wrong glasses or have a condition such as glaucoma or cataracts that limits your vision. Poor vision can increase your chances of falling.

Source: CDC 2004.

kit contains "What You Can Do to Prevent Falls," an informational brochure, and "Check for Safety," a home safety checklist designed to help older adults and caregivers identify and correct home hazards. It also contains four fact sheets and other relevant materials, and is available at http://www.cdc.gov/injury.

Other Aspects of a Bone-Healthy Lifestyle

In addition to having a healthy diet, sufficient physical activity, and avoiding falls, there are some other bone-healthy behaviors that can help protect the skeleton throughout life:

- Maintain a healthy body weight.
- Avoid smoking.
- If one drinks alcoholic beverages, do so in moderation (i.e., one drink per day for women and two drinks per day for men).
- For women, see a health care provider if menstrual periods stop for three months.
- For those who have a medical condition or who use medications that can affect the skeleton (listed in Tables 3-1 and 3-2 in Chapter 3), talk to a health care provider about ways to safeguard the skeleton.

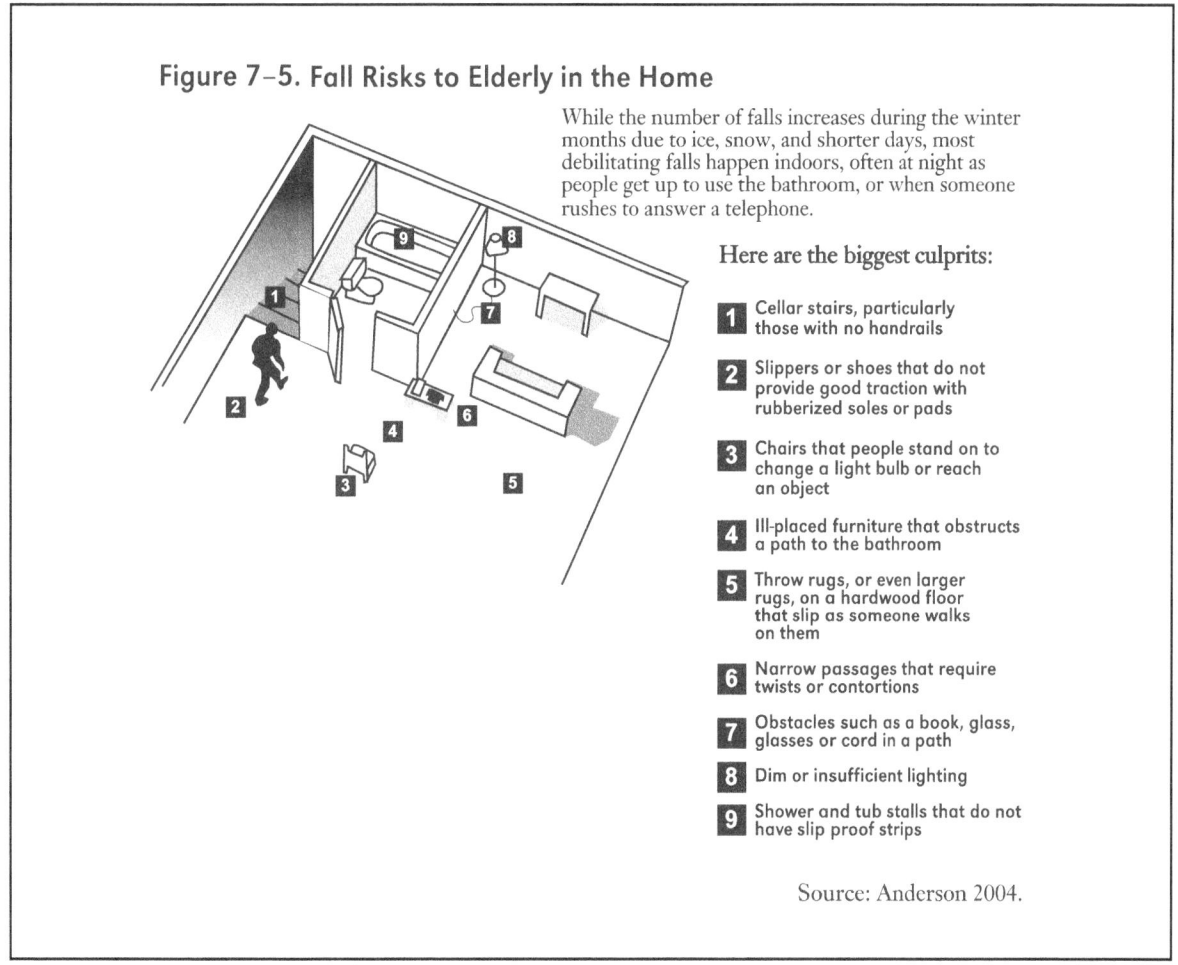

Figure 7–5. Fall Risks to Elderly in the Home

While the number of falls increases during the winter months due to ice, snow, and shorter days, most debilitating falls happen indoors, often at night as people get up to use the bathroom, or when someone rushes to answer a telephone.

Here are the biggest culprits:

1 Cellar stairs, particularly those with no handrails

2 Slippers or shoes that do not provide good traction with rubberized soles or pads

3 Chairs that people stand on to change a light bulb or reach an object

4 Ill-placed furniture that obstructs a path to the bathroom

5 Throw rugs, or even larger rugs, on a hardwood floor that slip as someone walks on them

6 Narrow passages that require twists or contortions

7 Obstacles such as a book, glass, glasses or cord in a path

8 Dim or insufficient lighting

9 Shower and tub stalls that do not have slip proof strips

Source: Anderson 2004.

Summary

Following the suggestions outlined in this chapter on diet, physical activity, and other lifestyle behaviors can help ensure good skeletal health throughout life. For more specific information on how to adopt a bone-healthy lifestyle, see the resources listed in Appendix C. It is never too late for individuals, even frail elders, to start following a bone-healthy lifestyle.

Key Questions for Future Research

Research questions related to lifestyle approaches that promote bone health are included in the questions identified in Chapter 6 on page 141.

References

[a]American College of Sports Medicine Position Stand. Exercise and physical activity for older adults. Med Sci Sports Exerc. 1998 Jun;30(6):992-1008.

[b]American College of Sports Medicine Position Stand. The recommended quantity and quality of exercise for developing and maintaining cardiorespiratory and muscular fitness, and flexibility in healthy adults. Med Sci Sports Exerc. 1998 Jun;30(6):975-91.

American Geriatrics Society; British Geriatrics Society; and American Academy of Orthopaedic Surgeons Panel on Falls Prevention. Guideline for the prevention of falls in older persons. J Am Geriatr Soc 2001 May; 49(5):664-72.

Anderson V. Fear of falling: senior citizens face serious injury, death from losing their balance. Atlanta Journal-Constitution 2004 Jan 6. Available from: http://www.ajc.com/health/content/health/0104/06falls.html.

Centers for Disease Control and Prevention [homepage on the Internet]. Growing stronger: strength training for older adults. [Atlanta(GA)]: The Center; [updated 2003 Nov 6; cited 2004 Feb 25]. Available from: http://www.cdc.gov/nccdphp/dnpa/physical/growing_stronger/.

Centers for Disease Control and Prevention [homepage on the Internet]. Preventing falls among seniors. [Atlanta(GA)]: The Center; [reviewed 2002 Aug 28; cited 2004 Feb 25]. Available from: http://www.cdc.gov/ncipc/duip/spotlite/falltips.htm.

Cook AJ, Friday JE. Food mixture or ingredient sources for dietary calcium: shifts in food group contributions using four grouping protocols. J Am Diet Assoc 2003 Nov;103(11):1513-9.

Fitzpatrick L, Heaney RP. Got soda? J Bone Miner Res 2003 Sep;18(9):1570-2.

Food and Drug Administration; U.S. Department of Health and Human Services Guidance on how to understand and use the nutrition facts panel on food labels [monograph on the Internet]. Internet ed. Rockville (MD): Food and Drug Administration; 200 Jun[updated Jul 2003;cited 2004 Jan 15]. Available from: http://www.cfsan.fda.gov/~dms/foodlab.html.

Heaney RP, Saville PD, Recker RR. Calcium absorption as a function of calcium intake. J Lab Clin Med. 1975 Jun;85(6):881-90.

Heaney RP, Dowell MS, Rafferty K, Bierman J. Bioavailability of the calcium in fortified soy imitation milk, with some observations on method. Am J Clin Nutr 2000 May;71(5): 1166-9.

Heaney RP, Weaver CM. Calcium and vitamin D. Endocrinol Metab Clin North Am 2003 Mar; 32(1):181-94, vii-viii. Review.

Institute of Medicine. Dietary reference intakes for calcium, phosphorus, magnesium, vitamin D, and fluoride. Washington, DC: National Academy Press; 1997. 432p.

Institute of Medicine. Dietary reference intakes for vitamin A, vitamin K, arsenic, boron, chromium, copper, iodine, iron, manganese, molybdenum, nickel, silicon, vanadium, and zinc. Washington, DC: National Academy Press; 2000. 800p.

Institute of Medicine. Dietary reference intakes for energy, carbohydrate, fiber, fat, fatty acids, cholesterol, protein and amino acids. Washington, DC: National Academy Press; 2002. 936p.

Jarvis JK, Miller GD. Overcoming the barrier of lactose intolerance to reduce health disparities. J Natl Med Assoc 2002 Feb;94(2):55-66. Review.

Keller JL, Lanon AJ, Barnard ND. The consumer cost of calcium from food and supplements. J. Am Diet Assoc 2002 Nov;102(11): 1669-71.

Kraemer WJ, Adams K, Cafarelli E, Dudley GA, Dooly C, Feigenbaum MS, Fleck SJ, Franklin B, Fry AC, Hoffman JRet al. American College of Sports Medicine position stand. Progression models in resistance training for healthy adults. Med Sci Sports Exerc. 2002 Feb;34(2):364-80.

McBean LD, Miller GD. Allaying fears and fallacies about lactose intolerance. J Am Diet Assoc 1998 Jun;98(6):671-6.

National Digestive Diseases Information Clearinghouse (NDDIC) [homepage on the Internet]. Bethesda (MD): National Institute of Diabetes and Digestive and Kidney Diseases (NIDDK) c2004 [cited 2004 June 24]. Lactose intolerance. Available from http:// digestive.niddk.nih.gov/ddiseases/pubs/ lactoseintolerance.

National Institutes of Health, Osteoporosis and Related Bone Diseases~National Resource Center. Other nutrients and bone health at a glance. Bethesda (MD): National Institutes of Health 2004. [revised 2001 Oct]. Fact Sheet. Available from: http://www.osteo.org/ orelatdis.asp.

National Institute on Aging. Exercise: a guide from the National Institute on Aging [monograph on the Internet]. Internet ed. Bethesda(MD): The Institute; [revised 2001 Jun; cited 2004 Jan 15]. [86p.] Available from: http://www.niapublications.org/ exercisebook/index.asp.

National Institute on Child Health and Human Development [homepage on the Internet]. Weight-bearing exercise for kids and teens. Bethesda (MD): The Institute; [cited 2004 Feb 15]. Available from: http://www.nichd.nih.gov/ milk/whycal/exercises.cfm.

National Osteoporosis Foundation. Boning up on osteoporosis: a guide to prevention and treatment. Washington, D.C.: National Osteoporosis Foundation; 2003. 74 p.

[a]Nelson, ME. Balance, muscle, bone, fractures. Slide presentation at the Surgeon General's Workshop on Osteoporosis and Bone Health; 2002 Dec 12-13; Washington, D.C.

[b]Nelson, ME. Global recommendations: physical activity in middle-aged and older adults (50+ years of age). In: Report of the Surgeon General's workshop on osteoporosis and bone health; 2002 Dec 12-13; Washington, D.C.

Seguin R, Nelson ME. The benefits of strength training for older adults. Am J Prev Med. 2003 Oct;25(3 Suppl 2):141-9.

Suarez FL, Saviano D, Arbisi P, Levitt MD. Tolerance to the daily ingestion of two cups of milk by individuals claiming lactose intolerance. Am J Clin Nutr 1997 May;65(5): 1502-6.

U.S. Department of Agriculture; U.S. Department of Health and Human Services. Nutrition and your health: dietary guidelines for Americans. 5th ed. Washington, D.C.: The Departments; 2000. 44p. (Home and Garden Bulletin No. 232).

USDA Nutrient Database for Standard Reference [database on the Internet]. U.S. Department of Agriculture (US); [release 15], 2002. Available from: http://www.nal.usda.gov/ fnic/foodcomp/.

U.S. Department of Health and Human Services; National Institutes of Health; National Heart Lung and Blood Institute; National High Blood Pressure Program. Facts about the DASH eating plan. Bethesda (MD): The Institute; 2003. 24p. (NIH Publication No. 03-4082).

U.S. Department of Health and Human Services. Physical activity and health: a report of the Surgeon General. Atlanta (GA): U.S. Department of Health and Human Services, Centers for Disease Control and Prevention, National Center for Chronic Disease Prevention and Health Promotion, President's Council on Physical Fitness and Sports, 1996. 300p.

Weaver CM, Proulx WR, Heaney R. Choices for achieving adequate dietary calcium with a vegetarian diet. Am J Clin Nutr 1999 Sep;70(3 Suppl):543S-548S.

Weinberg LG, Berner LA, Groves JE. Nutrient contributions of dairy foods in the United States, Continuing Survey of Food Intakes by Individuals, 1994-1996, 1998. J Am Diet Assoc 2004 Jun;104(6):895-902.

Whiting SJ, Healey A, Psiuk S, Mirwald R, Kowalski K, Bailey DA. Relationship between carbonated and other low nutrient dense beverages and bone mineral content of adolescents. Nutr Res 2001 Aug;21 (8):1107-15.

Wright JD, Wang CY, Kennedy-Stephenson J, Ervin RB. Dietary intake of ten key nutrients for public health, United States: 1999-2000. Adv Data 2003 Apr 17;(334):1–4.

Part Four

WHAT CAN HEALTH CARE PROFESSIONALS DO TO PROMOTE BONE HEALTH?

This part of the report describes what health care professionals can do with their patients to promote bone health. It seeks to dispel the belief among some health professionals that bone disease and fractures are a natural consequence of aging and that little can be done about it.

Chapter 8 emphasizes the need for health professionals to evaluate potential risk factors for bone disease and to promote bone-healthy behaviors in all patients. The chapter stresses, however, that comprehensive assessments that include diagnostic testing should be focused on those deemed at high risk of bone disease. To assist in this process, the chapter examines the potential risk factors for bone disease, highlights red flags that signal the need for further assessment, and reviews the use of formal assessment tools to determine who should get a bone density test and who is at risk of fracture. It includes real-life vignettes that highlight the need for the medical profession to become aware of the potential for severe osteoporosis to develop in younger men and women.

Chapter 9 focuses on preventive and therapeutic measures for those who have or are at risk for bone disease. It reviews a "pyramid approach" to treating bone diseases and to preventing falls and fractures, with maintenance of bone health through calcium, vitamin D, physical activity, and fall prevention representing the base of the pyramid for all individuals, including those with bone disease. This chapter also covers the second and third levels of the pyramid, which relate to addressing and treating secondary causes of osteoporosis and use of pharmacotherapy in appropriate individuals. One of the key messages of the chapter is that there are effective treatments available that can increase bone mass and/or reduce the risk of fractures for most patients who have or who are at high risk of getting osteoporosis. The chapter reviews the evidence and provides guidance on currently available anti-resorptive therapies, anabolic therapies, and hormone therapies, and offers a glimpse into future directions for treatment of osteoporosis. Finally, the chapter highlights treatment options for other bone diseases that are related to osteoporosis.

Chapter 10 "puts it all together" for health care professionals by translating the research into practical advice for preventing, diagnosing, and treating bone disease in patients of all ages. All health care professionals, especially primary care practitioners, have the opportunity and responsibility to dedicate themselves to promoting awareness of factors that influence bone health, identifying patients at risk of bone disease, and providing lifestyle and pharmacologic interventions where appropriate.

Chapter 8: Key Messages

- Much of the burden of bone disease can potentially be avoided if at-risk individuals are identified and appropriate interventions (both preventive and therapeutic) are made in a timely manner. The evidence suggests that health care providers frequently fail to identify and treat individuals at high risk for future osteoporosis or other disorders of bone, even those who have already had a fracture.

- It is important to evaluate the risks for poor bone health at all ages. Therefore, assessment of calcium and vitamin D intake, physical activity, and adverse behaviors such as smoking should be a routine part of health care for all individuals.

- Those in greatest need should receive a full assessment of bone health. Diagnostic methods are available that can help to identify those in the population who are at highest risk of fracture.

- Both the public and health care professionals need to be aware of a number of known, easy-to-identify risk factors for osteoporosis and other bone diseases.

- Providers should be aware of a number of red flags that might signal potential problems with an individual's bone health at different ages. One of the most important flags is a previous fragility-related fracture.

- While osteoporosis is clearly the most common bone disease, health care providers must also actively look for other bone diseases. Diseases such as hyperparathyroidism, rickets, osteomalacia, and Paget's disease can often be identified by being aware of the warning signs and/or through simple biochemical measurements. Early identification of such diseases is critical, since treatment at an early stage can often be highly effective.

- Bone mineral density or BMD testing should be performed on any patient for whom risk factor analysis indicates a strong potential for osteoporosis. Formal guidelines have been developed recommending BMD testing in certain populations, including postmenopausal women over age 65, younger women with multiple risk factors, and men and women with fragility fractures or who have other diseases or take medications that can greatly increase the risk of fracture.

- Individuals who are diagnosed with osteoporosis should be further assessed for secondary, treatable causes of the disease, particularly men and premenopausal women who suffer a fragility fracture.

Chapter 8

ASSESSING THE RISK OF BONE DISEASE AND FRACTURE

While individuals undoubtedly can do a great deal to enhance their bone health through appropriate lifestyle choices, health care professionals play an important supporting role in helping their patients to maintain strong, healthy bones throughout life. In addition to providing education about nutrition, physical activity, and other bone-healthy behaviors, health care professionals also need to assess the risks of bone disease and fracture in their patients and to identify and intervene with those at greatest risk.

In an optimal health care environment, expensive diagnostic tools and treatment interventions should be targeted at those who are at increased risk of a particular disease or condition. The challenge is to find simple ways to identify individuals in greatest need of more careful assessment. Thus, in contrast to the public health approaches to bone health in areas like nutrition and physical activity (which can be aimed at the entire population), this chapter discusses the tools available to identify and intervene with those in the population who are at highest risk of fracture.

As discussed in previous chapters, osteoporosis and other bone disorders represent a large burden for society and for individuals. Billions of dollars are spent each year to treat bone-disease-related fractures that often result in reduced function and quality of life. At worst, fractures start a downward spiral in health that can ultimately lead to severe disability or even death. Much of this burden can potentially be avoided if individuals who are at risk of bone disease are identified and appropriate interventions (both preventive and therapeutic) are made in a timely manner. Yet there has been relatively little focus on these strategies in this country. There are many studies documenting the failure to identify and treat individuals at high risk for fractures or other disorders of bone, even those who have already had a fracture (Solomon et al. 2003, Andrade et al. 2003, Kiebzak et al. 2002, Kamel et al. 2000, Feldstein et al. 2003). In a recent study of four well-established midwestern health systems, only one-eighth to a quarter of patients who had a hip fracture were tested for their bone density, fewer than a quarter were given calcium and vitamin D supplements, and fewer than one-tenth were treated with effective antiresorptive drugs (Harrington et al. 2002). The failure to diagnose and treat bone disease in many high-risk patients has serious implications, as the risk of future fractures is greatly increased in patients who have had a previous fragility fracture, especially in the first year or two after the fracture (Johnell et al. 2004).

Management of bone disease requires the appropriate application of current knowledge concerning the prevention, diagnosis, and treatment. Those patients who have "healthy" bones should be advised about appropriate steps to take with respect to prevention. Those who are "at risk" for bone disease (e.g., those with low bone mass and other risk factors) should be evaluated further, advised about appropriate prevention, and considered for treatment. Those with established bone disease should be advised about secondary prevention (e.g., ways to avoid first or repeat fractures) and be put on appropriate treatment. They should also be evaluated for so-called "secondary causes"—that is, diseases and drugs that can aggravate or even cause osteoporosis.

None of these activities can occur without implementation of strategies for assessing the risk of bone disease in a given patient. This assessment process helps to "sort" patients into different categories of risk, which in turn helps to determine appropriate next steps with respect to prevention, further diagnosis, and treatment. This chapter describes this assessment process, providing details on the best approaches to assessing bone health and diagnosing bone disease. It is important to remember that all of the many factors that can increase fracture risk should be considered in evaluation of the individual patient.

Step 1: Identify At-Risk Individuals Who Require Further Evaluation

The first step for health care providers in assessing individuals is to identify the relatively small number of younger individuals (out of the majority of individuals who do not have bone disease) who require further evaluation. This initial assessment ensures that more extensive

(and expensive) testing is reserved for those who likely need it. This multi-pronged process is described below.

Consider Potential Risk Factors for Bone Disease

Although there is a great deal more that needs to be discovered about which risk factors are most important for deciding to measure bone mineral density (BMD) in younger men and women (i.e., those for whom BMD is not recommended because of age alone), enough information already exists to dramatically improve diagnosis, prevention, and treatment of bone disease. That information needs to be applied more broadly by health care professionals.

Both the public and health care professionals need to be aware of a number of known, easy-to-identify risk factors for osteoporosis and other bone diseases. These factors relate to either the intrinsic strength of bone or the propensity to suffer injurious falls. Yet it is remarkable how often these signals are ignored in busy practice settings. All individuals, young and old, should be assessed to determine how many (if any) of these risk factors they have, and then those with a sufficient degree of risk need to undergo further evaluation (often a BMD test) to determine the appropriate next course of action (e.g., changes to lifestyle, pharmacologic treatment). If these steps are taken, much can be done to decrease the burden of bone disease in the population, and much illness and suffering can be avoided. This risk factor analysis is also critical in ensuring the efficient use of health care resources, helping to identify those at-risk individuals in need of BMD testing and potentially treatments without the need for expensive, universal screening. Finally, it is important to remember that bone

"Twelve thousand people come through our [health system's] doors with osteoporosis and we never notice them."—Health system physician

Men Can Get Osteoporosis, Too

This story demonstrates the importance of not forgetting that men can also get osteoporosis, even at a relatively young age. It also highlights the need for the medical profession to become aware of the potential for severe osteoporosis to develop in younger men.

This college professor first fractured his ankle as a young man. The doctor told him he might have "a little osteoporosis" and recommended that he take calcium to strengthen his bones, but did not test for osteoporosis. It was not until years later, after many warning signs, that he finally received a bone density test that showed severe osteoporosis. At that time he was placed on bisphosphonates, a treatment that he continues today. The bisphosphonates have helped him to regain some bone density. His BMD is presently stable, albeit at a very low level. Osteoporosis has had a profound effect on his life. He is constantly afraid of falling, and as a result seriously curtails his activities (e.g., he gave up running).

"Where in the heck were the doctors? I had a slew of warning signs but no one picked them up." —Male with severe osteoporosis

Not Just a Disease of the Elderly

This woman's story illustrates the need of the medical profession to be aware of the warning signs of bone disease in younger individuals and to be aware of appropriate treatments for the disease in this population.

This woman began suffering bone fractures while still in her 30s. Even as pain levels increased and her quality of life suffered, her doctor blamed her problems on clumsiness. After she turned 40, her internist attributed her problems to being a natural consequence of "getting old." Finally, after breaking her ankle at age 43, an orthopedist diagnosed osteoporosis. At this point she had lost bone mass and was shorter than earlier in life, probably due to spine fractures. The doctor told her there was no treatment available for osteoporosis. He advised her to take calcium supplements and to exercise, although he provided no guidance on what types of exercises would be helpful and safe. While she had a long list of "don'ts" with respect to her life, she did find that exercise made her feel better. Yet she remained paralyzed with fear, particularly after her physician gave her the following advice: "above all else, don't fall." Today, at age 55, she has finally turned the corner on the disease. Thanks to medical treatment, calcium supplements, and exercise, her bone mass has improved. She is no longer considered to have osteoporosis, but rather is classified as osteopenic (i.e., she has low bone mass).

"People with osteoporosis do not just die; they slowly break apart."
—Long-time osteoporosis sufferer

health can be compromised at any age, and thus the risks for poor bone health should be evaluated in individuals of all ages. Assessment of calcium and vitamin D intake, physical activity, and adverse behaviors such as smoking should be part of health care for all.

Be Aware of "Red Flags" That Signal Need for Further Evaluation

There are a number of "red flags" that might signal potential problems with an individual's bone health at different ages. Specific problems at different stages of life are discussed in Chapter 10. These "red flags" apply to both men and women. Indeed they may be particularly important to keep in mind in men and Black women, since they are often not considered to be at high risk for bone disease. One of the most important flags is a previous fragility-related fracture, as such a fracture is one of the strongest indicators that an individual may have osteoporosis or some other metabolic bone disease (Ettinger et al. 2003, Haentjens et al. 2003). Any individual with a history of fractures related to only mild or moderate trauma (e.g., a fall from standing height or less) should be assessed further for the potential for bone disease. Yet most are not adequately evaluated today. Another important flag relates to family history of the disease, since there is a component of heredity not only in osteoporosis, but also in Paget's disease and hyperparathyroidism as well as congenital disorders such as osteogenesis imperfecta. Thus, both the public and health care professionals should be alert to looking for other family members who have bone disease. This type of family case finding can and should lead to earlier diagnosis and treatment. The presence of certain bone diseases (e.g., Paget's disease) should be a flag for other family members to be screened, or for screening for associated disorders

(e.g., a patient with hyperparathyroidism who has other family members with the disease should undergo genetic screening for other associated endocrine disorders, such as multiple endocrine neoplasia syndromes, familial conditions in which patients may develop tumors of several endocrine glands).

"Red Flags" That Warrant Further Assessment for Osteoporosis or Other Bone Diseases

- History of fractures related to mild or moderate trauma (e.g., a fall from standing height or less)
- Family history of bone disease
- Low body weight
- Weight loss of more than 1 percent per year in the elderly
- Late onset of sexual development
- Unusual cessation of menstrual periods
- Anorexia nervosa (often related to marked weight reduction)
- Athletic amenorrhea syndrome (related to intense physical activity)
- Patients being treated with drugs that affect bone metabolism (e.g., glucocorticoids)
- Patients with diseases linked to secondary osteoporosis (see Chapter 3)
- High levels of serum calcium or alkaline phosphatase in otherwise healthy patients
- Hyperparathyroidism, hyperthyroidism, or treatment with high doses of thyroid hormone
- Height loss or progressive spinal curvature

Low body weight is another important "red flag" signaling the potential for osteoporosis; low body weight is associated with lower BMD and greater bone loss, even in premenopausal women (Bainbridge et al. 2004). Moreover, weight loss of more than 1 percent per year in the elderly is associated with more rapid bone loss and increased risk of fracture (Hannan et al. 2000, Knoke et al. 2003, Ensrud et al. 2003).

There are other potential flags as well. While bone disease is rare in children, the possibility of congenital disorders should be considered when children fracture, particularly with little trauma. In adolescents, health care professionals should consider abnormalities of sex hormone function, particularly at puberty, to be a potential risk factor, along with late onset of sexual development or loss of sexual function with cessation of menstrual periods. This is often related to marked weight reduction, in anorexia nervosa, or to intense physical activity, in the athletic amenorrhea syndrome. Individuals of all ages with calcium and vitamin D deficiency or prolonged immobilization and paralysis should also be carefully evaluated, as should those who have other diseases that increase the risk of bone loss and fractures, including gastrointestinal and kidney disorders and arthritis. Those patients being treated with drugs that affect bone metabolism (e.g., glucocorticoids) should also be considered as potentially being at risk. Finally, patients already diagnosed with osteoporosis should be screened for secondary, treatable causes of the disease, especially in men or premenopausal women who suffer fragility fractures. Diseases linked to secondary osteoporosis (see Chapter 3) are relatively uncommon in the population, but they can have a devastating effect on the bone health of the patients with these conditions and consequently may require specific treatment.

It is important to remember that not all the "red flags" point to osteoporosis, and that some may be an indicator of other types of bone disease. It is important to look for these diseases. For example, increased levels of serum calcium and alkaline phosphatase in blood are often found by routine screening, yet abnormal values are often ignored (Murff et al. 2003). High serum calcium concentration in an otherwise healthy patient most often indicates primary hyperparathyroidism, although many other causes of hypercalcemia need to be considered. Low serum calcium concentrations are less common but can occur in individuals with vitamin D deficiency and malabsorption. Hypocalcemia is also commonly seen in seriously ill patients and frequently is associated with increased severity of illness or death. Apparent hypocalcemia can be due to low serum protein concentrations, and hypercalcemia can be masked by such low concentrations. Patients with Paget's disease are often identified by the finding of a high serum alkaline phosphatase before there is evidence of bone pain or before the skeletal lesions have actually been detected. (Elevated serum alkaline phosphatase levels are often caused by other problems, particularly liver disease.) Such findings are important because treatment can be highly effective for these and other bone disorders if they are diagnosed early.

Suspicion of vitamin D deficiency (e.g., due to low intake, little exposure to sunshine) is another "red flag" that signals the need for further evaluation. This deficiency is common in the elderly, particularly individuals living in northern latitudes. Assessment of vitamin D deficiency can be accomplished by measuring the most abundant circulating form, 25-hydroxy vitamin D. This measurement should be carried out in individuals who are at high risk of deficiency, including those with evidence of gastrointestinal disorders that might result in malabsorption. Measurement of serum phosphorus is generally not critical in assessing bone health, but if the levels are low this may be an indication of hyperparathyroidism or vitamin D deficiency. Finally, high blood calcium levels can serve as a "red flag" that potentially indicates primary hyperparathyroidism, and PTH should be measured in all such patients. PTH measurements are also helpful in assessing the extent of secondary hyperparathyroidism in patients with calcium and/or vitamin D deficiency and in those with renal disease.

Consider Use of a Formal Assessment Tool to Determine the Need for BMD Testing

BMD testing still serves as the "gold standard" diagnostic test for identifying osteoporosis and fracture risk. As noted, population-wide BMD testing is not a cost-effective or practical method for assessing the risk of bone disease. While BMD testing has been recommended for some populations (women over age 65), BMD tests are not routinely used for other individuals, the vast majority of whom do not have and are not at risk for bone disease. Widespread BMD testing makes little economic or medical sense. Rather, as noted, the evidence supports the assessment of other risk factors first, in order to identify a subset of at-risk individuals who are most likely to benefit from the test (e.g., younger women with multiple risk factors and both men and women who have had fragility fractures or who have diseases that can greatly increase fracture risk). Some of these risk factors may act directly or indirectly to affect BMD levels, but others are independent of bone density (e.g., risk factors for falling).

Existing clinical recommendations (NOF 2003) already make use of universally accepted risk factors, such as gender, age, and history of spine fracture, in determining who should get BMD testing. Since age is a major determinant of fracture risk, many groups have recommended that BMD measurements be obtained in all White women over age 65 (age is a risk factor, see Figure 8-1) and for younger postmenopausal women with additional risk factors. It is interesting to note that treatment recommendations are also based on these risk factors, as treatment is recommended not only for those with low BMD, but also for those with an existing (especially recent) low-trauma spine fracture, regardless of BMD.

There is great interest in developing a screening tool or "clinical prediction rule" based on risk factors that can easily be assessed clinically (e.g., height and weight) or by patient report (e.g., personal or family history of fracture). The goal of a risk factor assessment tool is to produce a more individualized approach to diagnosis and treatment for all age, gender, and ethnic groups. Ideally, nurses and other nonphysician health care professionals should be able to administer the tool (e.g., by having a patient fill out a short questionnaire) and interpret the results, thus allowing someone other than the busy physician to play a lead role in identifying at-risk individuals.

A number of risk-factor assessment tools are in various stages of development. While there are some problems and limitations with each of these tools (see text box), progress is being made. The National Osteoporosis Foundation (NOF) checklist, for example, may be suitable for individual self-assessment. Individuals can use this checklist and discuss any concerns about their bone health at their next medical encounter. The Osteoporosis Risk Assessment Instrument (ORAI) calculates scores based on age, weight, and current estrogen use; it has a sensitivity of 93 percent—i.e., it identifies 93 percent of the people with low BMD—and specificity of 39 percent—i.e., 61 percent of the people identified

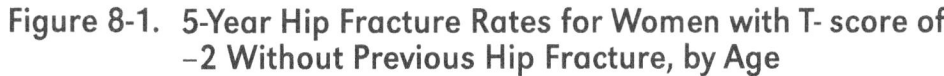

Figure 8-1. 5-Year Hip Fracture Rates for Women with T- score of
–2 Without Previous Hip Fracture, by Age

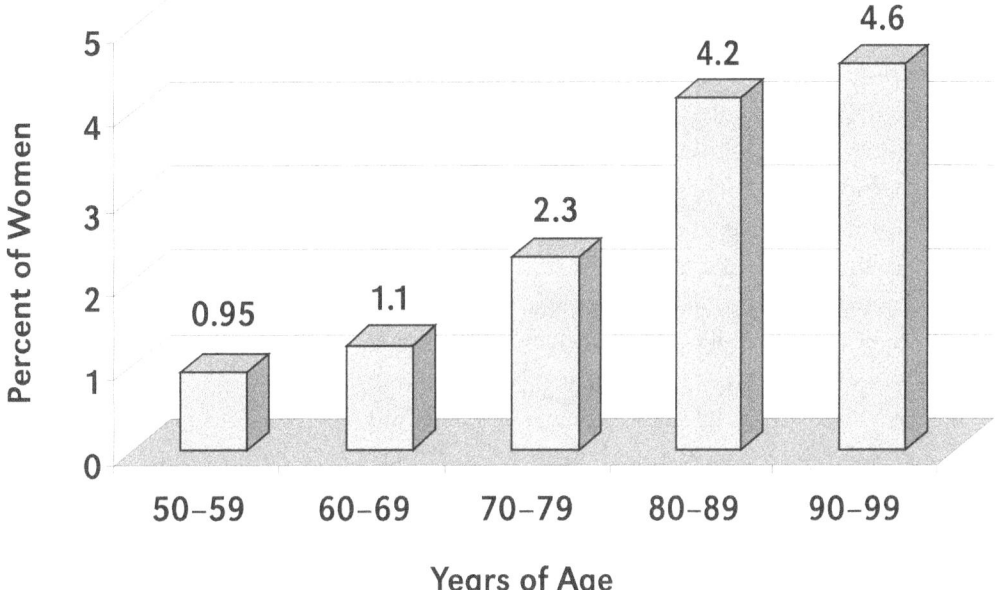

Note: This figure shows that a 90-year-old woman with a T- score of –2 has a 4.6-fold higher risk of having a hip fracture than a 50-year-old woman with the same T-score. Age is an important and independent determinant of fracture risk.

Source: Adapted from Nelson et al. 2001.

do not have low BMD (Cadarette et al. 2000; Cadarette et al. 2004). The Simple Calculated Osteoporosis Risk Estimation (SCORE) considers six risk factors—age, race, weight, estrogen use, rheumatoid arthritis, and personal fracture history—and has a sensitivity of 91 percent and specificity of 40 percent (Lydick et al. 1998), results that are quite similar to the ORAI tool. The Osteoporosis Self-Assessment Tool (OST) uses only two risk factors—age and weight—and also has similar sensitivity (92 percent) and higher specificity (46 percent) (Geusens et al. 2002, Richy et al. 2004, Cadarette et al. 2004). A score based on age, body weight, and fracture history was recently developed from the Dubbo Osteoporosis Epidemiology Study; it performed well in predicting low BMD, but not fractures (Nguyen et al. 2004). Finally, NOF

Problems and Limitations With Existing Tools

Some problems and limitations have slowed the development and widespread application of risk-factor assessment tools. One important issue relates to limitations of current medical knowledge about risk factors for bone health. While epidemiologic (large population) studies have established the importance of age, gender, and ethnic characteristics as important clinical predictors, there is still considerable uncertainty about which clinical characteristics to include in a risk-factor assessment tool. An important problem stems from limitations in the studies evaluating risk factors; they have been relatively well studied in older (over age 65) White women, but less well studied in other groups. It is possible that the importance of particular factors may differ between women and men, people of different races, and younger and older individuals. To date, the generally accepted risk factors for bone loss account for only one-third to one-fifth of the differences in BMD between individuals (Orwoll et al. 1996). Thus, it is clear that important risk factors remain to be discovered. In fact, one potential risk factor that has not been included in any of these instruments is height loss. While loss of height and curvature of the spine may not be related to bone health (they can be caused by poor posture, decreased muscle strength, or narrowing of the intervertebral discs (Ettinger et al. 1994, Coles et al. 1994, Balzini et al. 2003), they could be a sign of osteoporosis. Substantial height loss (more than one inch) and new spinal curvature should serve as a red flag that alerts health care providers to the possibility of vertebral compression fractures (Huang et al. 1996, Ensrud et al. 1997, Vogt et al. 2000). Providers should also consider tracking changes in height as a means of monitoring the impact of preventive and therapeutic measures for osteoporosis. One problem with this approach is that height loss is difficult to assess because an individual's memory of previous height can often be inaccurate, as can current height measurements. To overcome this problem, the use of specific devices for accurate measurement of height and spinal curvature (stadiometers and kyphometers) may be appropriate in specialty clinics.

practice guidelines consider age, weight, current cigarette smoking status, family history of fracture, and personal fracture history, but have not defined any specific scoring system (Johnston et al. 1998). Any of these approaches might be used in clinical practice to determine who would benefit from BMD testing. Examples of some of the most simple and useful of these tools appear in Chapter 10, including those that a busy clinician or patient could use to assess risk factors and determine if a BMD test is indicated.

Efforts have also begun to expand clinical risk assessment tools beyond the question of who should get a BMD test. Tools are being developed to assess not just the risk of low BMD, but also the risk for fractures (which is ultimately what we are trying to prevent). Individuals identified as having a high risk of fracture can be targeted for early intervention. A recently developed tool allows for a more global assessment of risk factors. The risk factors used to develop this tool were derived from the large "Study of Osteoporotic Fractures" (Cummings et al. 1995). This study identified numerous risk factors for hip fracture in elderly White women that are independent of BMD or personal fracture history (see Table 8-1). These risk factors relate to genetic influences on bone size (e.g., maternal fracture history) and bone turnover, lifestyle issues (e.g., exercise), height loss, weight changes, and other factors. These risk factors have been proven to be important in identifying fracture risk. For example, patients whose BMD was in the lowest third of the study population had about 4.6 times the risk of suffering a hip fracture risk as did women whose BMD was in the highest third. However, hip fracture risk was 17 times greater among the 15 percent of the women who had five or more risk factors (exclusive of bone density) than the 47 percent of the women with two or fewer risk factors (Cummings et al. 1995) (Figure 8-2).

Black et al. (2001) turned the most prevalent risk factors derived from the SOF study into a questionnaire that can be administered to patients (see Table 8-2). By assigning a point value to each of the answers, a summary FRACTURE score is developed. The usefulness of this questionnaire was tested in a large, prospective European study known as EPIDOS. As shown in Figure 8-3, individuals with a higher FRACTURE score had a much higher risk of suffering a hip fracture. It is important to remember, however, that this and other approaches to measuring the risk of fracture may not work as well in certain populations; some of the predictors of fracture for nursing home residents are different than those living in the community. For example, the risk of falling is especially critical in elderly nursing home residents, most of whom have fragile bones (Girman et al. 2002).

Table 8-1. Risk Factors for Hip Fracture Among Elderly White Women

Variable	Percent Increased Risk
Age (per 5 yr)	40%
History of maternal hip fracture	80%
Height at age 25 (per 6 cm loss)	30%
Previous hyperthyroidism	70%
Current use of long-acting benzodiazepines	60%
Current use of anticonvulsant drugs	100%
Inability to rise from chair	70%
Lowest quartile for depth perception (in vision)	40%
Resting pulse rate greater than 80 beats/min	70%
Any fracture since age of 50	50%

Note: The increases in risk for fracture listed here are from the Study of Osteoporotic Fractures and are all significant. The numbers indicate how much greater the chance of having a fracture is likely to be when these factors are present. Other risk factors have been identified in subsequent studies, for example, weight loss increases the risk of fracture in the elderly (Ensrud et al. 2003).

Source: Based on Cummings et al. 1995.

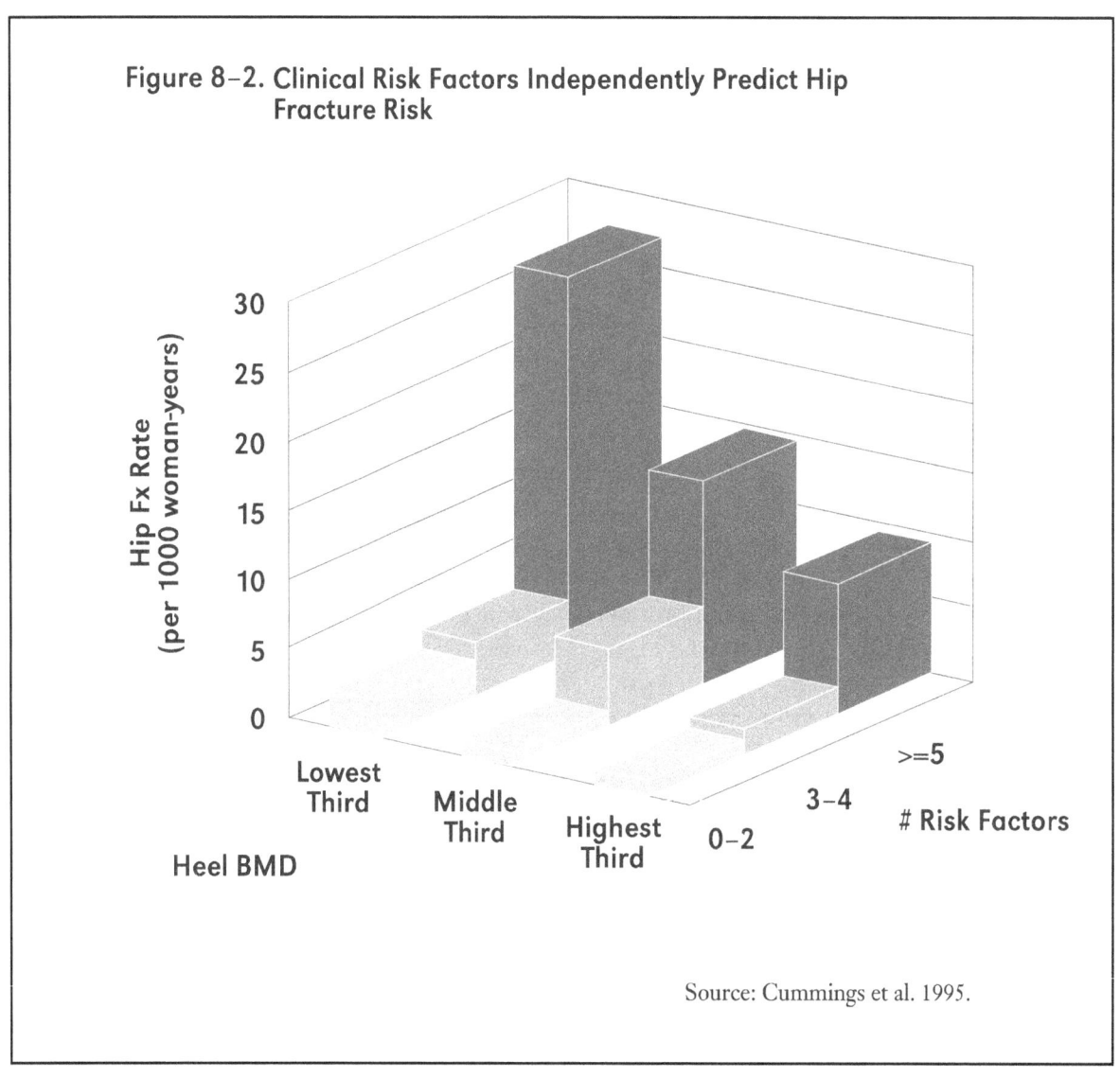

Figure 8–2. Clinical Risk Factors Independently Predict Hip Fracture Risk

Source: Cummings et al. 1995.

One of the most important needs going forward with respect to risk assessment tools is to incorporate the risk of falling into the system, since so many fragility-related fractures occur as a direct result of a fall. Risk factors for falling include visual or cognitive impairment, use of specific medications, and gait and balance disorders. Poor vision is a particularly important risk factor for the elderly (even those with glasses), since many elderly individuals do not have their eyes and glasses checked regularly.

Although high-technology testing of gait and balance are available, these have not been found to be clinically useful as a way to assess the risk of falling. Rather, clinicians rely on patient reports (e.g., prior falls [Nevitt et al. 1991], fear of falling [Tinetti et al. 1994]) and objective examination (e.g., Performance-Oriented Mobility Assessment [Tinetti 1986], Functional Reach [Duncan et al. 1992]). It is important to remember that while any fall should be investigated carefully, those falls

Table 8–2. FRACTURE Index Questions and Scoring

Figure 8–3. Five-Year Risk of Hip Fracture by Quintiles of FRACTURE Index

	Point Value
1. What is your current age?	
Less than 65	0
65–69	1
70–74	2
75–79	3
80–84	4
85 or older	5
2. Have you broken any bones after age 50?	
Yes	1
No/Don't know	0
3. Has your mother had a hip fracture after age 50?	
Yes	1
No/Don't know	0
4. Do you weigh 125 pounds or less?	
Yes	1
No	0
5. Are you currently a smoker?	
Yes	1
No	0
6. Do you usually need to use your arms to assist yourself in standing up from a chair?	
Yes	2
No/Don't know	0

If you have a current bone density (BMD) assessment, then answer the next question.

7. BMD results: Total Hip T-score	
T–score >-1	0
T–score between –1 and –2	2
T–score between –2 and –2.5	3
T–score <-2.5	4

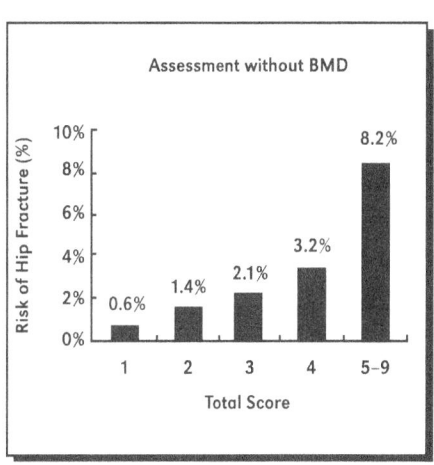

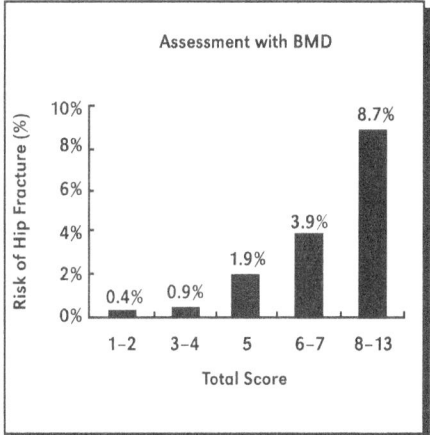

Note: This FRACTURE Index scoring system places a quantitative value on an individual's risk of fracture; the higher the score, the greater the fracture risk. It was developed from the data of 9704 U.S. white women in the Study of Osteoporotic Fractures and then tested against the EPIDOS database of 7575 French women. As shown in Figure 8-4, the index was predictive of fracture even without BMD, although adding BMD improved the discrimination to some extent. When applied to the EPIDOS data, the discrimination was even greater, for example, the five year fracture risk went from 0.6% for scores of 2–5 to 14.1% for scores of 11-14.

Source: Black et al. 2001.

that lead to fractures are the biggest concern. Individuals who have sustained a fracture as a result of minimal trauma likely do not need further evaluation by BMD testing to be considered in the high-risk category for bone disease and future fractures.

Those individuals who are identified as being both at risk of bone disease and at high risk of a fall might become candidates for further intervention, including exercise programs to improve strength and balance, modifications to the home environment, changes in medications that might make one prone to fall, and use of hip protectors to "cushion the blow" from a fall. (See Chapter 9 for more on hip protectors.)

Step 2: Measuring Bone Mineral Density (BMD) for Individuals at Risk of Osteoporosis

Once a high-risk patient is identified (step 1), further evaluation of that patient is warranted. This section deals with this evaluation process for those at risk of osteoporosis—the most common bone disease.

Why Measure BMD?

BMD testing remains the "gold standard" test for those at risk of osteoporosis. The reason for this is relatively straightforward—in the laboratory, bone strength is strongly related to BMD. More importantly, BMD remains a strong independent predictor of fracture risk. In fact, there is a clear relationship between BMD and fracture risk in older women. For each standard deviation decrease in BMD (in the spine, a one-standard deviation drop represents a loss of 10–12 percent of BMD), the risk of fracture increases by 1.5–2.5 times. The relationship between BMD and fracture is stronger than the relationship between cholesterol and heart attack, and as strong as the relationship between blood pressure and stroke (Marshall et al. 1996).

BMD measurement can be used to assess fracture risk and to establish the diagnosis and severity of osteoporosis. BMD testing can be used to assess changes over time (monitoring) in treated and untreated individuals. (It is important to note that while standard x-rays are used to diagnose fractures, they are not useful for measuring bone mass. It is estimated that one must lose 30 percent of BMD for bone loss to be noted on x-ray; furthermore, an improperly performed x-ray in a normal person may have the appearance of bone loss.)

Who Should Have a Bone Density Test and When

As noted earlier, an analysis of risk factors can be helpful in determining who should or should not get a BMD. Risk factors for bone disease and fractures are still not fully understood, especially for younger individuals, males, and non-Whites. In an effort to summarize general conclusions about what is and is not known, a variety of organizations, including government agencies and professional societies, have made attempts to develop guidelines on who should have a bone density test and when. This section reviews those recommendations.

Recommendations for Osteoporosis Screening and for Other Bone Diseases

There is general consensus that all women age 65 and older should have a BMD test, and that women at-risk of bone disease who are under age 65 should also be screened (although there is not universal agreement on what defines "at-risk" status). At present there are no differences in these recommendations across racial and ethnic groups. The U.S. Preventive Services Task Force (USPSTF) recommends bone density screening for all women age 65 and older and for younger postmenopausal women age 60–64 who are at high risk (body weight less than

70 kilograms, no current use of estrogen) (U.S. Preventive Services Task Force 2002). Risk factors that should also be considered include smoking, weight loss, family history, decreased physical activity, alcohol or caffeine use, or low calcium and vitamin D intake. The NOF also recommends testing women age 65 and older, and emphasizes four common and easily assessable risk factors that would justify screening in younger postmenopausal women:

- a family history of osteoporosis;
- a personal history of low-trauma fracture after age 45;
- current cigarette smoking; and
- low body weight (under 127 pounds) (NOF 2003).

The NOF also recommends BMD testing for men who present with fractures or are receiving treatment with a GNRH agonist for prostate cancer, as well as for all individuals who have primary hyperparathyroidism or are on long-term glucocorticoid treatment (National Osteoporosis Foundation 2002). The ISCD agrees with screening all women age 65 and older and also recommends screening healthy men starting at age 70, with earlier testing for men who are at high risk of osteoporosis or fracture (Binkley et al. 2002).

BMD testing should also be performed on any individual who has other potential risk factors for osteoporosis, especially anyone who has had a low-trauma fracture or who exhibit another clinical indication of osteoporosis (e.g., x-ray evidence of low bone mass), as well as those who have diseases or conditions known to cause increased bone loss (e.g., hyperthyroidism [increased activity of the thyroid gland in the neck], hyperparathyroidism [increased activity of the parathyroid gland in the neck], rheumatoid arthritis, certain diseases of the stomach or intestines, long-term menstrual irregularities,

Who Should Have a BMD Test?
- U.S. Preventive Services Task Force Guidelines
  ~ All women age 65 and older
  ~ Women between age 60–64 who are at high risk (body weight less than 70 kilograms, no current hormone therapy)
- National Osteoporosis Foundation Guidelines
  ~ All women age 65 and older
  ~ Postmenopausal women under age 65 with:
  ~ Family history of osteoporosis
  ~ Personal history of low-trauma fracture after age 45
  ~ Current cigarette smoking
  ~ Low body weight (less than 127 pounds)
- Other Clinical Recommendations
  ~ Low-trauma fractures as an adult
  ~ Hyperthyroidism
  ~ Hyperparathyroidism
  ~ Vitamin D deficiency (osteomalacia)
  ~ Rheumatoid arthritis
  ~ Medications that cause bone loss (glucocorticoids, excessive doses of thyroid hormone, medications used to treat seizures, medications that block sex hormone production)
  ~ Diseases that cause poor intestinal absorption

cessation of menstrual bleeding) and those who are using a medication that may cause increased bone loss (e.g., glucocorticoids, excessive doses of thyroid hormone, certain blood thinners, certain drugs that treat seizures, drugs that block sex hormone production) (Leib et al. 2004).

Methods for Measuring BMD

The most widely accepted method for measuring BMD is dual x-ray absorptiometry (DXA). DXA is very safe, as it involves levels of radiation that are lower than that derived from daily background radiation from the sky when taking a trans-Atlantic airplane flight, and much lower than those from undergoing an x-ray of the back. DXA measures BMD in the spine and hip, sites that are likely to fracture in patients who have osteoporosis (see Figures 8-4 and 8-5). These central skeletal sites are also most appropriate for monitoring the effectiveness of therapy, as they are more likely than peripheral sites to show an increase in BMD in response to treatment. DXA is precise and permits monitoring of patients over time. DXA also can be used to measure bone density in the forearm and whole body.

Several other techniques are available for bone mass measurement and are described briefly below (Genant et al. 1996, Grampp et al. 1997) (Table 8-3). While these methods do assess bone density and may provide an indication of fracture risk, it is important to note that the WHO recommendations and other guidelines for using BMD and interpreting BMD results for diagnosis (see next section for more details)

Figure 8-4. Bone Mineral Density (BMD) Measurements at Spine and Hip

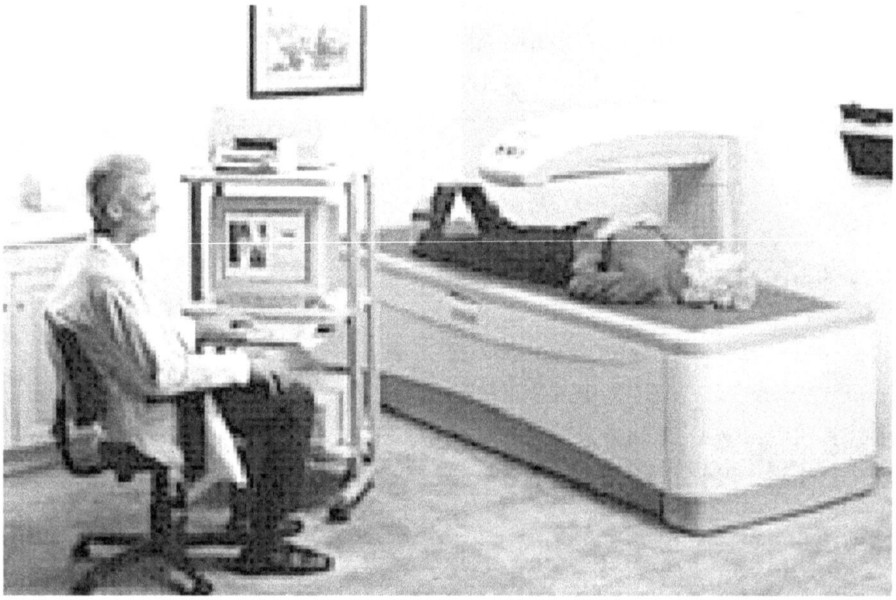

Source: Black 2002.

are based on DXA measurements of the hip or spine. In the future, these alternative tests may be further refined and others may be developed, thus improving the ability to identify individuals at risk of osteoporosis.

- Peripheral DXA (pDXA) uses scaled-down DXA instrumentation to measure peripheral sites such as the forearm, heel, or finger. These tests can help to identify

at-risk individuals who are most likely to benefit from further BMD testing. Using the test for this purpose is tricky, requiring the setting of a proper threshold for determining who needs further evaluation. A too-low threshold could prove ineffective in screening, with the result being that many healthy individuals undergo further (expensive)

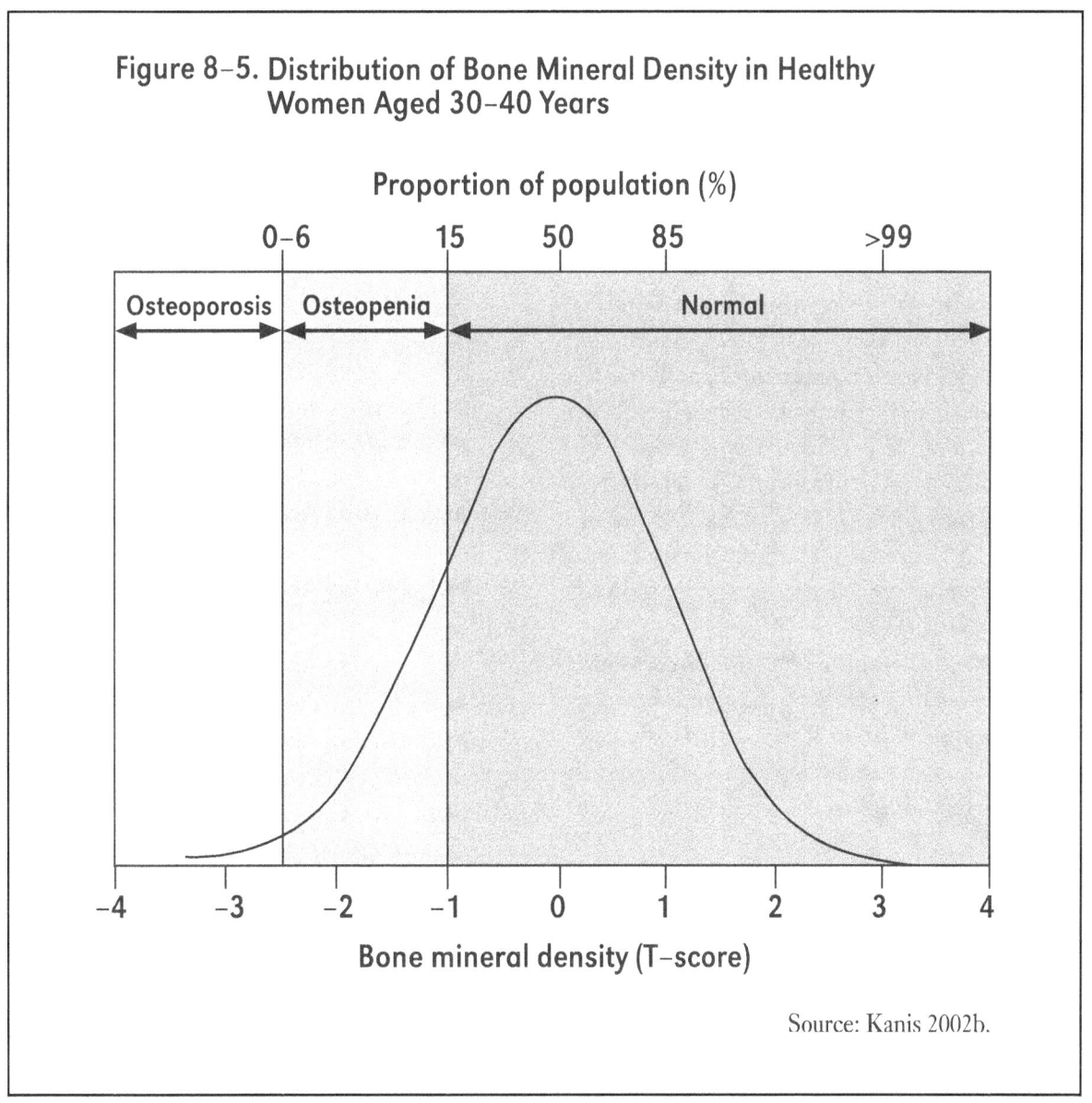

Figure 8–5. Distribution of Bone Mineral Density in Healthy Women Aged 30–40 Years

Source: Kanis 2002b.

evaluation. A too-high threshold could result in at-risk individuals being "screened out" and thus failing to receive further evaluation that could have resulted in timely diagnosis and treatment of bone disease. At present there is no scoring system for peripheral DXA that has been found to be preferable to using risk factor analysis as a means of determining who should and should not undergo DXA of the spine and hip.

- Peripheral quantitative computed tomography (pQCT) uses specialized equipment to measure cortical bone (the outer, more solid shell of bone) and cancellous bone (the inner, honeycomb-like bone) in the forearm. This technique is used primarily for research.

- Quantitative computed tomography (QCT) uses standard computed tomography equipment, usually with a phantom that must be scanned with the patient. It provides a true volumetric measurement of cancellous bone density in the spine. Although it involves greater radiation exposure, it may be used as an alternative to spine and hip DXA measurements.

- Quantitative ultrasound (QUS) uses sound waves to assess bone mass and thus does not use radiation. It can be used to measure bone in a variety of peripheral sites, such as the heel, tibia (leg), radius (wrist), and finger. Ultrasound devices measure the speed of sound (SOS), as well as specific changes in sound waves (i.e., broadband attenuation or BUA) as the sound waves pass through bone. Most devices use a formula to calculate a bone density equivalent or "T-score equivalent."

- Radiogrammetry uses measurements derived from standard x-rays of the hand to determine an index that compares cortical thickness with the total bone width in the mid-shaft of at least two metacarpal (palm) bones.

- Radiographic absorptiometry (RA), also called photodensitometry, uses a standard x-ray of the hand to measure density in the middle bones of the second, third, and fourth fingers. Specialized equipment is used to scan the film at high resolution, and special software is used to calculate bone volume and bone density. The cortical thickness of the bones also can be measured.

- Single x-ray absorptiometry (SXA) is used to measure peripheral sites such as the heel and forearm. The body part being measured is immersed in a water bath or water equivalent device. The SXA picture is similar to that obtained with DXA technology.

Incorporating these techniques for bone assessment into future clinical trials and observational studies will help in better understanding their appropriate use as a means of predicting the risk of bone disease and fracture.

Using and Interpreting BMD Measurements

BMD in young healthy adults is normally distributed as shown in Figure 8-5. An individual's BMD can be compared to the mean value in a reference population, such as young healthy adults. The difference between an individual's BMD and the mean BMD for the reference population can be expressed in standard deviation (SD) units; a score of 0 indicates BMD equal to the mean; a score of $+1$ indicates one standard deviation above the mean,

Table 8-3. Techniques for Bone Mass Measurement

Technique	Skeletal sites that can be measured	Time to measure	Radiation exposure (μSv)
DXA	Lumbar spine (PA view) Lumbar spine (lateral view) Proximal femur (hip) Forearm Total body	5–10 minutes	1–7
pDXA	Forearm, heel	<5 minutes	<1
pQCT	Forearm	< 5 minutes	<1
QCT	Lumbar spine	5–10 minutes	50–60
QUS	Heel, forearm, finger, tibia	< 5 minutes	none
Radiogrammetry	Finger	< 5 minutes	< 1
RA	Finger	< 5 minutes	< 1
SXA	Forearm, heel	< 5 minutes	1

Abbreviations: μSv, microsieverts; DXA, dual x ray absorptiometry; pDXA, peripheral dual x ray absorptiometry; pQCT, peripheral quantitative computed tomography; QCT, quantitative computed tomography; QUS, quantitative ultrasound; RA, radiographic absorptiometry; SXA, single x ray absorptiometry.

and a score of -1 is one standard deviation below. When an individual's BMD is compared to the mean BMD score in a young healthy population, this standard deviation measurement is referred to as a T-score. The T-score is calculated using the following formula:

T-Score

$$\frac{\text{Patient's BMD} - \text{Young Normal Mean}}{\text{Standard Deviation of Young Normal Mean}}$$

In 1994, a working group of the World Health Organization developed a classification system for osteoporosis based on BMD using the known gradient of the risk of fracture in the population as a whole. They sought to define osteoporosis using BMD so that the proportion of individuals identified as having osteoporosis by this method would be related to the lifetime risk of fracture in the population. Four general diagnostic categories were proposed for assessments done with DXA (Kanis 1994, Kanis 2002b):

- Normal: Hip BMD that is no more than 1 standard deviation below the young adult female reference mean (T-score greater than -1).
- Low bone mass (osteopenia): Hip BMD that is between 1–2.5 standard deviations below the young adult female mean (T-score less than -1 and greater than -2.5).
- Osteoporosis: Hip BMD that is 2.5 standard deviations or more below the young adult female mean (T-score less than -2.5).
- Severe osteoporosis (established osteoporosis): Hip BMD that is 2.5 standard deviations or more below the young adult mean in the presence of one or more fragility fractures.

In the young healthy population shown in Figure 8-5, about 15 percent of the women have a T-score of less than -1 and thus have low bone mass or osteopenia, while about 0.5 percent of women fall into the osteoporotic range, with a T-score of -2.5 or less. The proportion of women affected by osteoporosis increases with age as average bone density declines (Figure 8-6) and risk of fracture increases.

If there were only a single device for measuring BMD, and only a single skeletal site that was measured, absolute BMD, in g/cm2, could be used. However, it is difficult for clinicians to remember ideal or threshold cut-off points for absolute BMD levels as measured by a single type of machine at various locations, including the spine and hip, let alone remember the values for different types of machines that are calibrated (standardized) differently. The T-score provides a way to use a single set of numbers for all devices and all skeletal sites.

Another way of expressing BMD is the Z-score, which compares an individual with age-, gender-, and ethnicity-matched norms. Z-scores are not used for diagnosis because a person's Z-score can remain constant throughout life, even as BMD declines with age. However, the Z-score is useful in determining how an individual's BMD compares with what is expected for a person of a given age and body size. Although all patients with osteoporosis deserve at least a limited evaluation for secondary causes (i.e., not age-related) of bone loss, patients with a low Z-score (i.e., BMD significantly lower than expected for age and size) are particularly in need of an in-depth evaluation for secondary causes of osteoporosis. Z-scores are also useful in children to determine how their bone density compares to that of their peers. Since they have not reached adult peak bone mass, T-scores should not be used for children. Figure 8-7 is a graphical illustration of T-scores and Z-scores.

Figure 8–6. Distribution of Bone Mineral Density in Women of Different Ages, and the Prevalence of Osteoporosis (Shaded Area). T–score Below –2.5 = Osteoporosis

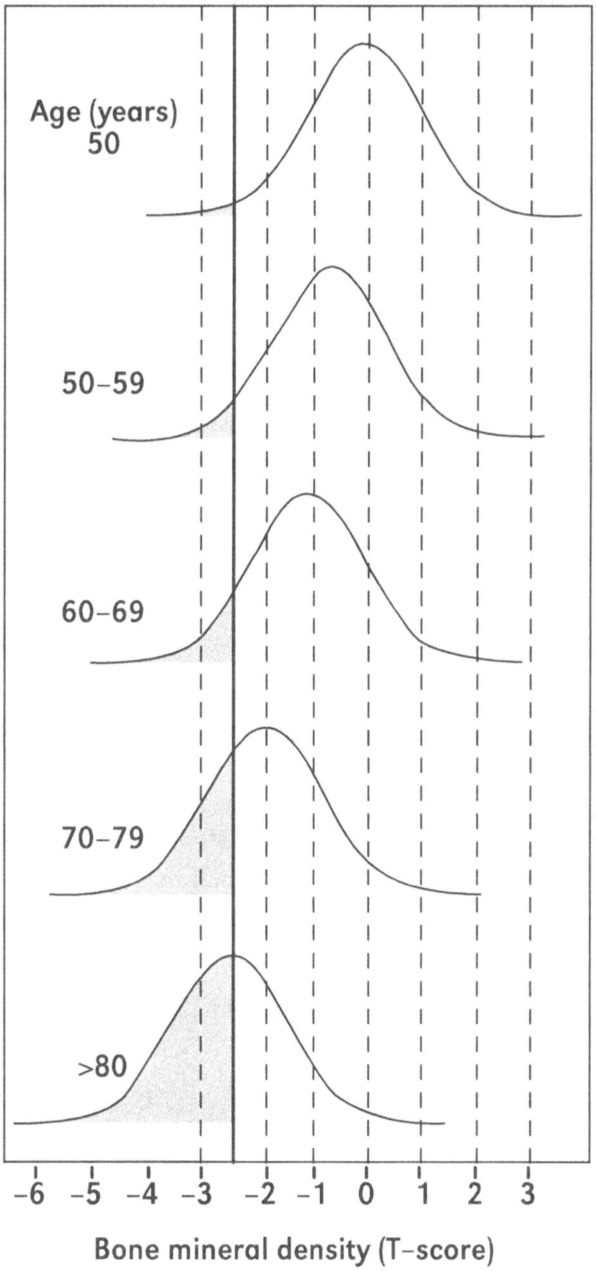

Source: Kanis 2002b.

The WHO classification was derived from studies of White postmenopausal women and applies to them, but not for men, premenopausal women, or non-White postmenopausal women. In general, men have a higher bone mass than do women of the same age, and Black men and women have higher bone mass do White men and women of the same age (Finkelstein et al. 2002, Looker 2002). Although controversial, the International Society for Clinical Densitometry (ISCD) recommends use of a single normative database (i.e., not adjusted for ethnicity) to calculate T-scores in non-White as well as White postmenopausal women, and use of a male normative database to calculate T-scores for men (Binkley et al. 2002). There are no official recommendations for the BMD standard deviation values that should be used to diagnose osteoporosis in men, premenopausal women, or children. The ISCD emphasizes that the diagnosis of osteoporosis in men, premenopausal women, and children should not be made on the basis of BMD alone (Leib et al. 2004). In fact, a Canadian panel of ISCD has developed guidelines for the diagnosis of osteoporosis in premenopausal women, men, and children (Kahn et al. 2004). This panel recommended that BMD measurements be used only in patients with fragility fractures or major secondary causes of bone loss. The panel also recommended that Z-scores, not T-scores, be used in children and pre-menopausal women. Finally, the panel recommended that the terms osteopenia and osteoporosis not be used for children, since the WHO criteria do not apply to them.

Not everyone with low BMD has osteoporosis; osteomalacia and other bone disorders should also be considered. In addition, as noted previously, low bone density is not the only risk factor for fracture; other factors include age, risk of falling, risk of injury, previous low-trauma fracture, family history of osteoporosis, etc. (see section on Risk Factor Analysis).

The National Osteoporosis Foundation (NOF) and the ISCD recommend using DXA to measure BMD in both the hip and spine and classifying the patient based on the lowest T-score of these measurements (Hamdy et al. 2002, NOF 2003). ISCD recommends using the mean score for the L-1 to L-4 vertebrae to calculate spine BMD and that vertebrae affected by local structural artifacts be excluded from this calculation (Leib et al. 2004). The U.S. Preventive Services Task Force and the Agency for Healthcare Research and Quality (Nelson et al. 2002) state that BMD at the femoral neck is the best predictor of hip fracture and is comparable to spine or forearm BMD for predicting fractures at other sites. ISCD recommends using forearm BMD for obese patients in whom the spine and hip measurements cannot be obtained (Leib et al. 2004).

Finally, when interpreting scores, it is important to remember that DXA measures areal density by calculating grams per square centimeter (bone mineral content divided by area), in contrast to "true" measures of density, which involve volumetric measurement). As a result, DXA underestimates the density of small bones and overestimates the density of large bones. Therefore, the size of the bone should be taken into account when deciding whether or not to medicate.

Use of DXA for Monitoring

DXA cannot only be used for making an initial diagnosis and treatment decision, but central DXA is also precise enough to be used for monitoring patients over time, provided the interval between measurements is tailored to the specific patient's situation (Lenchik et al. 2002). More research is needed on the best regimens for follow-up testing and for the best way to interpret changes in BMD in these follow-up tests. This section reports on the most appropriate approaches, given the current state of scientific evidence.

For individuals who are not currently receiving treatment, the timing of a repeat test should be based on the current BMD and the expected rate of bone loss (e.g., bone loss is faster during early menopause). For older individuals with above-average T-scores, repeat testing may not be necessary at all. For younger individuals who were initially screened due to risk factors but who have normal BMD values, repeating a test every 5–10 years may be helpful. For those with borderline low BMD and/or who may lose bone fairly rapidly (e.g., exposure to high doses of glucocorticoids), repeating the test in 2-3 years would be appropriate. For monitoring patients on treatment (which is the main reason for ongoing monitoring via BMD measurement), testing annually is inappropriate, and there is insufficient evidence to determine if testing every 2 years is useful (Nelson et al. 2002). Nonetheless, many practitioners repeat the test every 2 years for patients on treatment (Medicare covers testing every 2 years), while others wait longer. It is unlikely that repeated BMD

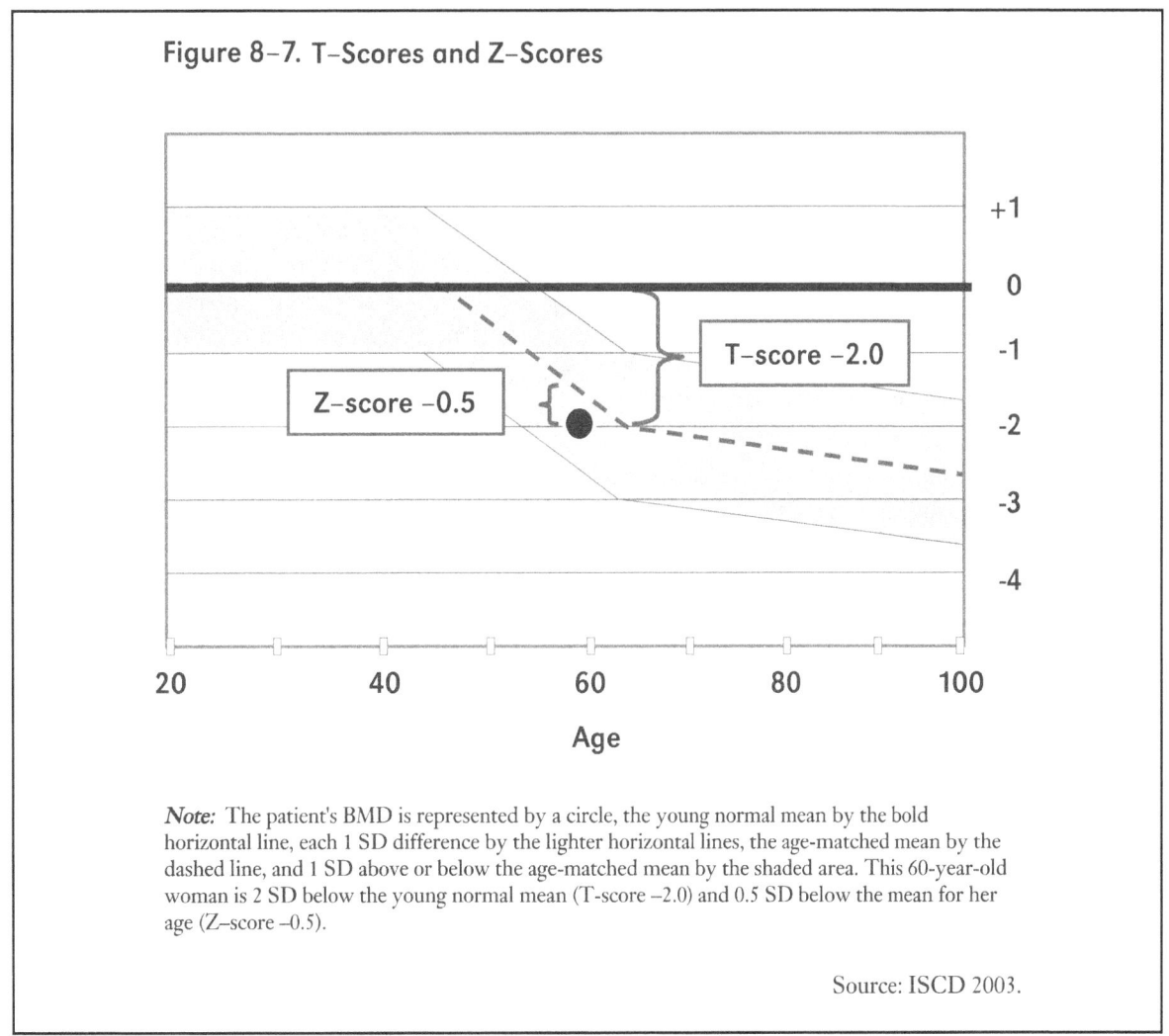

Figure 8–7. T–Scores and Z–Scores

Note: The patient's BMD is represented by a circle, the young normal mean by the bold horizontal line, each 1 SD difference by the lighter horizontal lines, the age-matched mean by the dashed line, and 1 SD above or below the age-matched mean by the shaded area. This 60-year-old woman is 2 SD below the young normal mean (T-score –2.0) and 0.5 SD below the mean for her age (Z–score –0.5).

Source: ISCD 2003.

measurements make a difference in patient compliance with treatment, as many patients who discontinue treatment do so after less than a year (before BMD would be repeated). One exception to the rules related to frequency of testing applies to patients receiving high-dose long-term glucocorticoid therapy, for whom monitoring is recommended every 6 months until BMD is shown to be stable or improved. When repeating BMD measurements, it is important to avoid over-interpretation of small changes as these can be due to differences in equipment or changes in positioning. Non-DXA techniques measuring peripheral sites, QCT, lateral spine DXA, and Ward's triangle DXA (the area of the hip with the lowest density) should not be used for monitoring osteoporosis.

Limitations of BMD Testing

As noted in various sections of this chapter, there are still a number of limitations with respect to BMD testing. Better guidelines are needed on which individuals should receive the test, how to interpret the results of initial and follow-up testing, and how to communicate those results to patients. Health care providers need clear, evidence-based approaches that will enable them to decide who should have BMD testing. They also need guidance in developing plans for treatment and prevention based on a combination of BMD data and other risk factors. More data on the outcomes of screening, prevention, and treatment programs should help to close the large current gap between evidence and practice (Bates et al. 2002, Cummings et al. 2002).

One important concern about the interpretation of results is the variability that exists across different types of BMD machines (even those made by the same manufacturer), and across similar types of machines made by different manufacturers. BMD measured on one type of machine cannot be accurately compared to BMD measured on a different type of machine, nor can BMD performed on the same type of machine at two different locations. There is also variability in the ability of technologists to perform the tests, in the training and ongoing certification of technologists, and in interpretations of results by physicians, each of which can undermine the comparability of results. As a result of all of these factors, daily equipment checks and a quality control system related to both the methodology and reporting of test results is critical to ensure the validity of DXA analysis. The ISCD has developed specific, detailed instructions for quality control as well as reporting of DXA measurements (Leib et al. 2004).

Depending on the skeletal site assessed, the prevalence of osteoporosis can be overestimated (e.g., by use of lateral spine DXA or spinal QCT) or underestimated (e.g., by heel ultrasound) compared to DXA of the spine or hip (Faulkner et al. 1999). There may be differences between the density of skeletal sites within an individual patient. For example, a patient may have a normal spine, but very low bone density at the hip, examination of multiple sites is more likely to result in a diagnosis of osteoporosis. It is important to remember that, despite these limitations, bone mineral density remains the single best predictor of fracture risk available today.

Looking to the Future: Potential Complements to BMD

Researchers in bone disease are developing new approaches that might one day serve as a standard complement to BMD tests. These approaches seek to incorporate additional information that can prove useful in identifying at-risk individuals who may be candidates for further evaluation and treatment, and/or in monitoring the effectiveness of therapy in patients already being treated. This section reviews these efforts.

Biochemical Markers of Bone Turnover

One major thrust relates to efforts to identify "markers" that reflect the rates at which bone breaks down and builds up. As noted in Chapter 2, bone is continuously remodeled in a process referred to as bone turnover whereby old bone is removed and replaced by new bone. Thus, bone resorption (the breaking down of bone) and formation (the building up of bone) are occurring throughout the skeleton at different sites and at different rates. Tests are now available that look for specific blood and urine markers that reflect the rate of each of these processes for the whole skeleton. While BMD measurements provide valuable information on fracture risk, they contribute no insight into the rate of bone turnover in a given patient. To the extent that the imbalance in the rate of bone resorption and formation may predict the rate of bone loss or enhance the ability to predict the risk of fracture, biochemical markers of bone turnover have the potential to complement the information provided by BMD measurements. As reviewed below, while current bone turnover markers have clear limitations, they do nonetheless have some role today in the management of the patient with osteoporosis, particularly to assess responses to therapy (Looker et al. 2000). With further refinement they are likely to play a more important role in the future.

Table 8-4 lists currently bone turnover markers that are currently available. These can be broadly separated into markers of bone resorption and formation; each of these markers is discussed briefly below.

Resorption Markers. Resorption markers are primarily based on measurement of collagen breakdown products that are released into the circulation as bone is resorbed. In recent years rapid and relatively inexpensive tests capable of measuring these breakdown products have been developed, representing a major advance in this area. Most commonly used are the tests for urine and, more recently, blood (serum) (Looker et al. 2000, Garnero et al. 1998, Miller et al. 1999). These markers measure cross-linked (connected) fragments of type I collagen that are released as bone collagen is broken down (Robins et al. 1994). While initially a sophisticated technique was re-

Table 8–4. Currently Available Bone Biochemical Markers

Resorption markers	Formation markers
N-telopeptide of type I collagen (NTX)	Osteocalcin
C-telopeptide of type I collagen (CTx)	Bone specific alkaline phosphatase (BSAP)
Free and total pyridinolines (Pyd)	Aminoterminal propeptide of type I collagen (PINP)
Free and total deoxypyridinolines (Dpd)	Carboxyterminal propeptide of type I collagen (PICP)

quired to measure these molecules, there are now a number of relatively easy to perform tests that can measure them in the blood and urine (Robins et al. 1995).

Formation Markers: Since bone resorption and formation are coupled processes, blood-based bone formation markers are also useful in assessing bone turnover. Osteocalcin and bone specific alkaline phosphatase (BSAP) can serve as such markers, as they are proteins that are made during the process of bone formation (Deftos et al. 1992, Garnero and Delmas 1993). In addition, since a major product of osteoblasts is type I collagen, tests have also been developed that can measure fragments of the collagen precursor chain that are removed and released into the circulation during the processing of the collagen precursor molecule in bone.

Extensive research studies of bone biochemical markers have uncovered potential clinical uses for these markers. These uses, along with current limitations, are reviewed briefly below.

Estimation of Bone Mass. Bone biochemical markers cannot and should not be used to diagnose osteoporosis or to estimate bone mass; direct measurement of BMD is most effective for these tasks.

Estimation of Fracture Risk. There is evidence to suggest that increased bone turnover may be an independent predictor of fracture risk. In a prospective study of elderly (those over age 75) French women, excess excretion of urinary C–terminal collagen crosslinked peptides (CTx) and free deoxypyridinoline crosslinks (Dpd), two of the commonly used biochemical markers of resorption, was associated with an increased risk of hip fracture, even after adjusting for femoral neck BMD (Garnero et al. 1996). Moreover, in a meta-analysis (combination analysis of multiple studies) of trials using antiresorptive drugs (drugs that slow the breakdown of bone), investigators showed that the change in

resorption markers brought on by these agents was related to the reduction in non-spine fracture risk (Hochberg et al. 2002). Specifically, they found that, on average, a drug that reduced bone resorption by 70 percent would decrease the risk of non-spine fractures by 40 percent, independent of effects on BMD. However, while estimation of fracture risk independently of BMD remains an intriguing and potentially important use of bone turnover markers, their routine use for this purpose in individual patients cannot be recommended at this time, largely due to the variability of the measurements.

Estimation of Rate of Bone Loss. Several studies indicate that, at least for groups of individuals, bone biochemical markers can be used to estimate the rate of bone loss. For example, a 4-year study by Garnero et al. (Garnero et al. 1999) found that women with normal bone turnover lost less than 1 percent BMD over 4 years, while those in the high turnover group lost 3–5 times that amount of bone. Here again, the variability of measurements is such that markers may not provide an accurate estimate of bone loss in an individual patient (Nelson et al. 2002).

Selection of Individuals for Therapy. There are reports indicating that individuals with the highest levels of bone turnover appear to have the best response to antiresorptive therapy. In a two-year study of estrogen/progestin treatment, Chesnut and colleagues found that individuals in the highest quartiles for initial excretion of urinary NTx (a biochemical marker) had the greatest gain in BMD in response to hormone treatment (Chesnut et al. 1997). However, the review by the Agency for Healthcare Research and Quality (AHRQ) concluded that studies relating marker results and bone loss had no obvious trend and markers were not useful for patient selection (Nelson et al. 2002). Further studies are needed to evaluate these issues, particularly with respect to more accurate measurements and better quality control.

Monitoring Effectiveness of Therapy. Perhaps the most important use for bone markers today is in monitoring the effectiveness of ongoing therapy. A number of studies indicate that a significant reduction in bone resorption markers occurs within four to 6 weeks after initiation of antiresorptive therapy, followed by a decrease in bone formation markers in 2-3 months (Garnero et al. 1994). Thus, bone turnover markers could theoretically be used to quickly learn when therapy is not working, certainly much more quickly than could a follow-up BMD test 2 years after initiation of therapy. Markers have been used for this purpose for many years for monitoring the response to treatment in Paget's disease. Failure to show the expected reduction in resorption markers could indicate that the patient is not taking the medication in the prescribed manner or that the dose or type of therapy needs to be changed. However, the review by the AHRQ concluded that no marker could accurately determine if an individual would respond to therapy as confirmed by subsequent BMD measurements (Nelson et al. 2002). Work is ongoing to determine the clinical usefulness of following markers in patients being treated with antiresorptive drugs for osteoporosis.

Summary. To summarize, bone biochemical markers may have a potential future role in the identification and management of the patient with osteoporosis. The remodeling rate itself may play a central role in bone fragility rather than just as a marker of bone loss and future declines in bone mass. When the remodeling rate is high, many of the material qualities of bone that contribute to fragility and inability to resist fracture are sub-optimal (Heaney 2003).

Continued improvements in these markers may lead to their use as independent estimators of fracture risk, of rates of bone loss, and perhaps for optimal selection of patients for specific therapies as well as for monitoring of response to these therapies.

Next-Generation Models for Assessment

Advances in understanding of biochemical markers and genetic factors related to bone disease are leading to the potential for more sophisticated tools for assessing the risk of bone disease in individuals. With that goal in mind, an effort to develop a system that estimates a patient's fracture risk over the next 5–10 years is now underway as a joint activity of the International Osteoporosis Foundation and the National Osteoporosis Foundation of the United States (Kanis et al. 2002a and 2000c). Data from most of the world's epidemiology studies are being merged in order to identify consistent risk factors for fracture and to develop a clinical prediction rule that utilizes this information, plus BMD measurements if available, to estimate an individual's personal fracture risk over the next decade of his or her life. In this scheme the risk of all types of osteoporotic-related fractures (not just hip fractures) would be assessed, so that the entire burden of the disease can be recognized. A patient's personal fracture risk could provide a much better basis for individualized treatment decisions. However, it will be important to validate this approach in the community.

Looking ahead, the evolution of risk factor analysis will likely involve the expansion of generally accepted risk factors such as age, gender, race, and fracture history, all of which are well-established as validated estimators. Other potential risk factors are being studied and may play a larger role in the future. The most promising include biochemical markers of bone metabolism and genetic risk factors, which represents an evolving area of research. Candidate genes include receptors (proteins in a cell or on its surface that bind specific substances such as hormones and are necessary for these substance to act on the cell) such as the vitamin D or estrogen receptor genes, and components of bone itself, such as the collagen gene. In the future, the characterization of gene subtypes and further clarification of the roles that these and many other genes that regulate bone cells play may allow for the development of assessment tools that are able to identify at an early age individuals at high risk of developing osteoporosis later in life. Additional research on biochemical markers, genetic factors, and other clinical risk factors is needed, especially related to groups other than older White women and to the prediction of fracture risk over the very long term.

Key Questions for Future Research

Assessing the risk of bone disease and fracture remains a challenge. Not all of the risk factors have been identified, and the relative importance of those that are known remains unclear. The answers to the following research questions can help in meeting this challenge:

- What strategies would be most effective in promoting the cost-effective use of bone densitometry more broadly to the at-risk population?

- Given the limitations of bone densitometry, what tests and/or tools are most effective in predicting the risk of fracture and/or deformity in an individual? Which tools are most practical in different clinical settings? What existing and yet-to-be-identified risk factors are most effective at predicting this risk?

- What practical methods are most effective at assessing the other part of the definition of osteoporosis—"micro-architectural deterioration" (changes that occur in bone because of deterioration of its fine structure)—especially at high-risk sites such as the vertebral bodies and proximal femur. New imaging techniques will be important not only in analyzing skeletal microarchitecture, but also in detecting early skeletal lesions (e.g., in those who have Paget's disease or cancer).

- How can biochemical markers best be used in assessing fracture risk? One key requirement will be the standardization and quality control of current assays of bone remodeling.

- Are there new, as yet undiscovered biochemical markers of bone resorption and formation that could be useful in assessing fracture risk? Can these markers be identified through detailed studies of proteins produced by bone cells and deposited in bone matrix?

References

Andrade SE, Majumdar SR, Chan KA, Buist DS, Go AS, Goodman M, Smith DH, Platt R, Gurwitz JH. Low frequency of treatment of osteoporosis among postmenopausal women following a fracture. Arch Intern Med. 2003 Sep 22;163(17):2052-7.

Bainbridge KE, Sowers M, Lin X, Harlow SD. Risk factors for low bone mineral density and the 6-year rate of bone loss among premenopausal and perimenopausal women. Osteoporos Int 2004 Jan 22.

Balzini L, Vannucchi L, Benvenuti F, Benucci M, Monni M, Cappozzo A, Stanhope SJ. Clinical characteristics of flexed posture in elderly women. J Am Geriatr Soc 2003 Oct;51(10):1419-26.

Bates DW, Black DM, Cummings SR. Clinical use of bone densitometry: Clinical applications. JAMA 2002 Oct 16;288 (15):1898-1900.

Binkley NC, Schmeer P, Wasnich RD, Lenchik L. What are the criteria by which a densitometric diagnosis of osteoporosis can be made in males and non-Whites? J Clin Densitom 2002;5(Suppl):S19-27.

Black DM, Steinbuch M, Palermo L, Dargent-Molina P, Lindsay R, Hoseyni MS, Johnell O. An assessment tool for predicting fracture risk in postmenopausal women. Osteoporos Int 2001;12(7):519-28.

Black DM. BMD measurements. Slide presentation at the Surgeon General's Workshop on Osteoporosis and Bone Health; 2002 Dec 12-13; Washington, DC.

Cadarette SM, Jaglal SB, Kreiger N, McIsaac WJ, Darlington GA, Tu JV. Development and validation of the Osteoporosis Risk Assessment Instrument to facilitate selection of women for bone densitometry. CMAJ 2000 May 2;162(9):1289-94.

Cadarette SM, McIsaac WJ, Hawker GA, Jaakkimainen L, Culbert A, Zarifa G, Ola E, Jaglal SB. The validity of decision rules for selecting women with primary osteoporosis for bone mineral density testing. Osteoporos Int 2004 Jan 17.

Chesnut CH 3rd, Bell NH, Clark GS, Drinkwater BL, English SC, Johnston CC, Jr., Notelovitz M, Rosen CJ, Cain DF, Flessland KA,et al. Hormone replacement therapy in postmenopausal women: Urinary N-telopeptide of type I collagen monitors therapeutic effect and predicts response of bone mineral density. Am J Med 1997;102(1):29-37.

Coles RJ, Clements DG, Evans WD. Measurement of height: Practical considerations for the study of osteoporosis. Osteoporos Int 1994 Nov;4(6):353-6.

Cummings SR, Nevitt MC, Browner WS, Stone K, Fox KM, Ensrud KE, Cauley J, Black D, Vogt TM. Risk factors for hip fracture in white women. Study of Osteoporosis Fractures Research Group. N Engl J Med 1995 Mar 23;332(12):767-73.

Cummings SR, Bates D, Black DM Clinical use of bone densitometry: scientific review. JAMA 2002 Oct 16;288(15):1889-1897.

Deftos LJ, Wolfert RL, Hill CS, Burton DW. Two-site assays of bone Gla protein (osteocalcin) demonstrate immunochemical heterogeneity of the intact molecule. Clin Chem 1992 Nov;38(11):2318-21.

Duncan PW, Studenski S, Chandler J, Prescott B. Functional reach: Predictive validity in a sample of elderly male veterans. J Gerontol 1992 May;47(3):M93-8.

Ensrud KE, Black DM, Harris F, Ettinger B, Cummings SR. Correlates of kyphosis in older women. The Fracture Intervention Trial Research Group. J Am Geriatr Soc 1997 Jun;45(6):682-7.

Ensrud KE, Ewing SK, Stone KL, Cauley JA, Bowman PJ, Cummings SR; Study of Osteoporotic Fractures Research Group. Intentional and unintentional weight loss increase bone loss and hip fracture risk in older women. J Am Geriatr Soc 2003 Dec;51(12):1740-7.

Ettinger B, Black DM, Palermo L, Nevitt MC, Melnikoff S, Cummings SR. Kyphosis in older women and its relation to back pain, disability and osteopenia: The study of osteoporotic fractures. Osteoporos Int 1994 Jan;4(1):55-60.

Ettinger B, Ray GT, Pressman AR, Gluck O. Limb fractures in elderly men as indicators of subsequent fracture risk. Arch Intern Med 2003 Dec 18-22;163(22):2741-7.

Faulkner KG, von Stetten E, Miller P. Discordance in patient classification using T-scores. J Clin Densitom. 1999 Fall;2(3):343-50.

Feldstein AC, Nichols GA, Elmer PJ, Smith DH, Aickin M, Herson M. Older women with fractures: Patients falling through the cracks of guideline-recommended osteoporosis screening and treatment. J Bone Joint Surg Am 2003 Dec;85-A(12):2294-302.

Finkelstein JS, Lee MT, Sowers M, Ettinger B, Neer RM, Kelsey JL, Cauley JA, Huang MH, Greendale GA. Ethnic variation in bone density in premenopausal and early perimenopausal women: Effects of anthropometric and lifestyle factors. J Clin Endocrinol Metab 2002 Jul; 87(7):3057-67.

Garnero P, Delmas PD. Assessment of the serum levels of bone alkaline phosphatase with a new immunoradiometric assay in patients with metabolic bone disease. J Clin Endocrinol Metab 1993 Oct; 77(4):1046-53.

Garnero P, Shih WJ, Gineyts E, Karpf DB, Delmas PD. Comparison of new biochemical markers of bone turnover in late postmenopausal osteoporotic women in response to alendronate treatment. J Clin Endocrinol Metab 1994 Dec; 79(6):1693-700.

Garnero P, Hausherr E, Chapuy MC, Marcelli C, Grandjean H, Muller C, Cormier C, Breart G, Meunier PJ, Delmas PD. Markers of bone resorption predict hip fracture in elderly women: The EPIDOS Prospective Study. J Bone Miner Res 1996 Oct; 11(10):1531-8.

Garnero P, Delmas PD. Biochemical markers of bone turnover. Applications for osteoporosis. Endocrinol Metab Clin North Am 1998 Jun; 27(2):303-23. Garnero P, Sornay-Rendu E, Duboeuf F, Delmas PD. Markers of bone turnover predict postmenopausal forearm bone loss over 4 years: The OFELY study. J Bone Miner Res 1999 Sep; 14(9):1614-21.

Genant HK, Engelke K, Fuerst TP, Gluer CC, Grampp S, Harris ST, Jergas M, Lang T, Lu Y, Majumdar S, et al. Noninvasive assessment of bone mineral and structure: State of the art. J Bone Miner Res 1996 Jun; 11(6):707-30.

Geusens P, Hochberg MC, van der Voort DJ, Pols H, van der Klift M, Siris E, Melton ME, Turpin J, Byrnes C, Ross P. Performance of risk indices for identifying low bone density in postmenopausal women. Mayo Clin Proc 2002 Jul;77(7):629-37.

Girman CJ, Chandler JM, Zimmerman SI, Martin AR, Hawkes W, Hebel R, Sloane PD, Magaziner J. Prediction of fracture in nursing home residents. J Am Geriatr Soc 2002 Aug;50(8):1341-7.

Grampp S, Genant HK, Mathur A, Lang P, Jergas M, Takada M, Gluer CC, Lu Y, Chavez M. Comparisons of noninvasive bone mineral measurements in assessing age-related loss, fracture discrimination, and diagnostic classification. J Bone Miner Res 1997 May; 12(5):697-711.

Greenspan SL, Myers ER, Maitland LA, Resnick NM, Hayes WC. Fall severity and bone mineral density as risk factors for hip fracture in ambulatory elderly. JAMA 1994 Jan;271(2):128-33.

Haentjens P, Autier P, Collins J, Velkeniers B, Vanderschueren D, Boonen S. Colles fracture, spine fracture, and subsequent risk of hip fracture in men and women. A meta-analysis. J Bone Joint Surg Am 2003 Oct;85-A(10): 1936-43.

Hamdy RC, Petak SM, Lenchik L; International Society for Clinical Densitometry Position Development Panel and Scientific Advisory Committee. Which central dual x-ray absorptiometry skeletal sites and regions of interest should be used to determine the diagnosis of osteoporosis? J Clin Densitom 2002;5(Suppl):S11-8.

Hannan MT, Felson DT, Dawson-Hughes B, Tucker KL, Cupples LA, Wilson PW, Kiel DP. Risk factors for longitudinal bone loss in elderly men and women: The Framingham Osteoporosis Study. J Bone Miner Res 2000 Apr;15(4): 710-20.

Harrington JT, Broy SB, Derosa AM, Licata AA, Shewmon DA. Hip fracture patients are not treated for osteoporosis: A call to action. Arthritis Rheum Dec 15;47(6):651-4.Heaney RP. Remodeling and skeletal fragility. Osteoporos Int. 2003 Sep;14(Supplement 5):12-15.

Hochberg MC, Greenspan S, Wasnich RD, Miller P, Thompson DE, Ross PD. Changes in bone density and turnover explain the reductions in incidence of nonvertebral fractures that occur during treatment with antiresorptive agents. J Clin Endocrinol Metab 2002 Apr; 87(4):1586-92.

Huang C, Ross PD, Lydick E, Davis JW, Wasnich RD. Contributions of vertebral fractures to stature loss among elderly Japanese-American women in Hawaii. J Bone Miner Res 1996 Mar;11(3):408-11.

International Society for Clinical Densitometry, Inc. ISCD Bone Densitometry Clinician Course. Version 5.3. Lecture 5 "Use of bone densitometry for the diagnosis of osteoporosis." Graph courtesy of Steven M. Petak, MD, JD, FACE. West Hartford(CT): The ISCD; 2003.

Johnell O, Kanis JA, Oden A, Sernbo I, Redlund-Johnell I, Petterson C, De Laet C, Jonsson B. Fracture risk following an osteoporotic fracture. Osteoporos Int 2004 Mar;15(3):175-9.

Kahn AA, Bachrach L, Brown JP, Hanley DA, Josse RG, Kendler DL, Leib ES, Lentle BC, Leslie WD, Lewiecki M, et al.; Canadian Panel of the International Society of Clinical Densitometry. Standards and guidelines for performing central dual-energy x-ray absorptiometry in premenopausal women, men, and children. J Clin Densitom 2004 Spring; 7(1):51-64.

Kamel HK, Hussain MS, Tariq S, Perry HM, Morley JE. Failure to diagnose and treat osteoporosis in elderly patients hospitalized with hip fracture. Am J Med. 2000 Sep;109(4):326-8.

Kanis JA, Melton LJ 3rd, Christiansen C, Johnston CC, Khaltaev N. The diagnosis of osteoporosis. J Bone Miner Res 1994 Aug;9(8):1137-41.

[a]Kanis JA, Johnell O, Oden A, De Laet C, Jonsson B, Dawson A. Ten-year risk of

osteoporotic fracture and the effect of risk factors on screening strategies. Bone 2002 Jan;30(1):251-8.

[b]Kanis, JA. Osteoporosis III: Diagnosis of osteoporosis and assessment of fracture risk. Lancet 2002 June;359(9321):1929-36.

[c]Kanis JA, Black D, Cooper C, Dargent P, Dawson-Hughes B, De Laet C, Delmas P, Eisman J, Johnell O, Jonsson B, et al. A new approach to the development of assessment guidelines for osteoporosis. Osteoporosis Int 2002 Jul;13(7):527-36.

Kiebzak GM, Beinart GA, Perser K, Ambrose CG, Siff SJ, Heggeness MH. Under-treatment of osteoporosis in men with hip fracture. Arch Intern Med. 2002 Oct 28;162(19):2217-22.

Knoke JD, Barrett-Connor E. Weight loss: A determinant of hip bone loss in older men and women. The Rancho Bernardo Study. Am J Epidemiol 2003 Dec 15;158(12):1132-8.

Leib ES, Lewiecki M, Binkley N, Hamdy RC; International Society for Clinical Densitometry. Official positions of the International Society for Clinical Densitometry. J Clin Densitom 2004 Spring;7(1):1-6.

Lenchik L, Kiebzak GM, Blunt BA;International Society for Clinical Densitometry Position Development Panel and Scientific Advisory Committee. What is the role of serial bone mineral density measurements in patient management? J Clin Densitom 2002; 5(Suppl):S29-38.

Looker AC, Bauer DC, Chesnut CH 3rd, Gundberg CM, Hochberg MC, Klee G, Kleerekoper M, Watts NB, Bell NH. Clinical use of biochemical markers of bone remodeling: Current status and future directions. Osteoporos Int 2000; 11(6):467-80.

Looker AC. The skeleton, race, and ethnicity [editorial]. J Clin Endocrinol Metab 2002 Jul; 87(7):3047-50.

Lydick E, Cook K, Turpin J, Melton M, Stine R, Byrnes C. Development and validation of a simple questionnaire to facilitate identification of women likely to have low bone density. Am J Manag Care 1998 Jan;4(1):37-48.

Marshall D, Johnell O, Wedel H. Meta-analysis of how well measures of bone mineral density predict occurrence of osteoporotic fractures. BMJ 1996 May 18;312(7041):1254-9.

Miller PD, Baran DT, Bilezikian JP, Greenspan SL, Linday R, Riggs BL, Watts NB. Practical clinical application of biochemical markers of bone turnover: consensus of an expert panel. J Clin Densitom 1999 Fall; 2(3):323-42.

Murff HJ, Gandhi TK, Karson AK, Mort EA, Poon EG, Wang SJ, Fairchild DG, Bates DW. Primary care physician attitudes concerning follow-up of abnormal test results and ambulatory decision support systems. Int J Med Inf. 2003 Sep;71(2-3):137-49.

National Osteoporosis Foundation. America's bone health: The state of osteoporosis and low bone mass in our nation. Washington (DC): National Osteoporosis Foundation; 2002.

National Osteoporosis Foundation. Physician's guide to prevention and treatment of osteoporosis. Washington (DC); 2003.

Nelson HD, Morris CD, Kraemer DF, Mahon S, Carney N, Nygren PM, Helfand MH (Oregon Health & Science University Evidence-based Practice Center, Portland, OR). Osteoporosis in postmenopausal women: diagnosis and monitoring Evidence Report/Technology Assessment No. 28. Rockville (MD): Agency for Healthcare

Research and Quality; 2001 Nov. Publication No.: 01-E032. Contract No.:290-97-0018

Nevitt MC, Cummings SR, Hudes ES. Risk factors for injurious falls: A prospective study. J Gerontol 1991 Sep;46(5):M164-70.

Nguyen TV, Center JR, Pocock NA, Eisman JA. Limited utility of clinical indices for the prediction of symptomatic fracture risk in postmenopausal women. Osteoporos Int 2004 Jan;15(1):49-55.

Orwoll ES, Bauer DC, Vogt TM, Fox KM. Axial bone mass in older women. Study of Osteoporotic Fractures Research Group. Ann Intern Med 1996 Jan 15;124(2):187-96.

Richy F, Gourlay M, Ross PD, Sen SS, Radican L, De Ceulaer F, Ben Sedrine W, Ethgen O, Bruyere O, Reginster JY. Validation and comparative evaluation of the osteoporosis self-assessment tool (OST) in a Caucasian population from Belgium. QJM 2004 Jan;97(1):39-46.

Robins SP, Woitge H, Hesley R, Ju J, Seyedin S, Seibel MJ. Direct enzyme-linked immunoassay for urinary deoxypyridinoline as a specific marker for measuring bone resorption. J Bone Miner Res 1994 Oct;9(10):1643-9.

Solomon DH, Finkelstein JS, Katz JN, Mogun H, Avorn J. Underuse of osteoporosis medications in elderly patients with fractures. Am J Med. 2003 Oct 1;115(5):398-400.

Tinetti ME. Performance-oriented assessment of mobility problems in elderly patients. J Am Geriatr Soc 1986 Feb;34(2):119-126.

Tinetti ME, Mendes de Leon CF, Doucette JT, Baker DI. Fear of falling and fall-related efficacy in relationship to functioning among community-living elders. J Gerontol 1994 May;49(3):M140-7.

U.S. Preventive Services Task Force. Screening for osteoporosis in postmenopausal women: recommendations and rationale. Ann Intern Med 2002 Sep 17;137(6):526-8.

Vogt TM, Ross PD, Palermo L, Musliner T, Genant HK, Black D, Thompson DE. Vertebral fracture prevalence among women screened for the Fracture Intervention Trial and a simple clinical tool to screen for undiagnosed vertebral fractures. Fracture Intervention Trial Research Group. Mayo Clin Proc. 2000 Sep;75(9):888-96.

Chapter 9: Key Messages

- There have been important advances in the ability to prevent and treat fractures in the last 10 years, especially in those with skeletal fragility. Just as with the use of diagnostic measures, there has been a failure in the United States to apply appropriate preventive and treatment measures to many persons at risk for bone disease.

- Everyone should be informed of the basic elements of maintaining bone health and preventing bone disease. Paying attention to the basics—appropriate physical activity, nutrition, and smoking—is critical for everyone, especially those who have, or who are at risk of developing, osteoporosis.

- Any individual who is diagnosed with osteoporosis should be evaluated for potential secondary causes of the disease, including the presence of other disorders or the use of medications that can cause harm to bone. If secondary causes are present, actions should be taken to minimize their impact.

- For the most common bone diseases, drugs that prevent bone breakdown (antiresorptives) have been shown to be effective in reducing the risk of future fractures. These drugs not only slow any further deterioration of the skeleton, but also allow for some repair and restoration of bone mass and strength.

- When antiresorptive therapy is not enough, anabolic therapy is available to help build new bone and further reduce the risk of fracture. While this approach has been developed for the prevention and treatment of osteoporotic fractures, it can also be applied to other bone diseases.

- For individuals who remain at high risk of fracture, an extensive fall prevention program should be developed. This program should aim to minimize the risk of falls in the home and community; avoid the use of drugs that increase the risk of bone disease or falls; and protect those who do fall through the use of hip protectors.

- Specific, effective treatments exist for a number of bone diseases other than osteoporosis, including hyperparathyroidism, rickets, and osteomalacia. Treatment is also available for some congenital bone disorders and for bone disease associated with kidney failure. For all of these conditions, early detection and treatment are critical to avoiding crippling deformities and fractures.

Chapter 9

PREVENTION AND TREATMENT FOR THOSE WHO HAVE BONE DISEASES

Just as there have been great advances in the ability to identify individuals at risk of fracture (see Chapter 8), there have been equally important advances in the ability to prevent and treat fractures in these individuals, especially those with skeletal fragility. In particular the introduction of bisphosphonates and selective estrogen receptor modulators (SERMs) has given health care providers new approaches to therapy.

Just as for the use of diagnostic measures, numerous studies indicate that there has been a failure in the United States to apply preventive and treatment measures to many persons at risk for bone disease. As a result, most high-risk individuals (e.g., those who have suffered a fragility fracture) do not get the testing and treatment that they need. Use of bone mineral density (BMD) testing in this population ranges from 3–23 percent, while use of calcium and vitamin D supplementation ranges from 11–44 percent, and use of antiresorptive therapy ranges from 12–16 percent (Morris et al. 2004, Smith 2001 et al.). In fact, most physicians fail to discuss osteoporosis with their patients, even after a fracture (Pal 1999). In a large study of older adults, four out of five hip or wrist fracture patients did not receive any treatment after the fracture. The same study also found that certain groups of patients, including men, older persons, non-Whites, and those with comorbid conditions, were less likely than White women to receive treatments (Solomon et al. 2003). Even when physicians do suggest therapy, it often does not conform with recommended practice, as many patients with low BMD are not treated while others with high BMD are (Solomon et al. 2000). In other words, the gap between clinical knowledge and its application in the community remains large.

It is also important to recognize that the ideal drugs for the treatment of osteoporosis or other bone disorders have yet to be developed. Inexpensive, effective agents with few side effects are needed so that they can be used broadly to prevent fractures and deformities in the enormous number of individuals who will be at risk of bone disease as the population ages. (See Chapter 4 for more details on the large at-risk population.)

This chapter reviews the latest evidence on the prevention and treatment of fractures in individuals with or at high risk for bone disease. As the box below indicates, the use of the terms "prevention" and "treatment" can be confusing, since the goal of many treatments is the prevention of disease or fractures. At the same time, prevention is often considered a treatment for those with or at risk for bone disease. Nonetheless, it is important to recognize the critical role of prevention in all individuals, including (and perhaps especially) in those known to have bone disease and/or to be at high risk of fracture.

Treatment as Prevention, and Prevention as Treatment

The concept of prevention within the area of bone health is complex, and often encompasses measures that may be more commonly considered as treatments. In fact, in the field of bone health, the terms treatment and prevention are often used in an interchangeable manner, since the major goal of treatment is the prevention of fractures.

Within both bone health and general health care, prevention can be thought of as taking anticipatory actions designed to reduce the possibility that an event or condition will occur that could lead an individual to a state of dependency. Within this broad definition are three different types of preventive activities.

- *Primary* prevention refers to actions that prevent a disease or injury (e.g., osteoporosis) that could lead to a state of impairment.

- *Secondary* prevention refers to activities that block the progression of an existing impairment (e.g., bone disease) to a disability (e.g., fracture); interventions within this area are often also considered to be treatments.

- *Tertiary* prevention refers to actions that block or slow the progression of a disability (e.g., fracture) to a state of dependency. In some cases these actions may also be considered treatments.

Preventive measures within the area of bone health span all three types. For example, certain measures to achieve optimal bone mass can be considered primary prevention, including encouraging adequate intake of calcium and vitamin D, appropriate physical activity, and other bone-healthy lifestyle behaviors.

Other measures that are commonly considered treatments for osteoporosis, such as using antiresorptive and anabolic agents, should also be thought of as secondary prevention, since they are designed to retard the progression of the disease to prevent disability. Fall prevention in this population may also be seen as secondary prevention, since its purpose is to prevent disability in an individual who already has bone disease.

Appropriate and comprehensive treatment of a fracture is considered tertiary prevention, because such treatment attempts to prevent a person with a disability from becoming dependent. Drugs prescribed to individuals who have already sustained a fracture are also a part of this tertiary prevention effort. From a public health perspective, physical therapy and other forms of rehabilitation are considered methods of tertiary prevention in this population.

This paradigm also fits the management of other bone diseases. For example, early treatment of Paget's disease can prevent fractures and hence can be considered as either secondary or tertiary prevention, depending on the status of the patient when the treatment is given. The bottom line is that a spectrum of preventive activities exists within the area of bone disease, and treatment is a part of that spectrum. Assuring bone health requires that preventive measures be implemented in all its aspects: to optimize peak bone mass;, to block excessive resorption; to increase bone formation; to decrease skeletal fragility; to decrease the severity and frequency of falls; and to accelerate recovery from fracture. In fact, this entire spectrum of prevention is central to promoting bone health in all populations.

Treatment of Osteoporosis = Prevention of Fractures

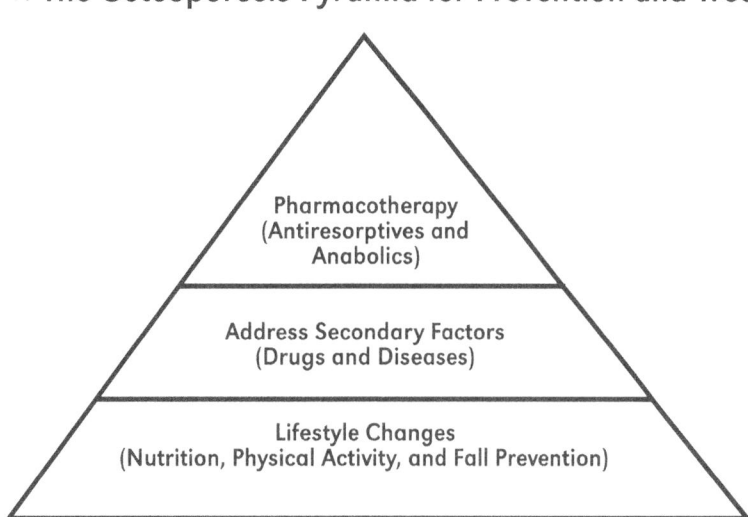

Figure 9-1. The Osteoporosis Pyramid for Prevention and Treatment

Pharmacotherapy
(Antiresorptives and
Anabolics)

Address Secondary Factors
(Drugs and Diseases)

Lifestyle Changes
(Nutrition, Physical Activity, and Fall Prevention)

Note:
The Base of the Pyramid: The first step in the prevention and treatment of osteoporosis and the prevention of fractures is to build a foundation of nutrition and lifestyle measures that maximize bone health. The diet should not only be adequate in calcium and vitamin D, but should have a healthy balance of other nutrients. A weight-bearing exercise program should be developed. Cigarette smoking and excessive alcohol use must be avoided. In the older individual, at high risk for fractures, the changes in lifestyle would include a plan not only to maximize physical activity, but also to minimize the risk of falls. The use of hip protectors can be considered in some high-risk patients. Diseases that increase the risk of falls by causing visual impairment, postural hypotension (a drop in blood pressure on standing, which leads to dizziness), or poor balance should be treated. Drugs that cause bone loss or increase the risk of falls should be avoided or given at the lowest effective dose.

The Second Level of the Pyramid: The next step is to identify and treat diseases that produce secondary osteoporosis or aggravate primary osteoporosis. These measures are the foundation upon which specific pharmacotherapy is built and should never be forgotten.

The Third Level of the Pyramid: If there is sufficiently high risk of fracture to warrant pharmacotherapy, the patient is usually started on antiresorptives. Anabolic agents are used in individuals in whom antiresorptive therapy is not adequate to prevent bone loss or fractures. Chapter 9 summarizes the indications for antiresorptive and anabolic therapy.

A Pyramid Approach

One of the primary goals in the treatment of osteoporosis and other bone diseases is to maintain bone health by preventing bone loss and perhaps even by building new bone. Another goal is to minimize the risk and/or impact of falls, since they are typically the precursor to the most devastating consequence of bone disease: fractures. The best way to realize these goals is to employ a combination of various prevention and treatment strategies. In fact, maintaining bone health and preventing fractures and deformities requires a "pyramid" approach (Figure 9-1).

The building blocks of physical activity and good nutrition (particularly with respect to adequate intake of calcium and vitamin D) represent measures are not enough there are now additional treatments that can be given to build new bone (anabolics) and further reduce fracture risk. While this approach has been developed for the prevention and treatment of osteoporotic fractures, it can also be applied to other bone diseases.

For those individuals who remain at high risk of fracture even after treatment (e.g., the frail elderly), the base of the pyramid should include an extensive program to minimize the risk of falls in the home and community, to avoid the use of drugs that increase the risk, and to provide hip protectors that reduce the risk of fracture in those who do fall.

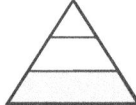

The Base of the Pyramid: Maintaining Bone Health and Preventing Fractures

Prevention is, by far, the most effective way to promote bone health, and thus represents the base of the pyramid (Figure 9-1a). Everyone should be informed of the basic elements of maintaining bone health. Everyone should strive for adequate levels of calcium and vitamin D intake. Everyone should engage in regular weight-bearing exercise and avoid behaviors that impair bone health such as smoking. Everyone should understand the basics about how to avoid falling. These elements serve as the foundation of prevention of bone disease and fractures. They may be all that are required in individuals at low risk of bone disease, but they are critically important for high-risk patients as well.

The remainder of this section provides a very brief overview of the key elements of prevention that every individual and provider should know. Much more detail about each of these areas is provided in Chapters 6 and 7.

Calcium: For postmenopausal women, the recommended total daily calcium intake is 1,200 mg per day in two or more doses. These levels of intake can be achieved through dietary sources of calcium, including both dairy and non-dairy products. A detailed list of these foods and beverages appears in Chapter 7, while another list ranked by calcium content can be found in Chapter 10. In addition, calcium supplements (e.g., calcium carbonate, calcium citrate, other calcium salts) are available in the form of pills, chewable tablets, and liquids, as discussed in Chapter 7. The total daily calcium intake should not exceed 2,500 mg (IOM 1997).

Vitamin D. Vitamin D is important for absorption of calcium and mineralization (hardening) of bone. As discussed in Chapter 6, vitamin D is synthesized in the skin through sunlight exposure, or it may be taken as a supplement. However, the skin of older individuals does not synthesize vitamin D as well as the skin of younger individuals, and in some parts of the country, the winter sun does not produce vitamin D in the skin of all individuals. In addition, vitamin D is not available in many foods other than fortified milk, which contains 100 IU (international units) per cup. Thus, many individuals will need to take a supplement, especially those who avoid sun exposure, use sun block, or do not drink milk. The recommended dose of vitamin D is 200 to 600 IU daily, with the dose dependent on age, as shown in Table 7-1 (IOM 1997). However, many experts are recommending more vitamin D for the frail elderly (Heaney and Weaver 2003). The total daily vitamin D intake of persons who are not vitamin D deficient should not exceed 2,000 IU (IOM 1997). Many calcium supplements contain vitamin D. Most multivitamins contain 400 IU of vitamin D. Vitamin D supplements can be taken on their own, or with calcium or food.

Patients who are vitamin D insufficient (low levels of vitamin D in the blood) or deficient (very low levels of vitamin D in the blood) require treatment with higher doses of vitamin D. Vitamin D deficiency can lead to secondary hyperparathyroidism (see below) with normal levels of blood calcium. Severe cases lead to osteomalacia or rickets (see Chapter 3). It should be noted that the optimal range for 25-hydroxyvitamin D is higher than the "normal" ranges reported from clinical laboratories, since these ranges are obtained from a population that includes individuals with sub-optimal levels. Patients can be treated with vitamin D supplementation of 50,000 IU once a week for up to 3 months with follow-up blood tests of vitamin D, calcium, and PTH levels. Some patients may require longer courses of treatment (Pettifor 2003).

Physical Activity. Weight-bearing, strength, and balance-training exercises are also an important part of any osteoporosis prevention and treatment program, regardless of age. They can help increase or preserve bone mass and may also help reduce the risk of falling. As discussed in Chapter 6, all types of physical activity can contribute to bone health. Activities that are weight bearing or involve impact are most useful for increasing or maintaining bone mass. Activities that are not weight bearing or are low impact may help improve balance and coordination and maintain muscle mass, which can help prevent falls. To encourage increased levels of physical activity among all age groups, "Physical Activity and Health: A Surgeon General's Report" recommends a "minimum of 30 minutes of physical activity of moderate intensity (such as brisk walking) on most, if not all, days of the week" (USDHHS 1996). Since the skeleton responds preferentially to strength training and short bouts of high-load impact activity (such as skipping or jumping), the same report recommends that adults supplement their cardiorespiratory endurance activity with strength-developing exercise at least two times per week. Chapter 7 addresses specific ways to incorporate strength and loading activities into an overall habit of physical activity.

For those who cannot engage in regular physical activity due to disability, mechanical stimulation of the skeleton might prove beneficial. Recent, small studies found that use of vibrating platforms increased BMD and slowed bone loss (Rubin 2004 et al., Verschueren et al. 2004, Ward et al. 2004). This may provide another way to reduce fracture risk both in the elderly and in younger individuals with disabling conditions that limit their ability to exercise. However, the long-term safety and efficacy of such approaches remain to be determined, and therefore specific rehabilitation and exercise programs aimed at increasing activity and function remain critically important in the frail elderly and in younger individuals with neuromuscular disabilities.

Fall Prevention. Falls represent perhaps the biggest threat to the bone health and the functional independence of older individuals. Falls are common and frequently are the precipitating event that leads to a fracture or fractures in an individual. Thus, fall prevention offers another important opportunity to protect the bones throughout life, but particularly in those over age 60. Falls occur for a variety of reasons, with multiple factors often contributing to a single fall. These factors include problems with balance, mobility, vision, lower extremity weakness, and/or blood pressure or circulation. Often these problems are compounded by an acute illness (e.g., infection, fever, dehydration, arrhythmia), a new medication, or an environmental stress (e.g., standing or walking on an unsafe surface, poor lighting) that leads to the fall. To reduce the risk of falls, a variety of fall prevention measures should be encouraged for frail, elderly individuals. These include regular vision checks; elimination (where possible) of medications and/or dosages that may cause dizziness, low blood pressure, or confusion; and addressing environmental problems or obstacles that can lead to falls, including removing throw rugs, installing night lights, installing railings on stairs and grab bars in showers, encouraging use of rubber-soled shoes and slippers, and attaching phone cords and other wires to the baseboard of the wall. Hip protectors or hip pads might also be useful in reducing the impact of those falls that do occur. More information on fall prevention strategies can be found in Chapter 7.

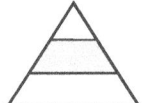

The Second Level of the Pyramid: Assessing and Treating Secondary Causes

The first level of the pyramid applies to all individuals whether or not they have low bone mass or multiple risk factors for osteoporotic fractures. The second level (Figure 9-1b), which is important for patients at high risk for fractures, involves determining whether there are secondary causes or aggravating factors for the osteoporosis and addressing them therapeutically if they exist.

The vast majority of older postmenopausal women with osteoporosis will have the primary form of the disease, with secondary factors likely playing only a limited role. However, there can be considerable therapeutic benefit from uncovering such factors and dealing with them appropriately if they exist. In men and younger women with osteoporosis, secondary factors often play a major role, and the diagnosis and treatment of these factors may be the most important part of managing their bone disease. For a complete list of secondary factors that can cause or contribute to osteoporosis, see Chapter 3.

One important reason for dealing with secondary factors is that the therapeutic response to specific treatment can be substantial. For example, large increases in BMD have been observed after treatment of hyperparathyroidism (Silverberg 1995) and epidemiologic studies have shown that fracture rates decrease substantially when glucocorticoid therapy is discontinued (van Staa 2000).

A careful history can suggest possible secondary factors and guide the health care provider in carrying out appropriate tests. At a minimum, serum calcium concentration should be measured. In populations and geographic areas where vitamin D deficiency is common, measurement of 25-hydroxy vitamin D is another useful screening test. Measurement of calcium and creatinine in fasting, second-voided morning urines or 24-hour urines may be useful in detecting high or low calcium excretion. High calcium excretion may be associated with bone loss while low calcium excretion may be associated with malabsorption and vitamin D deficiency. Patients with gluten-sensitive enteropathy or sprue may present with osteoporosis yet have few gastrointestinal symptoms. Weight loss is often a key sign of this disorder or of other underlying diseases such as malignancy. Many physicians recommend screening for thyroid disease, which is relatively inexpensive. Because screening for Cushing's syndrome can be difficult and costly, it should be reserved for patients in whom the history and physical examination strongly suggest the possibility of this disorder.

Treatment of most secondary causes of bone loss and fractures is generally well established and is described later in this chapter. In patients with severe osteoporosis the treatment of secondary factors should be carried out together with pharmacotherapy for the bone itself, as this approach helps to improve bone strength and

Study Design Issues Related to Treatment

Many studies have focused on the effectiveness and safety of treatments for bone disease, and consequently many issues must be considered in examining and comparing the results of these studies. First, therapeutic effectiveness is best examined with interventions that have been assessed in randomized (i.e., treatment is randomly given to patients), double-blinded (i.e., patients and physicians are not told what treatment the patients are on), placebo-controlled (i.e., some participants take an inactive pill to control for expectations) trials. Second, a study duration of at least 3 years is preferable in order to see meaningful results. In recent years, the FDA has required organizations that apply for FDA approval for drugs to treat osteoporosis to conduct randomized, double-blind, placebo-controlled trials of at least 3 years' duration to test the drug's effectiveness with respect to fracture reduction. Studies of fracture reduction can focus on clinical fractures (fractures that are painful), spine fractures assessed by standard x-rays (two-thirds of these fractures are *not* painful), non-spine fractures, and hip fractures. Although the most important study outcome is fracture risk reduction, changes in BMD or markers of bone turnover (see Chapter 8) can be used as supportive evidence of the effectiveness of treatment. Another study outcome relates to how quickly the medication will work in improving BMD or reducing risk of fractures.

In addition, it is important to consider the duration of therapies (to help in determining the recommended length of treatment) and to know what happens when therapies are discontinued.

Despite the multitude of good studies, it is not possible to compare the effectiveness of different therapies by comparing the results from separate investigations. This is because the inclusion and exclusion factors for patient enrollment in the various studies are different; the duration, intensity of daily physical activity, outcome measures, and statistical analyses vary; and the amount or type of calcium/vitamin D supplements varies. Therapies can only be compared if they have been given to patients in the same trial. For this reason, the differences in effects on fracture reduction and BMD that are reported for medications from different studies may not represent true differences in the efficacy of the drug being used, but rather differences in the populations being tested. Because comparative studies require unrealistically high numbers of patients, it is unlikely they will be funded.

A meta-analysis is a summary of multiple studies evaluating the same type of treatment. Because it incorporates many studies, such analysis often provides the best available evidence on the effectiveness of a given treatment. Several meta-analyses have been conducted that help to better understand the value of treatments, including for calcium and vitamin D. The results of these studies are reported in Chapter 6.

minimize fracture risk as quickly as possible. BMD measurements, which are ordinarily done every 2 yearss during the treatment of primary osteoporosis, may be done more frequently for

some individuals with secondary osteoporosis, including those with glucocorticoid-induced osteoporosis, which can cause relatively rapid changes in BMD.

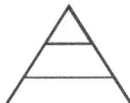

The Third Level of the Pyramid: Treatment

Treatment represents the third level of the pyramid (Figure 9-1c). This section reviews treatment options for bone disease, with an emphasis on osteoporosis, the disease for which the most treatment options exist.

Drug Therapy for Osteoporosis

There are two primary types of drug therapy for osteoporosis. The first is use of antiresorptive agents, which are drugs that *reduce* bone loss, while the second involves use of anabolic agents, which are drugs that *build* bone. Antiresorptive therapies include use of bisphosphonates, estrogen, selective estrogen receptor modulators (SERMs), and calcitonin. Antiresorptive therapies reduce bone loss, stabilize the microarchitecture of the bone, and decrease bone turnover—all leading to fracture reduction. They increase BMD because the resorption spaces in bone get refilled with new bone and the amount of mineral in the bone increases. Antiresorptive therapies act by decreasing the activity of the osteoclasts, the cells responsible for bone resorption (breakdown). Antiresorptive therapy should be considered for all patients with the diagnosis of osteoporosis as well as for some other bone disorders. This therapy is effective in reducing the risk of future fractures, although, as discussed below, different forms of antiresorptive therapy vary in their safety and efficacy. At present, the Food and Drug Administration has approved two bisphosphonates, alendronate and risedronate, for prevention or treatment of osteoporosis for either daily or weekly oral administration. Another bisphosphonate, ibandronate, is being considered and additional agents (see below) are under investigation, including intravenous forms. Only one SERM, raloxifene, is FDA-approved. Many estrogen preparations are approved for prevention of bone loss. Nasal and injectable calcitonin are also approved for treatment of osteoporosis.

Anabolic therapy is now available for those individuals who continue to fracture or lose bone on an adequate program of general prevention and antiresorptive therapy. The only FDA-approved anabolic agent is a synthetic form of parathyroid hormone known as teriparatide. Teriparatide, which is given as a daily subcutaneous injection, costs substantially more than does antiresorptive therapy.

In some situations individuals with osteoporosis have been treated with a combination of two antiresorptive agents or with an antiresorptive and an anabolic agent. Sometimes the two agents are given simultaneously while other times they are given sequentially. The effectiveness of these types of combination therapies is currently being studied.

The remainder of this section reviews the evidence to date on the effectiveness of the different types of antiresorptive and anabolic agents that are available and of therapies that combine two antiresorptive agents or an antiresorptive agent with an anabolic agent.

Antiresorptive Therapy

Bisphosphonates. Bisphosphonates are phosphate-based, non-hormone compounds that have been shown to increase BMD and decrease fractures (Fleisch 2001). At present, there are two bisphosphonates that are FDA-approved and readily available for osteoporosis prevention and treatment: alendronate (Fosamax®) and risedronate (Actonel®). These medications bind to the bone surface and then are taken up by osteoclasts (cells that break down bone) as these cells attempt to resorb that bone. They block the pathway that leads to production of certain essential lipid compounds inside the osteoclast, thus leading to earlier cell death and therefore a diminished ability for osteoclasts to cause bone loss.

The effectiveness of this approach has been well documented. For example, alendronate has been shown to increase BMD by 6–8 percent at the spine and by 3–6 percent at the hip over a three-year period in postmenopausal women with osteoporosis (Black et al. 1996, Liberman et al. 1995). These seemingly modest increases in BMD are associated with significant reductions in fracture risk—roughly 50 percent, in fact, for spine, hip, and wrist fractures (Black et al. 1996, Cranney et al. 2002a). These agents show benefits quickly, as evidence of a reduced risk of fracture can be seen as early as a year for spinal fractures and in 18 months for hip fractures (Black et al. 2000). In addition, approximately 95 percent of postmenopausal women who take alendronate maintained or increase their bone mass (Black et al. 2000, Liberman et al. 1995).

Alendronate has been shown to prevent bone loss in a diverse array of patients, including younger postmenopausal women without osteoporosis and elderly, frail residents of long-term care facilities (Fleisch 2001). The drug has been studied in clinical trials and appears to be safe and effective for up to 10 years (Bone et al. 2004). Furthermore, the benefits of alendronate appear to continue after the therapy is stopped; for example, when older postmenopausal women discontinue therapy after several years of treatment, BMD appears to be maintained for 2 yearss (Tonino et al. 2000). Alendronate also appears to work for men, and it is therefore approved for the treatment of male osteoporosis. In one study, BMD of the spine increased approximately 5 percent at the end of 2 years in men with osteoporosis (Orwoll et al. 2000). In another 3-year study of men with primary osteoporosis, alendronate was compared to alfacalcidol, an active vitamin D analog, and found to reduce vertebral fractures by 57 percent and increase spine BMD by 11.5 percent, as compared to the alfacalcidol-treated group (Ringe et al. 2004). Alendronate and calcitriol were found to slow the rapid bone loss that occurs after heart transplantation, but calcitriol was found to cause an excessive increase in urine calcium excretion in many patients (Shane et al. 2004). Finally, alendronate is approved for the prevention of steroid-induced osteoporosis (Saag et al. 1998) and for the treatment of Paget's disease (Lyles et al. 2001) and has also been shown to be helpful for patients with osteoporosis imperfecta and bone loss due to hyperparathyroidism (Chow et al. 2003) (see below and Chapter 3).

Alendronate is currently approved for all women for *prevention* of postmenopausal osteoporosis at a dose of 5 mg daily or 35 mg if taken once a week. It is approved for the *treatment* of postmenopausal osteoporosis at a dose as compared to the alfacalcidol-treated group (Ringe et al. 2004). Alendronate and calcitriol were found to slow the rapid bone loss that occurs after heart transplantation, but calcitriol wasof 10 mg daily or 70 mg if taken once a week. Alendronate is well-tolerated (Liberman et al. 1995, Black et al. 1996, Cranney et al. 2002a); the most common side effects include pain in osteoporosis, alendronate was compared to alfacalcidol, an active vitamin D analog, and found to reduce vertebral fractures by 57 percent and increase spine BMD by 11.5 percent, the stomach or esophagus and swallowing difficulties. Esophageal ulcers have occurred in some patients on these types of daily bisphosphonates. Alendronate should not be used in patients with abnormalities of the esophagus that delay esophageal emptying, such as stricture (narrowing) or achalasia (muscle spasm).

Like alendronate, risedronate has also been shown to increase BMD and reduce fracture risk significantly. Studies have found that risedronate increases spine BMD by approximately 5 percent and hip BMD by 2–3 percent over 3 years in postmenopausal women with osteoporosis (Harris et al. 1999). Treatment with risedronate is associated with a 41 percent reduction in spine fractures (Harris et al. 1999), a 39 percent reduction in non-spine fractures (Harris et al. 1999), and a 30 percent reduction in hip fractures (McClung et al. 2001). Like alendronate, the benefits of risedronate can be seen relatively quickly. For example, reductions in spine fractures can occur after 1 year of therapy (Harris et al. 1999). Studies have examined the safety and effectiveness of risedronate for up to 5 years and have shown persistent reduction in fractures without adverse effects (Sorensen et al. 2003). Risedronate also has been shown to prevent bone loss at the hip and spine in postmenopausal women with low bone mass who do not have osteoporosis but have low bone mass (as indicated by BMD). Risedronate is approved for both the prevention *and* treatment of steroid-induced osteoporosis in men and pre- and post-menopausal women (Reid et al. 2000), and for the treatment of Paget's disease (Lyles et al. 2001) (see below and Chapter 3). Risedronate is approved at a dose of 5 mg per day or 35 mg once per week. The most common side effects include pain in the stomach or esophagus and difficulties in swallowing.

Ibandronate is another bisphosphonate that is currently FDA-approved for the treatment and prevention of osteoporosis in postmenopausal women at a dose of 2.5 mg daily; however, it is not readily commercially available. Over a 3-year period, ibandronate has been shown to decrease the incidence of new spine fractures by 52 percent and to increase BMD at the spine by 5 percent (Delmas et al. 2002), with no abnormalities found on bone histology (Recker et al. 2004). Ibandronate has also been shown to prevent bone loss in early postmenopausal women who are not yet osteoporotic (McClung et al. 2004).

Etidronate is a bisphosphonate that is not FDA-approved for the prevention and treatment of osteoporosis in the United States, although it is approved in Canada and other countries. It is approved in the United States for the treatment of Paget's disease (see below). Several small studies in postmenopausal women with osteoporosis have shown that etidronate increases BMD by 4–5 percent at the spine over 2–3 years and decreases spine fractures by approximately 50 percent (Watts et al. 1990, Hanley et al. 2000). It also has been shown to prevent bone loss in patients who start or are on chronic steroid therapy. In contrast to the other bisphosphonates that are taken daily, etidronate is taken on an intermittent schedule of 400 mg per day for 2 weeks every 3 months which is repeated for 2 years or more. A generally well-tolerated drug (Hanley et al. 2000), etidronate acts differently than do other bisphosphonates. When it is removed from the bone surface by osteoclasts, it forms toxic products inside the cell, thus resulting in early death of osteoclasts. However, it is not as potent as the newer bisphosphonates and can also impair the laying down of mineral during new bone formation if given in high doses.

All bisphosphonates are poorly absorbed and therefore should be taken alone first thing in the morning on an empty stomach with a full glass of water. Food should not be eaten for at least 30 minutes after taking the drug. Patients should not lie down during this period, to prevent irritation of the esophagus. Physicians should proceed cautiously when prescribing amino-bisphosphonates (alendronate or risedronate) to patients with a known history of narrowing or ulcers of the esophagus or long-term problems with stomach ulcers and heartburn that require medication. Bisphosphonates are incorporated into bone and, therefore, may continue to provide benefits for a long period of time after treatment is discontinued (unlike hormone therapy, as discussed earlier). Bisphosphonates should not be given to pregnant women or patients with poor kidney function, since good kidney function is required to clear this drug from the blood. Little information is available on the use of bisphosphonates in children. Bisphosphonates that need only be administered once a year on an intravenous basis are currently under investigation (see Future Agents). This approach would circumvent the problems of poor absorption and gastrointestinal irritation and might also improve compliance.

Hormone Therapy. As noted in earlier chapters, estrogen is a hormone that is important throughout life to bone development and maintenance in both men and women. Unlike the bisphosphonate drugs discussed earlier in this chapter, estrogen acts on many reproductive and non-reproductive tissues in the body. Therefore, the use of exogenous forms of estrogen as a drug for the prevention or treatment of osteoporosis necessarily involves consideration of how the form and dose of estrogen might affect other tissues. Of particular importance is whether there are any risks that might limit its use.

• *Background on Hormone Therapy.* Fuller Albright, a clinical researcher in the 1930s, observed that most of his patients with osteoporosis were postmenopausal women.

Given this, Albright proposed that estrogen triggers a buildup of calcium reserves in bone during adolescence to provide for later reproductive needs (pregnancy and lactation), and that bone is lost after menopause when estrogen levels decrease (Riggs et al. 2002). Many subsequent observations have confirmed the theory that "replacing" estrogen in postmenopausal women prevents bone loss, and thus this approach naturally seemed to be an effective way to stave off the effects of menopause on bone.

The FDA approved estrogen in 1942 in the form of conjugated equine estrogens (CEE), derived from the urine of pregnant horses, for the relief of menopausal symptoms. The use of hormone therapy by postmenopausal women increased dramatically during the 1960s, and, in 1972, the FDA approval was extended to postmenopausal osteoporosis. This latter approval was based on evidence from trials that evaluated the impact of estrogen therapy on bone mass, not on fracture reduction. However, by the early 1970s it also became clear that estrogen alone (without progestin) was associated with an increased risk of endometrial (uterine) cancer. Since this time only women who have had their uterus removed by hysterectomy are prescribed estrogen alone; others receive estrogen combined with some form of progesterone, another hormone, to protect the uterus.

• *The Evidence on Estrogen and Combination Hormone Therapy.* Randomized, placebo-controlled studies have been conducted on the impact of hormone therapy on BMD, including the Postmenopausal Estrogen/Progestin Interventions (PEPI) trial (Writing Group 1996) and the Women's Health, Osteoporosis, Progestin, Estrogen (HOPE) study (Lindsay et al. 2002). These trials and a recent meta-analysis

(Wells et al. 2002) show that postmenopausal hormone therapy has a consistent and favorable effect on BMD at all sites, including increases at the spine (3.5–7 percent), hip (2–4 percent), and forearm (3–4.5 percent). These studies also suggest that increases in BMD become apparent within the first year of hormone therapy. Both the PEPI trial and the meta-analysis, which included different forms of estrogen (CEE as well as estradiol, the natural form of estrogen in humans) and combination therapy, found no significant differences in the effects of different formulations of estrogen on bone density.

Research evaluating the impact of hormone therapy on fracture rates, however, is more limited. Studies comparing women who had taken postmenopausal hormones over a long period of time with women who had never taken hormones indicate that there are fewer fractures in the hormone users (Kiel et al. 1987, Cauley et al. 1995). These types of "observational" studies, which observe what people decide to do or take on their own, are subject to biases. For example, women who take hormones are also more likely to take other measures to enhance their health. In fact, up until the mid-1990s, there had been very few randomized clinical trials of estrogen focusing on fracture as an outcome, and these trials tended to be quite small.

Nevertheless, Torgerson and Bell-Syer attempted to fill this evidence gap by systematically reviewing those randomized trials of estrogen therapy that did include fractures as an outcome to be evaluated. Their meta-analyses suggest that estrogen reduces the risk of non-spine fractures by 27 percent (Torgerson and Bell-Syer 2001a) and spine fractures by 33 percent (Torgerson and Bell-Syer 2001b).

The WHI Hormone Trials, which were designed and initiated in the early 1990s to address the primary question of whether postmenopausal HT decreased the risk of heart disease, have provided answers on a range of chronic disease outcomes in older women, including fractures. Two separate trials were conducted. One enrolled women with an intact uterus and evaluated the effects of an estrogen-progestin combination or E+P (0.625 mg conjugated equine estrogen, CEE, and 2.5 mg medroxyprogesterone, MPA, daily) (Rossouw et al., 2002), while the second evaluated the effect of estrogen (0.625 mg CEE) alone in women who have had hysterectomies (Anderson et al. 2004). The WHI trial of combined continuous hormone therapy confirmed for the first time the effects of these hormones on osteoporotic fracture reduction at several sites, including the hip (Cauley et al., 2003). Hip and spine fractures were reduced by at least one-third in both of the trials and total fractures fell by 24–30 percent. Thus, these two large trials, which included 16,608 women in the E+P study and 10,739 women in the estrogen-only study, confirmed the anti-fracture efficacy of postmenopausal HT, and they are consistent with observational studies of hormone users and the results of trials evaluating the effect of HT on BMD.

The clear benefits of postmenopausal HT to the skeleton must be tempered by the other results from the WHI trials, which were discontinued early because of the deleterious effects encountered. Both trials found an increased risk of stroke, cognitive impairment, and deep vein thrombosis in the women taking HT (Rossouw et al. 2002, Anderson et al. 2004, Shumaker et al. 2003; Shumaker et al. 2004). The trials also found no clear cardiovascular benefit to HT. Breast cancer risk was increased in women taking the combined continuous therapy (E+P) during the 5.2 years of the study, a finding that is consistent with observational studies (Collaborative Group 1997, Lagro-Janssen 2003). This increase in breast cancer was not observed in the estrogen-only trial after 6.6 years of use. Extended follow-up of all WHI hormone trial participants is planned, and may provide further insight into this discrepancy.

• *The Future for Hormone Therapy and Bone Health.* Any decision to use hormone therapy must take into consideration its impact on the overall risk of negative health outcomes, including not only its potential to reduce the risk of fractures, but also its potential to increase the risk of other health problems. The Food and Drug Administration (FDA 2003) has advised that postmenopausal women who use or are considering using estrogen or estrogen with progestin discuss the therapy's benefits and risks with their physicians. These products are approved therapies for relief from moderate to severe hot flashes and symptoms of vulvar and vaginal atrophy. Although HT is effective for the prevention of postmenopausal osteoporosis, it should only be considered for women at significant risk of osteoporosis who cannot take non-estrogen medications. The FDA recommends that estrogens and progestins should be used at the lowest possible doses for the shortest amount of time needed to achieve treatment goals. It is not yet clear whether following this advice will lead to long term benefits for bone health. Lower doses of estrogen or combination hormones can help to preserve bone density in the short term in postmenopausal women. For example, the Women's HOPE study, a randomized, placebo-controlled study that investigated the efficacy of various lower doses of CEE and CEE/MPA found that doses as low as 0.3 mg per day of CEE or the combination significantly increased spine and hip BMD from baseline within 2 years of therapy (Lindsay et al. 2002). Prestwood et al. (2003) showed that low dose estradiol also preserves bone. Unfortunately, at this point, the long-term effects of different doses, formulations (including estrogens or progesterone), and modes of administration (e.g., transdermal administration) on bone and other tissues have simply not been studied.

These results raise the question as to whether there might be some benefit to using hormone therapy for a short period of time and then terminating its use (so as to reduce the likelihood of negative health outcomes). Two randomized clinical trials shed some light on this issue, as they followed women who stopped hormone use at the end of a clinical trial. These studies indicate that bone loss begins again when hormones are withdrawn (Greendale et al. 2002, Greenspan et al. 2002b). Moreover, the long-term observational studies (Kiel et al. 1987, Cauley et al. 1995) suggest that even long-term hormone therapy users (including those on therapy for more than 10 years) who terminate therapy do not enjoy a lower risk of hip fractures many years later. In fact, a recent study (Yates et al. 2004) found that there was a higher rate of hip fracture in those who discontinued hormone therapy than in those who never used it. Another study, a large prospective trial of 5,200 fractures among 140,000 postmenopausal women in the United Kingdom, found that while there was a decrease in fracture risk at all sites in patients currently on estrogen, there was no decrease in risk in past users of hormone therapy, even those who had discontinued use within the past year (Banks et al. 2004). Thus, the bottom line is that taking hormone therapy during early menopause is unlikely to have a long-term effect on the risk of fractures.

Despite all the negatives that have been raised recently about HT, it is important to remember that natural estrogen (i.e., that which is produced by the body) is still critical to bone health, even for postmenopausal women (and older men). The evidence suggests that postmenopausal women with extremely low endogenous estrogen levels face an increased risk of both spine and hip fractures when compared with postmenopausal women with average levels of estrogen (Cummings et al. 1998). Very low doses of hormone therapy for these individuals may be a promising treatment (Prestwood et al. 2003).

The goal of this type of an approach is to capture the positive effects of estrogen on bone without incurring any of the deleterious effects on other tissues. In fact, this is the principle that has driven research into the selective estrogen receptor modulators or SERMS that are discussed in the next section; these agents selectively act on the estrogen receptors in bone, breast, and other tissues.

> "In the final analysis very little is known about anything, and much that seems true today turns out to be only partly true tomorrow."
>
> —Fuller Albright, reflecting on the state of affairs of medicine in general and of endocrinology in particular in 1948 (Albright and Reifenstein 1948).

Selective Estrogen Receptor Modulators. Selective estrogen receptor modulators (SERMs) interact with estrogen receptors located throughout the body (McDonnell 2003). Estrogen receptors are the "switches" that turn cell activity on and off (see Chapter 2 for more details). SERMs bind to the estrogen receptors, altering the way they interact with other proteins and DNA. Different SERM medications may have different actions on cholesterol, breast and uterine tissue, clotting, BMD, and hot flashes. They have been shown to provide some of the benefits of estrogen (improvement of BMD and cholesterol) without some of the negative side effects (such as breast tenderness and menstrual bleeding or spotting) (Ettinger et al. 1999). In fact, in large-scale clinical trials of postmenopausal women with osteoporosis, raloxifene (Evista®), the only FDA-approved SERM, has been shown to increase spine BMD by 2–3 percent and hip BMD by approximately 2.5 percent after 3 years (Ettinger et al. 1999). Spine fractures were reduced by approximately 50 percent, but there was no effect on hip or other non-spine fractures (Ettinger et al. 1999, Cranney et al. 2002b). Spine fracture reduction is evident at 1 year (Maricic et al. 2002) and is sustained for up to at least 4 years if patients remain on therapy (Delmas et al. 2002). When therapy is discontinued, bone turnover (breakdown) can return to its previous state, resulting in bone loss. Other potential benefits include a decrease in total cholesterol and low density cholesterol; there is no change in high density cholesterol. Although studies have not been specifically designed to examine prevention of breast cancer with raloxifene, investigators from the study mentioned above found that there was a decreased incidence of breast cancer in the women who took raloxifene for 3 years (Cummings et al. 1999). There are now studies ongoing to examine raloxifene's effect on breast cancer and cardiovascular disease prevention.

Raloxifene is FDA-approved for the prevention *and* treatment of postmenopausal osteoporosis at a dose of 60 mg daily. There are some side effects, including the potential for a return of hot flashes, blood clots in the legs, or blood clots in the lungs. Therapy with SERMs must be discontinued for patients who are immobilized or inactive for long periods of time (e.g., during hospitalizations).

Another SERM, tamoxifen, is used for the prevention of breast cancer, but it is not approved for the prevention and treatment of osteoporosis. Small clinical trials in premenopausal and postmenopausal women participating in a breast cancer prevention study demonstrated that tamoxifen maintains or improves BMD in postmenopausal women but causes bone loss in premenopausal women (Powles et al. 1996). Information on fracture reduction from clinical trials is not available.

Newer SERMs under development may be more beneficial to the bones, heart, and breast tissue. They may also decrease hot flashes and improve cholesterol. There are no data to suggest that SERMs would be beneficial in the treatment of male osteoporosis, Paget's disease, or childhood osteoporosis.

Calcitonin. Calcitonin is a hormone secreted by the parafollicular (non-thyroid) cells found within the thyroid gland (Silverman 2003). Its effect on bone is to inhibit bone resorption by acting directly on the osteoclasts. Its ability to inhibit osteoclast activity has been known for more than four decades. At one time in the 1970s, calcitonin was the only drug available to treat hypercalcemia of malignancy and Paget's disease of the bone. Calcitonin was also one of the first drugs available for the treatment of osteoporosis.

In the 1970s and 1980s, calcitonin was administered as a subcutaneous (under the skin) injection. More recently, nasal calcitonin replaced the injection form of this hormone. Although originally very popular as an alternative for postmenopausal women who could not tolerate bisphosphonates, estrogen, or raloxifene, its use has declined with the advent of newer treatments for postmenopausal

osteoporosis. Oral and inhaled forms of calcitonin are currently under development.

There are only a few randomized controlled trials for nasal calcitonin. The Prevent Recurrence of Osteoporotic Fractures (PROOF) trial, the largest RPCT of nasal calcitonin, reported that spine fractures declined by 33 percent for those individuals taking a 200 IU dose per day, but there was no significant decline for those receiving 100 or 400 IU per day. Furthermore, there were no significant differences in non-spine fracture rates after 5 years (Chesnut et al. 2000).

The PROOF trial has come under scrutiny for a number of reasons, including the somewhat surprising finding that those individuals taking a higher dose did not see a reduction in fractures. In addition, a large number of the subjects did not complete the study. Hence flaws in the study methods used do not allow a firm conclusion about calcitonin's impact on spine and non-spine spine fractures (Chesnut et al. 2000). Calcitonin may have a somewhat unique benefit in providing pain relief, particularly for women who have just sustained a spine fracture (Mehta et al. 2003). Studies looking at this potential benefit also do not provide a clear-cut answer. Nasal calcitonin has very few side effects, namely, nasal stuffiness, nausea, and dry mouth. It is currently approved at 200 IU per daily spray for the treatment (not prevention) of osteoporosis in women who underwent menopause five or more years ago.

Combination Antiresorptive Therapy. Although bisphosphonates, hormone therapy, and SERMs are all antiresorptive drugs, they work through different mechanisms of action, implying that they could have an additive effect if used in combination (i.e., using both would be more beneficial than would either used alone).

Therefore, antiresorptive drugs have been studied in combination. One study compared 2-year use of two antiresorptive therapies together to similar use of estrogen and alendronate alone in postmenopausal women with a hysterectomy (Bone et al. 2000). BMD increased approximately 8 percent at the spine in those on combination therapy, compared to 6 percent in women taking alendronate or estrogen. Similar trends were noted in BMD at the hip, where combination therapy resulted in a 1–2 percent greater increase in BMD than either therapy alone. Importantly, participants in the combination therapy group did not have additional unexpected side effects. A recent 3-year study in women age 65 and older found that using hormone therapy and alendronate together resulted in greater increases in bone mass at the spine and hip than did therapy with either agent alone (Greenspan et al. 2003).

Hormone therapy has also been used in combination with risedronate in a short-term study. At the end of a year, the hip BMD (but not the spine BMD) of participants on combination therapy was greater than that of participants receiving hormone therapy or risedronate alone (Harris et al. 2001). In another 1-year study, hip BMD was greater in participants taking a combination therapy of alendronate and raloxifene than in those taking either agent alone (Johnell et al. 2002). The study also found that BMD of the spine and hip in participants taking alendronate alone was significantly higher than in participants taking raloxifene alone; however, the study was not large enough to determine whether there was any difference in fracture reduction.

Studies have also examined another important issue—whether combination therapy is better than single-agent therapy at maintaining BMD after discontinuation of the treatment. Investigators who examined BMD in women on combination therapy (alendronate and estrogen replacement) and single therapy (alendronate or hormone therapy) followed them for an additional year after therapy was discontinued. Those who had taken combination therapy or alendronate alone during the first 2 years maintained BMD of the spine and hip following discontinuation of therapy. However, women who gained bone during 2 years on hormone replacement lost their BMD gains at the spine and hip during the year after therapy was discontinued (Greenspan et al. 2002).

Combination therapies (multiple drugs) are more expensive and, in principle, could cause more side effects than therapy with single drugs. Moreover, because these trials did not examine fracture reduction, it is unclear if combination therapy is a cost-effective strategy for reducing risk of fracture. Therefore, in clinical practice today, combination therapy is generally reserved for patients who have experienced a fracture while on therapy with a single drug, those who start out with a very low BMD and a history of multiple fractures, and those with very low BMD who lose more bone mass on therapy with a single drug. The combination of anabolic and antiresorptive agents is discussed below.

Anabolic Therapy. Over the last half century, antiresorptive therapy has been the primary treatment for osteoporosis. Recent research has discovered the potential of intermittent parathyroid hormone (PTH) as a therapeutic option for patients with severe osteoporosis. Unlike other available agents, bone-building therapy with PTH features stimulation of new bone formation (Rosen and Rackoff 2001). Eighteen months of PTH therapy causes thickening of the outer shell of bones, large increases in connections between bony islands within the skeleton, and an overall net increase in bone strength.

Every normal person has PTH. It is typically secreted at a low level, but secretion increases in response to reduced levels of serum calcium, a process that appears to contribute to bone breakdown. In fact, primary hyperparathyroidism, that is, uncontrolled overactivity of the parathyroid glands, has been known to contribute to bone loss, particularly of the cortical (outer shell) of bone (see Chapter 3). Intermittent injections of PTH as a therapy actually hold promise as a means of building up bone. Animal studies have demonstrated that PTH given intermittently as a daily subcutaneous injection leads to significant increases in BMD, restoration of the inner structure of bone, and increases in bone size (Lotinun et al. 2002). This paradox— the fact that PTH secreted continuously can break down bone while intermittent injections of the same hormone may actually build bone— has never been fully explained. It may be related to the intermittent nature of the exposure to the hormone that occurs during treatment, as opposed to the exposure to continuous, excessive levels of PTH that occur in individuals with hyperparathyroidism.

Human recombinant PTH (1-34), known as teriparatide, was developed in the 1980s, with the hope that it could promote bone building in humans. Clinical trials designed to test the impact on fracture rates in humans, which were originally designed to last 3 years, were stopped early because of animal data showing osteosarcoma (bone tumor) formation. Despite early discontinuation the studies demonstrated significant increases in BMD and reduction in fractures. For example, in a study with over 1,600 postmenopausal, osteoporotic women, spine BMD increased by 9.7 percent and hip BMD increased by 2.6 percent (Neer et al. 2001) after approximately 21 months on teriparitide. Spine fractures decreased by 65 percent and non-spine

fractures by 53 percent (Neer et al. 2001). Teriparatide also increases BMD in men; in an approximately 10-month study, spine BMD increased by 5.9 percent and hip BMD by 1.2 percent (Orwoll 1998). The effects on fracture risk have not been studied in men.

Because of these significant potential benefits, the FDA approved teriparatide for the treatment of osteoporosis in postmenopausal women and in men who are at high risk for fracture. The approved dose (20Fg daily by subcutaneous injection) and duration of treatment have not been found to be associated with an increased risk of osteosarcoma in humans.

While the PTH administered daily to postmenopausal women and men with osteoporosis may benefit some patients (particularly those with very severe disease), there are some limitations to use of the drug. First, it should not be prescribed to pediatric patients or adult patients with hypercalcemia (high levels of calcium in the blood), Paget's disease (see below), kidney disease, kidney stones, bone metastases (cancers that have traveled from another part of the body to bone), or bone cancer. Second, a small subset of patients may develop high blood calcium as well as leg cramps and dizziness. Third, it may increase serum uric acid, which could potentially lead to gout, although there is no evidence of an increase in clinical gout. Fourth, there may be issues related to compliance since a daily injection is required. Finally, it is much more expensive than antiresorptive therapy.

Additional forms of PTH therapy may be on the horizon. For example, PTH(1-84) has shown early promise as a treatment for osteoporosis in preliminary bone density studies (Hodsman et al. 2003).

Combination Antiresorptive/Anabolic Therapy. The idea of combining an anabolic agent with an anti-resorptive therapy has been around for more than a decade. With the advent of PTH, combination studies have been proposed to evaluate the impact of PTH therapy with antiresorptive therapies such as estrogen and alendronate. PTH plus estrogen has been shown to have a greater effect on spine and hip BMD than estrogen alone, but there are no trials comparing that combination to PTH alone, nor are there any studies that evaluate differences in the impact on fracture rates (Cosman et al. 2001). Two studies examining the effects of simultaneous PTH and alendronate treatment suggest that there may actually be smaller BMD increases with combination therapy than with PTH alone (Black et al. 2003, Finkelstein et al. 2003). Another recent study evaluated the impact of sequential treatment with PTH for a year followed by alendronate for a year in 66 women with postmenopausal osteoporosis year. This sequential treatment method resulted in substantial increases in spinal BMD (Rittmaster et al. 2000). The response to PTH treatment may be affected by prior treatment with different antiresorptive agents. Like those patients on estrogen therapy (Lindsay et al 1997), patients previously treated with raloxifene showed a rapid and complete response to PTH, while those previously treated with alendronate had a reduced response in terms of biochemical markers of bone formation and BMD (although they did show increases eventually) (Ettinger et al. 2004). No data on the relative impact of PTH treatment on fractures are available for these different groups.

Future Agents. There are several new antiresorptive and anabolic drugs on the horizon for the treatment of osteoporosis. Among antiresorptive agents, progress has been made both in developing new treatments and in improving the means of administering bisphosphonates. For example, intravenous pamidronate has been available for the treatment of Paget's disease and hypercalcemia of malignancy (high blood calcium due to cancer) for nearly a decade. Smaller studies have also demonstrated that it is effective in increasing bone mass when administered every 3 months to postmenopausal women with osteoporosis (Coleman et al. 2000). A newer drug, zoledronic acid, was recently approved for the treatment of metastatic breast cancer, myeloma (see below) and hypercalcemia (Coleman et al. 2000). It is administered intravenously is extremely effective in treating these conditions. A recent trial of this agent, given as a single intravenous dose once per year, was shown to increase spine BMD in women with osteoporosis (Reid et al. 2002). A large phase III trial is in progress to assess its effectiveness at reducing fractures.

Along with finding new uses for existing antiresorptive agents, researchers have also uncovered several potential new types of treatments during the drug discovery process. A newer class of antiresorptive drugs (known as integrin inhibitors) prevent osteoclasts from anchoring to bone surfaces and thereby absorbing the underlying bone (Hutchinson et al 2003). Early studies with this therapy are encouraging with respect to both safety and effectiveness. Agents that mimic the action of osteoprotegerin can also inhibit bone resorption and could become useful drugs (Onyia et al. 2004). Statins, the cholesterol-lowering drugs, have been found to stimulate bone formation and may also decrease bone resorption in animals. Some observational studies in humans suggest that statin users have fewer fractures, while other studies do not. Controlled cardiovascular trials did not confirm a reduction in fractures (Bauer et al. 2004). Finally, strontium ranelate is an element that has some antiresorptive as well as anabolic qualities, but the method of action is unclear. In initial studies, strontium has been shown to improve

Osteoporosis Drug Therapy

- Antiresorptive agents (reduce bone loss)
  - ~ Bisphosphonates (alendronate, risedronate)
  - ~ Hormone or estrogen replacement
  - ~ Selective estrogen receptor modulators (SERMs) (raloxifene)
  - ~ Calcitonin
- Anabolic agents (build bone)
  - ~ Parathyroid hormone (teriparatide)

spine bone density and reduce spine fractures (Meunier et al. 2002, 2004).

Other new anabolic agents are also being developed and tested. PTH-related peptide (PTHrP), a naturally occurring relative of PTH that is normally made in the breast, uterus, and pancreas, is undergoing clinical trials for the treatment of osteoporosis. PTHrP is best known as a secretion of certain cancers that produces severe hypercalcemia (high calcium levels in the blood) and bone resorption. However, when administered as a single dose intermittently, it has been shown to markedly increase BMD without causing hypercalcemia (Horwitz et al. 2003).

Treatment of Osteoporotic Fractures

For all osteoporotic fractures, the consistent goal is for patients to regain their pre-fracture level of function. All patients with low-trauma fractures should be evaluated for other bone diseases (see below) and secondary causes of bone loss (see Chapter 3). They should also be evaluated with respect to the need for additional preventive measures (calcium, vitamin D, exercise, fall prevention) and for drug therapy, as described earlier in this chapter. What follows is a review of the various available treatments for specific types of osteoporotic-related fractures, including fractures of the hip, spine, and wrist.

Hip Fractures. Surgery is the most common treatment for individuals who suffer a hip fracture. Virtually all intertrochanteric fractures (those in the major part of the hip) and most femoral neck fractures (those in the neck section of the hip) are surgically stabilized with the use of internal metal devices. A large percentage of displaced (unconnected) femoral neck fractures are treated with partial or total replacement of the hip because of the significant risk of healing complications (Zuckerman 1996).

Proper management of hip fracture patients begins before surgery, at the time of admission. Evaluation and management of pre-existing medical conditions is necessary before proceeding to surgery. When possible, management of pre-existing conditions and surgical repair within 24–48 hours of admission has been shown to decrease the incidence of post-surgery complications and the possibility of death within a year of surgery by more than 40 percent (Zuckerman et al. 1995). The procedure should be performed by a surgeon who has expertise in hip fracture stabilization, which will allow the initiation of mobilization immediately after surgery. The vast majority of hip fracture patients should be encouraged to become mobile by the first or second post-operative day. Mobility can help to avoid the medical problems associated with prolonged bed rest, such as muscle atrophy, blood clots in the legs or lungs, pressure sores, skin breakdown, and overall deconditioning.

The use of antibiotics for the first 24–48 hours after surgery is also advisable, as this practice has been shown to be effective in decreasing post-surgery infections. Use of techniques to thin the blood after surgery has also been shown to be effective in decreasing the incidence of blood clots, particularly in patients who are slow to mobilize (Todd et al. 1995). Adequate pre- and post-surgery pain control is also important, not only for patient comfort, but also to promote active participation in rehabilitation.

Since hip fractures generally occur in elderly patients with other, associated medical and psychosocial problems, the health care team should include professionals from many disciplines, including the orthopaedic surgeon, medical specialists (geriatricians, physiatrists [rehabilitation specialists], primary care physicians, and medical sub-specialists as necessary), nurses, physical and occupational therapists, nutritionists, and social workers. The in-hospital care of hip fracture patients should be guided, whenever possible, by the use of evidence-based clinical care pathways (clinical care based on medical studies) that make use of standardized evaluation and management approaches. This approach should also extend to the entire continuum of care, from the acute care hospital into the post-discharge setting, whether that setting is an acute or sub-acute rehabilitation facility, a skilled nursing facility, or a return home. Effective communication across health settings by health care providers is also important to effective care management (Morris and Zuckerman 2002). Discharge from acute care hospitals and independent rehabilitation facilities should be based on patient progress.

Spine Fractures. Spine fractures usually occur in the middle or lower section of the back as a result of minor strain, such as lifting a grocery bag. Some patients develop fractures without any identifiable trauma. Spine fractures due to osteoporosis result in the progressive collapse of bones in these areas, which typically cause increasing levels of spinal deformity and pain.

However, about two-thirds of spine fractures go undiagnosed because there is little or no pain, or the pain is attributed to one of the many other causes of back pain (Johnell et al. 2002). Similarly, other signs of a spine fracture, including deformities and height loss, are often accepted as a normal part of aging and thus not investigated further.

It is not unusual for patients to have prolonged pain and disability following spine fractures. Treatment of spine fractures typically focuses on pain control and progressive increases in levels of mobilization. Back braces are of limited benefit. More recently, procedures have been developed to treat patients who have prolonged pain. Vertebroplasty is a technique in which acrylic cement (or orthopedic cement mixture) is injected into the spine bone for the purpose of stabilizing the fracture (Evans et al. 2003). Kyphoplasty involves using a balloon to re-expand the collapsed bone and then filling the cavity with bone cement. This procedure has the potential to stabilize the fracture, prevent further collapse, and restore some degree of height to the bone (Lieberman et al. 2001). Both vertebroplasty and kyphoplasty have been shown to provide effective pain relief and stabilization of the fracture (Evans et al. 2003, Lieberman et al. 2001). Although complications from these procedures have been infrequent, they can be significant if the bone cement leaks out into the blood stream or into the spinal canal, causing nerve damage. Unfortunately, the potential benefit of these two procedures has not yet been accurately assessed in RPCTs, where they might be compared to each other and to nonsurgical management.

Wrist Fractures. Wrist fractures commonly occur as a result of osteoporosis. They include fractures of the radius and/or ulna (the two long bones in the forearm), as well as of the small bones of the wrist. The term Colles' fractures refers to fractures of the end of the radius, which has a large amount of trabecular bone. Wrist fractures are usually treated by either surgical repositioning and casting or placement of an external fixation device to prevent further fracture. Depending on the type of fracture, one of the following will be used to immobilize the wrist until an x-ray shows evidence of healing (usually in 4–8 weeks): a brace or splint, cast, external fixation, internal fixation, or combined external and internal fixation. Although most patients return to an adequate level of functioning, many do experience some loss of range of motion of the wrist.

Other Fractures. Osteoporotic fractures occur in other areas of the body, including the upper arm, thigh, shin, collar bone, and ribs. These fractures are treated by a variety of surgical and non-surgical measures.

Rehabilitation of Osteoporotic Fractures

Hip Fractures. As noted previously, hip fracture patients typically undergo surgery to reposition the hip through internal fixation (e.g., insertion of a metal pin or plate) or to replace the hip through joint replacement. Immediately following either type of surgery, in-hospital rehabilitation focuses on training the patient to safely move in bed, to get out of bed, and to begin walking with partial weight-bearing on the surgical side using either a walker or crutches. A physician specializing in rehabilitation medicine or a physical therapist evaluates the patient, administers or supervises the treatment sessions, and makes discharge recommendations. An occupational therapist also may evaluate the patient and provide training in performing activities of daily living (e.g., bathing, dressing) during recovery from the fracture. The occupational therapist may also provide the patient with assistive devices, such as long-handled shoe horns and devices that help the patients put on his or her socks.

Since the inpatient hospital stay typically is limited to 2–3 days after surgery, most patients require additional rehabilitation. Transfer to a rehabilitation facility (a specialty hospital or a skilled nursing home) is common, with length of stay in this setting ranging from several days to several weeks. Following discharge to home, rehabilitation is continued through in-home therapy with a physical therapist or visits to an outpatient facility. This phase of the rehabilitation focuses on general conditioning, strengthening of muscle, and walking longer distances on different terrains and with less assistance. The degree to which a patient progresses from relying on the support of assistive devices during walking to more complete weight-bearing on the fractured limb will depend on the type of surgery and implanted metal as well as the physical condition of the patient. The "typical" patient progresses from a walker to a four-footed cane to a single-point cane to no assistive device for walking. However, 85 percent of patients still use an assistive device for walking 6 months after the fracture (Marotolli et al. 1992).

Nutrition has been shown to be important during recovery from hip fracture. Supplementation with calcium, vitamin D, and protein (20 grams per day) have been reported to improve hospital and rehabilitation courses and to increase BMD a year after the fracture (Schurch et al. 1998).

6 months after hospital discharge, an evaluation should be performed to determine the patient's functional status and to set goals for the future. Many patients require further therapy to reach these goals, whereas others may have reached their potential.

Spine Fractures. As noted above, only about one-third of spine fractures come to clinical attention, but those that do usually are painful. Therefore, pain control is a high priority after the initial spine fractures and after multiple fractures, when chronic pain often becomes a problem. Bedrest should be partial (resting in bed interspersed with 30- to 60-minute periods of erect sitting, standing, and walking) and limited to 4 days or less. Individuals should be taught to position themselves (e.g., while sitting, standing, or lying down) and to move (e.g., when lifting, dressing, doing housework) while maintaining good posture, which reduces loads on the fracture and minimizes pain. To minimize pain and decrease risk of a new spine fracture, family members should be taught to assist patients in performing tasks without increasing the loads on the patient's spine (Bonner et al. 2003).

Walking should be encouraged even in frail individuals. A gradual progression starting at only 2–3 minutes and working up to twenty or more minutes can be achieved by adding a minute or two to walking sessions each week. Short-term use of a back brace is recommended when trunk weakness prevents a patient from maintaining an upright posture. An occupational therapist can fit the proper device. Weaning from the device, as muscle strength and endurance improve, will maximize recovery. However, in some patients with chronic pain and deformity, continued use of a flexible support device that helps maintain back strength and posture may be helpful in reducing pain and improving function (Pfeifer et al. 2004). If walking is limited due to pain, use of a rolling walker with four wheels and hand brakes may help the patient stay active during recovery, thus preventing loss of muscle strength and bone mass. This type of

walker allows the use of the arms to keep the trunk erect, thereby shifting the weight of the upper body away from the newly fractured bone. Individuals with a new spine fracture should avoid use of a standard walker, since each time the walker is lifted the loads on the vertebral bodies are increased.

Exercising in a way that safely challenges balance is also important for rehabilitation of spinal fracture patients, although this exercise must be accompanied by an assessment of the risk of falling and the addressing of modifiable risk factors for falling, such as vision problems, medications that cause dizziness, and hazards in the home. Active range of motion exercises should be continued during recovery, but resistance/strengthening exercises should not be initiated or resumed until the fracture has healed (in approximately 8 to 12 weeks). Since the risk of another spine fracture is high in patients who have had fractures, patients should be instructed to avoid exercises and activities that put high loads on the bones of the spine, such as flexing or rotating the spine (sit ups, toe touches). Exercises and activities done with good spine alignment and low to moderate amounts of weight should be gradually increased, with the goals of regaining muscle strength and promoting maintenance of bone mass. Abdominal strengthening (by tightening the muscles in the abdomen or belly without moving the back) is safe and important to reducing loads on the low back. Spinal extension exercise (i.e., stretching backwards) within a moderate range is safe and can improve hyperkyphosis (a spine that is bent excessively forward) and may help prevent new spine fractures (Sinaki et al. 2002).

Wrist Fractures. Rehabilitation of the wrist after the cast, brace, or surgical metal is removed requires about 3 months, but reaching maximum levels of recovery can take up to 24 months, and some problems may persist for years. During healing of a wrist fracture, all of the following are important: arm elevation; early mobilization of the hand, elbow, and shoulder; and control of swelling. Progressive exercises, taught by either a physical or occupational therapist, typically include active and passive range of motion and resistance and grip strengthening, such as squeezing a ball (Bonner et al. 2003). A small number of patients suffer from sympathetic dystrophy (complex regional pain syndrome) after a wrist fracture, resulting in swelling, weakness, and chronic pain in the wrist.

Treatment of Other Diseases of the Bone

There are specific, effective (and often curative) treatments for a number of bone diseases other than osteoporosis, including hyperparathyroidism, rickets, and osteomalacia. There is also treatment available for some congenital bone disorders and for bone disease associated with kidney failure. Early recognition and treatment of all of these conditions is the key to avoiding crippling deformities and fractures. What follows is a brief review of treatment options for the most common of these diseases.

Primary Hyperparathyroidism. Primary hyperparathyroidism is caused by an excessive release of PTH from one or more of the parathyroid glands. (See Chapter 3 for more a more detailed description.) Surgical removal of the parathyroid adenoma (benign tumor) or of three-and-a-half glands (if all four glands are enlarged) often cures the disease. In 2002, an NIH-sponsored workshop on the management of non-symptomatic primary hyperparathyroidism concluded that patients who are clearly symptomatic with bone disease or kidney stones should be advised to have surgery (Bilezikian et al. 2002, Bilezikian and Silverberg

2004). There is considerable controversy concerning the need for intervention in patients who have no clear signs or symptoms of the disease. Treatment guidelines for non-symptomatic patients relate to the degree of hypercalcemia (greater than 1 mg/dL serum calcium above the upper limits of normal), hypercalciuria (greater than 400 mg per day urine calcium), and age (under age 50). An independent panel of experts that convened after the end of the NIH workshop suggested that new guidelines for surgery for non-symptomatic patients with primary hyperparathyroidism should be based on levels of bone density that are in line with modern definitions of osteoporosis. If T-score measurements are below −2.5 at any site, surgery is now being recommended. The evidence suggests, moreover, that parathyroid surgery is effective; patients who undergo such surgery have increased their bone mass by 10 percent or more over the 3- to 4-year period following surgery, with the largest gains occurring in the spine (Silverberg et al. 1999). Parathyroid surgery patients have also experienced a decreased incidence of fractures (Vestergaard and Mosekilde 2004). Optimal parathyroid surgery requires exceptional expertise in being able to localize and identify abnormal parathyroid glands and remove them with minimal injury to other tissues. Recent advances have led to newer approaches such as minimally invasive parathyroidectomy for removal of a single parathyroid adenoma with a small incision and minimal trauma to other tissues (Udelsman 2002). This approach requires successful pre-surgery location of the abnormal parathyroid gland, usually by technetium-99m-sestamibi scanning and/or ultrasound imaging (Alexander et al. 2002). Many patients who are not candidates for surgery for parathyroidectomy appear to do very well when they are managed conservatively with appropriate measures to avoid dehydration and further bone loss (Silverberg et al. 1999).

Currently, there are no FDA-approved medications for primary hyperparathyroidism. However, medical therapy may be available in the future. Specifically, calcimimetic (calcium-mimicking) agents, which can inhibit parathyroid hormone secretion, offer a direct approach to the medical therapy of primary hyperparathyroidism (Silverberg et al. 1997). Antiresorptive therapy can be used in patients with primary hyperparathyroidism and low bone mass who refuse surgery or for whom surgery is contraindicated (Rubin et al. 2003, Parker et al. 2002, Chow et al. 2003).

Renal Osteodystrophy. Renal osteodystrophy is a complex bone disease that occurs because of chronic renal (kidney) failure; a more detailed description of the disease and its causes can be found in Chapter 3. Treatment of renal osteodystrophy depends on the type of abnormality in the bone and on the stage of the renal disease. An important aspect of prevention of renal osteodystrophy is the early implementation of dietary phosphate and protein restriction, oral 1,25-dihydroxy vitamin D (calcitriol) treatment, and adequate oral intake of calcium and vitamin D. A recent analysis of hemodialysis patients suggested that treatment with a vitamin D analog, paricalcitol, resulted in lower mortality than did treatment with calcitriol (Teng et al. 2003). All patients progressing to end-stage renal disease are offered treatment to control uremia (high levels of blood urea nitrogen) with dialysis. An increasing number of patients on dialysis are offered the option of kidney transplantation. The incidence of osteoporosis after transplantation (when bone loss can be aggravated by the drugs that are used to suppress the immune response and prevent rejection of the transplant) can be reduced by keeping the dose of corticosteroids and anti-transplant drugs to a minimum (Cohen and Shane 2003). However, osteoporosis in post-transplant patients may also be treated in its own right by anti-osteoporotic therapies such as bisphosphonates.

Paget's Disease of Bone. Paget's disease of bone is localized, excessive bone remodeling that leads to increased bone resorption and formation (see Chapter 3 for more details). The primary therapy involves use of bisphosphonates, which decrease bone resorption and slow bone turnover (Lyles et al. 2001). Alendronate, risedronate, tiludronate, and etidronate are bisphosphonates that are approved for the treatment of Paget's disease. The doses used for treatment of Paget's disease are generally higher than those used for osteoporosis treatment. Bisphosphonates lead to a decrease in alkaline phosphatase and often decrease the skeletal pain associated with the excessive bone turnover. Calcitonin (as an under-the-skin injection or nasal spray) has also been used to treat Paget's disease, but is less effective than bisphosphonates (Deal 2004). PTH should not be given to patients with Paget's disease.

Bone Metastases of Cancer. Bone metastases are common in a number of cancers, and they contribute heavily to morbidity and mortality, most prominently in prostate, breast, and multiple myeloma. Bone metastases are often associated with severe and frequently intractable pain (Mundy 2002). The relationship between prostate cancer and the bone is unique among cancers. Approximately 90 percent of advanced prostate cancer patients develop clinically significant bone metastasis,

Treatment of Other Bone Diseases

- Primary hyperparathyroidism
  - ~ Removal of parathyroid adenoma(s) by surgery if signs or symptoms meet guidelines
  - ~ Hormone therapy or bisphosphonates may be helpful
- Renal osteodystrophy (bone disease from kidney failure)
  - ~ Treatment of kidney problem (dialysis, transplantation)
  - ~ Special diets
  - ~ Calcitriol
- Paget's disease of bone
  - ~ Bisphosphonates (alendronate, risedronate, tiludronate, etidronate)
- Multiple myeloma
  - ~ Chemotherapy
  - ~ Stem cell transplantation
  - ~ Bisphosphonates
- Osteogenesis imperfecta
  - ~ Rehabilitation
  - ~ Physical therapy
  - ~ Bisphosphonates

causing osteoblastic remodeling of the bone that contributes to the morbidity and mortality of patients. Bone metastases are also frequent in breast cancer, often leading to both osteoblastic and osteoclastic lesions. Multiple myeloma can cause rapid bone loss with pain, fractures, and increased blood calcium (see Chapter 3 for more details). The major source of morbidity and mortality associated with MM are osteolytic lesions that form throughout the axial skeleton, resulting from increased osteoclastic bone resorption that occurs adjacent to the myeloma cells. New bone formation that normally occurs at the sites of bone destruction is also absent, as local factors produced by myeloma cells appear to induce extensive bone destruction and block new bone formation.

There are some treatments available to treat bone metastases caused by cancers. Bisphosphonates, which are potent inhibitors of bone resorption, significantly reduce skeletal morbidity in patients with advanced breast cancer and can reduce metastasis to bone by human breast cancer cells in an experimental model (Cancer Supplement 2003). Pamidronate, a second generation bisphosphonate, has recently been approved by the FDA for treatment of breast cancer osteolysis. Zoledronic acid, a third-generation bisphosphonate, has also been approved for treatment of cancer patients. Another inhibitor of bone resorption, the protein osteoprotegerin, has also been shown to be effective in reducing bone metastases in animal models of breast and prostate cancer and in reducing bone pain in patients (Cancer Supplement 2003). Although bisphosphonates significantly reduce skeletal morbidity associated with solid tumor metastases to bone, most studies indicate no improvement in survival (Cancer Supplement 2003). Thus, in order to improve therapy and ultimately prevent bone metastases, a more precise understanding of the pathophysiology of bone metastases is necessary, as the level of current understanding is very limited (Cancer Supplement 2003).

Osteogenesis Imperfecta. Osteogenesis imperfecta (OI) is an inherited skeletal disorder that results from several different genetic defects (see Chapter 3 for more details). Patients with OI have low bone mass and brittle bones that fracture easily. Treatment of patients is mainly oriented at preventing and treating fractures in these patients. It involves a team of health professionals that typically includes orthopedists, rehabilitation physicians, and physical therapists. Encouraging results have been reported with bisphosphonate therapy (Glorieux et al. 1998).

Key Questions for Future Research

There is good evidence that proper nutrition and lifestyle can promote bone health and that pharmacotherapy can slow bone loss or even build new bone. However, there is still no "cure" for osteoporosis or for most other bone disorders. Those drugs that do exist, moreover, are still not ideal in terms of their expense, ease of administration, and/or side effects. Answers to the following research questions would help to move the field closer to the development of "ideal" therapies that can prevent and/or cure bone disease:

- What are the relative risks and benefits of different types of drug therapies in different populations? When is it best to use bisphosphonates, SERMS, or anabolic agents?

- What is the effectiveness of pharmacotherapy in treating persons who have already sustained hip fractures?
- Are combination therapies more effective than single therapies? Is there any time when it is best to use a combination of anti-resorptive and anabolic therapy?
- What doses, schedules, and methods of administration are most effective in encouraging compliance and preventing fractures in the community (not just within the confines of a clinical trial)? Can lower doses, shorter courses, or wider spacing of treatment help?
- What is the efficacy and utility of vertebroplasty and kyphoplasty?
- How can we improve the therapy of other bone diseases, particularly osteogenesis imperfecta, hyperparathyroidism, and renal osteodystrophy?

References

Albright, Fuller; Reifenstein, Edward C. Jr. The parathyroid glands and metabolic bone disease: Selected studies. Baltimore (MD): Williams and Wilkins; 1948.

Alexander HR Jr, Chen CC, Shawker T, Choyke P, Chan TJ, Chang R, Marx SJ. Role of preoperative localization and introoperative localization maneuvers including intraoperative PTH assay determination for patients with persistent or recurrent hyperparathyroidism. J Bone Miner Res 2002 No;17 Suppl 2:N133-40.

Anderson GL, Limacher M, Assaf AR, Bassford T, Beresford SA, Black H, Bonds D, Brunner R, Brzyski R, Caan B, Chlebowski R, Curb D, Gass M, Hays J, Heiss G, Hendrix S, Howard BV, Hsia J, Hubbell A, Jackson R, Johnson KC, Judd H, Kotchen JM, Kuller L, LaCroix AZ, Lane D, Langer RD, Lasser N, Lewis CE, Manson J, Margolis K, Ockene J, O'Sullivan MJ, Phillips L, Prentice RL, Ritenbaugh C, Robbins J, Rossouw JE, Sarto G, Stefanick ML, Van Horn L, Wactawski-Wende J, Wallace R, Wassertheil-Smoller S; Women's Health Initiative Steering Committee. Effects of conjugated equine estrogen in postmenopausal women with hysterectomy: the Women's Health Initiative randomized controlled trial. JAMA. 2004 Apr 14;291(14):1701-12.

Banks E, Beral V, Reeves G, Balkwill A, Barnes I; Million Women Study Collaborators. Fracture incidence in relation to the pattern of use of hormone therapy in postmenopausal women. JAMA 2004 May 12;291(18):2212-20.

Bauer DC, Mundy GR, Jamal SA, Black DM, Cauley JA, Ensrud KE, van der Klift M, Polo HA. Use of statins and fracture: Results of 4 prospective studies and cumulative meta-analysis of observational studies and controlled trials. Arch Intern Med 2004 Jan 26;164(2):146-52.

Bilezikian JP, Potts JT, Fuleihan Gel-H, Kleerekoper M, Neer R, Peacock M, Rastad J, Silverberg SJ, Udelsman R, Wells SA. Summary statement from a workshop on asymptomatic primary hyperparathyroidism: A perspective for the 21st century. J Bone Miner Res 2002 Nov;17 Suppl 2:N2-11.

Bilezikian JP, Silverberg SJ. Clinical practice. Asymtomatic primary hyperparathyroidism. N Engl J Med 2004 Apr 22;350(17):1746-51.Black DM, Cummings SR, Karpf DB, Cauley JA, Thompson DE, Nevitt MC, Bauer DC, Genant HK, Haskell WL, Marcus R, et al. Randomised trial of effect of alendronate on risk of fracture in women with existing vertebral fractures. Fracture Intervention Trial Research Group. Lancet 1996 Dec 7;348(9041):1535-41.

Black DM, Thompson DE, Bauer DC, Ensrud K, Musliner T, Hochberg MC, Nevitt MC, Suryawanshi S, Cummings SR. Fracture risk reduction with alendronate in women with osteoporosis: The Fracture Intervention Trial. FIT Research Group. J Clin Endocrinol Metab 2000 Nov;85(11):4118-24.

Black DM, Greenspan SL, Ensrud KE, Palermo L, McGowan JA, Lang TF, Garnero P, Bouxsein ML, Bilezikian JP, Rosen CJ; PaTH Study Investigators. The effects of parathyroid hormone and alendronate alone or in combination in postmenopausal osteoporosis. N Engl J Med. 2003 Sep 25;349(13):1207-15.

Bone HG, Greenspan SL, McKeever C, Bell N, Davidson M, Downs RW, Emkey R, Meunier PJ, Miller SS, Mulloy AL, et al. Alendronate and estrogen effects in postmenopausal women with low bone mineral density. Alendronate/Estrogen Study Group. J Clin Endocrinol Metab 2000 Feb;85(2):720-6.

Bone HG, Hosking D, Devogelaer JP, Tucci JR, Emkey RD, Tonino RP, Rodriguez-Portales JA, Downs RW, Gupta J, Santora AC, et al.; Alendronate Phase III Osteoporosis Treatment Study Group. 10 years' experience with alendronate for osteoporosis in postmenopausal women. N Engl J Med 2004 Mar 18;350(12):1189-99.

Bonner FJ Jr, Sinaki M, Grabois M, Shipp KM, Lane JM, Lindsay R, Gold DT, Cosman F, Bouxsein ML, Weinstein JN, et al. Health professional's guide to rehabilitation of the patient with osteoporosis. Osteoporos Int 2003;14 Suppl 2:S1-22.

Cancer (Supplement). Third North American Symposium on Skeletal Complications of Malignancy. 2003 Feb 1;97(3):719-892.

Cauley JA, Seeley DG, Ensrud K, Ettinger B, Black D, Cummings SR. Estrogen replacement therapy and fractures in older women. Study of Osteoporotic Fractures Research Group. Ann Intern Med 1995 Jan 1;122(1):9-16.

Cauley JA, Robbins J, Chen Z, Cummings SR, Jackson RD, LaCroix AZ, LeBoff M, Lewis CE, McGowan J, Neuner J, et al.; Women's Health Initiative Investigators. Effects of estrogen plus progestin on risk of fracture and bone mineral density: The Women's Health Initiative randomized trial. JAMA 2003 Oct 1;290(13):1729-38.

Chesnut CH 3d, Silverman S, Andriano K, Genant H, Gimona A, Harris S, Kiel D, LeBoff M, Maricic M, Miller P, et al. A randomized trial of nasal spray salmon calcitonin in postmenopausal women with established osteoporosis: The Prevent Recurrence of Osteoporotic Fractures study. PROOF Study Group. Am J Med 2000 Sep;109(4):267-76.

Chow CC, Chan WB, Li JK, Chan MN, Chan MH, Ko GT, Lo KW, Cockram CS. Oral alendronate increases bone mineral density in postmenopausal women with primary hyperparathyroidism. J Clin Endocrinol Metab 2003 Feb;88(2):581-7.

Cohen A, Shane E. Osteoporosis after solid organ and bone marrow transplantation. Osteoporos Int. 2003 Aug;14(8):617-30.

Coleman RE. Optimising treatment of bone metastases by Aredia™ and Zometa™. Breast Cancer 2000;7(4):361-9.

Collaborative Group on Hormonal Factors in Breast Cancer. Breast cancer and hormone replacement therapy: Collaborative reanalysis of data from 51 epidemiological studies of 52,705 women with breast cancer and 108,411 women without breast cancer. Lancet. 1997 Oct 11;350(9084):1047-59.

Cosman F, Nieves J, Woelfert L, Formica C, Gordon S, Shen V, Lindsay R. Parathyroid hormone added to established hormone therapy: Effects on vertebral fracture and maintenance of bone mass after parathyroid hormone withdrawal J Bone Miner Res 2001 May;16(5):925-31.

[a]Cranney A, Wells G, Willan A, Griffith L, Zytaruk N, Robinson V, Black D, Adachi J, Shea B, Tugwell P, Guyatt G; Osteoporosis Methodology Group and the Osteoporosis Research Advisory Group. Meta-analyses of therapies for postmenopausal osteoporosis. II. Meta-analysis of alendronate for the treatment of postmenopausal women. Endocr Rev 2002 Aug;23(4):508-16.

[b]Cranney A, Tugwell P, Zytaruk N, Robinson V, Weaver B, Adachi J, Wells G, Shea B, Guyatt G; Osteoporosis Methodology Group and the Osteoporosis Research Ad-

visory Group. Meta-analyses of therapies for postmenopausal osteoporosis. IV. Meta-analysis of raloxifene for the prevention and treatment of postmenopausal osteoporosis. Endocr Rev 2002 Aug;23(4):524-8.

Cummings SR, Browner WS, Bauer D, Stone K, Ensrud K, Jamal S, Ettinger B. Endogenous hormones and the risk of hip and vertebral fractures among older women. Study of Osteoporotic Fractures Research Group. N Engl J Med 1998 Sep10;339(11):733-8.

Cummings SR, Eckert S, Krueger KA, Grady D, Powles TJ, Cauley JA, Norton L, Nickelsen T, Bjarnason NH, Morrow M, et al. The effect of raloxifene on risk of breast cancer in postmenopausal women: Results from the MORE randomized trial. JAMA 1999 Jun 16;281(23):2189-97.

Deal C. The use of intermittent human parathyroid hormone as a treatment for osteoporosis. Curr Rheumatol Rep. 2004 Feb;6(1):49-58.

Delmas PD, Ensrud KE, Adachi JD, Harper KD, Sarkar S, Gennari C, Reginster JY, Pols HA, Recker RR, Harris ST, et al.; Multiple Outcomes of Raloxifene Evaluation Investigators. Efficacy of raloxifene on vertebral fracture risk reduction in postmenopausal women with osteoporosis: Four-year results from a randomized clinical trial. J Clin Endocrinol Metab 2002 Aug;87(8):3609-17.

Ettinger B, San Martin J, Crans G, Pavo, I. Differential effects of teriparatide on BMD after treatment with raloxifene or alendronate. J Bone Miner Res 2004 May;19(5):745-51.

Ettinger B, Black DM, Mitlak BH, Knickerbocker RK, Nickelsen T, Genant HK, Christiansen C, Delmas PD, Zanchetta JR, Stakkestad J, et al. Reduction of vertebral fracture risk in postmenopausal women with osteoporosis treated with raloxifene:

Results from a 3-year randomized clinical trial. Multiple outcomes of Raloxifene evaluation (MORE) investigators. JAMA 1999 Aug 18;282(7):637-45.

Evans A, Jensen M, Kip K, DeNardo AJ, Lawler GJ, Negin GA, Remley KB, Boutin SM, Dunnagan SA. Vertebral compression fractures: Pain reduction and improvement in functional mobility after percutaneous polymethylmethacrylate vertebroplasty—retrospective report of 245 cases. Radiology 2003 Feb;226(2):366-72.

Finkelstein JS, Hayes A, Hunzelman JL, Wyland JJ, Lee H, Neer RM. The effects of parathyroid hormone, alendronate, or both in men with osteoporosis. N Engl J Med 2003 Sep 25;349(13):1216-26.

Fleisch H. Development of bisphosphonates. Breast Cancer Res. 2002;4(1):30-4.

Food and Drug and Administration. [homepage on the Internet]. Rockville (MD): Food and Drug Administration; 2003 Sep [cited 2004 Mar 12]. Menopause and hormones. Available from: http://www.fda.gov/womens/menopause/mht-FS.html.

Glorieux FH, Bishop NJ, Plotkin H, Chabot G, Lanoue G, Travers R. Cyclic administration of pamidronate in children with severe osteogenesis imperfecta. N Engl J Med 1998 Oct 1;339(14):947-52.

Greendale GA, Espeland M, Slone S, Marcus R, Barrett-Connor E; PEPI Safety Follow-Up Study (PSFS) Investigators. Bone mass response to discontinuation of long-term hormone replacement therapy: Results from the Postmenopausal Estrogen/Progestin Interventions (PEPI) Safety Follow-Up Study. Arch Intern Med 2002 Mar 25;162(6):665-72.

Greenspan SL, Emkey RD, Bone HG, Weiss SR, Bell NH, Downs RW, McKeever C,

Miller SS, Davidson M, Bolognese MA, et al. Significant differential effects of alendronate, estrogen, or combination therapy on the rate of bone loss after discontinuation of treatment for postmenopausal osteoporosis. A randomized, double-blind, placebo-controlled trial. Ann Intern Med 2002 Dec 3;137(11):875-83.

Greenspan SL, Resnick NM, Parker RA. Combination therapy with hormone replacement and alendronate for prevention of bone loss in elderly women: A randomized controlled trial. JAMA 2003 May 21;289(19):2525-33.

Hanley DA, Ioannidis G, Adachi JD. Etidronate therapy in the treatment and prevention of osteoporosis. J Clin Densitom 2000 Spring;3(1):79-95.

Harris ST, Watts NB, Genant HK, McKeever CD, Hangartner T, Keller M, Chesnut CH 3d, Brown J, Eriksen EF, Hoseyni MS, et al. Effects of risedronate treatment on vertebral and nonvertebral fractures in women with postmenopausal osteoporosis: A randomized controlled trial. Vertebral Efficacy with Risedronate Therapy (VERT) Study Group. JAMA 1999 Oct 13;282(14):1344-52.

Harris ST, Eriksen EF, Davidson M, Ettinger MP, Moffett AH Jr, Baylink DJ, Crusan CE, Chines AA. Effect of combined risedronate and hormone replacement therapies on bone mineral density in postmenopausal women. J Clin Endocrinol Metab 2001 May;86(5):1890-7.

Heaney RP, Weaver CM. Calcium and vitamin D. Endocrinol Metab Clin North Am. 2003 Mar;32(1):181-94, vii-viii. Review.

Hodsman AB, Hanley DA, Ettinger MP, Bolognese MA, Fox J, Metcalfe AJ, Lindsay R. Efficacy and safety of human parathyroid hormone-(1-84) in increasing bone mineral density in postmenopausal osteoporosis. J Clin Endocrinol Metab. 2003 Nov;88(11):5212-20.

Horwitz MJ, Tedesco MB, Gundberg C, Garcia-Ocana A, Stewart AF. Short-term, high-dose parathyroid hormone-related protein as a skeletal anabolic agent for the treatment of postmenopausal osteoporosis. J Clin Endocrinol Metab 2003 Feb;88(2):569-75.

Hutchinson JH, Halczenko W, Brashear KM, Breslin MJ, Coleman PJ, Duong le T, Fernandez-Metzler C, Gentile MA, Fisher JE, Hartman GD, Huff JR, Kimmel DB, Leu CT, Meissner RS, Merkle K, Nagy R, Pennypacker B, Perkins JJ, Prueksaritanont T, Rodan GA, Varga SL, Wesolowski GA, Zartman AE, Rodan SB, Duggan ME. Nonpeptide alphavbeta3 antagonists. 8. In vitro and in vivo evaluation of a potent alphavbeta3 antagonist for the prevention and treatment of osteoporosis. J Med Chem. 2003 Oct 23;46(22):4790-8.

Institute of Medicine. Dietary reference intakes for calcium, phosphorus, magnesium, vitamin D, and fluoride. Washington (DC): National Academy Press; 1997.

Johnell O, Scheek WH, Lu Y, Reginster J.Y., Need AG, Seeman E. Additive effects of raloxifene and alendronate on bone density and biochemical markers of bone remodeling in postmenopausal women with osteoporosis. J Clin Endocrinol Metab 2002 Mar;87(3):985-92.

Kiel DP, Felson DT, Anderson JJ, Wilson PW, Moskowitz MA. Hip fracture and the use of estrogens in postmenopausal women. The Framingham study. N Engl J Med 1987 Nov 5;317(19):1169-74.

Lagro-Janssen T, Rosser WW, van Weel C. Breast cancer and hormone-replacement therapy: Up to general practice to pick up the pieces. Lancet. 2003 Aug 9;362(9382):414-5.

Liberman UA, Weiss SR, Broll J, Minne HW, Quan H, Bell NH, Rodriguez-Portales J, Downs RW Jr, Dequeker J, Favus M. Effect of oral alendronate on bone mineral density and incidence of fracture in postmenopausal osteoporosis. The Alendronate Phase III Osteoporosis Treatment Study Group. N Engl J Med 1995 Nov 30;333(22):1437-43.

Lieberman IH, Dudeney S, Reinhardt MK, Bell G. Initial outcome and efficacy of "kyphoplasty" in the treatment of painful osteoporotic vertebral compression fractures. Spine 2001 Jul 15;26(14):1631-8.

Lindsay R, Nieves J, Formica C, Henneman E, Woelfert L, Shen V, Dempster D, Cosman F. Randomised controlled study of effect of parathyroid hormone on vertebral-bone mass and fracture incidence among postmenopausal women on estrogen with osteoporosis. Lancet 1997 Aug 23;350(9077):550-5.

Lindsay R, Gallagher JC, Kleerekoper M, Pickar JH. Effect of lower doses of conjugated equine estrogens with and without medroxyprogesterone acetate on bone in early postmenopausal women. JAMA 2002 May22-29;287(20):2668-76.

Lotinun S, Sibonga JD, Turner RT. Differential effects of intermittent and continuous administration of parathyroid hormone on bone histomorphometry and gene expression. Endocrine. 2002 Feb;17(1):29-36.

Lyles KW, Siris ES, Singer FR, Meunier PJ. A clinical approach to diagnosis and management of Paget's disease of bone. J Bone Miner Res 2001 Aug;16(8):1379-87.

Maricic M, Adachi JD, Sarkar S, Wu W, Wong M, Harper KD. Early effects of raloxifene on clinical vertebral fractures at 12 months in postmenopausal women with osteoporosis. Arch Intern Med 2002 May 27;162(10):1140-3.

Marottoli RA, Berkman LF, Cooney LM Jr. Decline in physical function following hip fracture. J Am Geriatr Soc 1992 Sep;40(9):861-6.

McClung MR, Geusens P, Miller PD, Zippel H, Bensen WG, Roux C, Adami S, Fogelman I, Diamond T, Eastell R, et al. Effect of risedronate on the risk of hip fracture in elderly women. Hip Intervention Program Study Group. N Engl J Med 2001 Feb 1;344(5):333-40.

McClung MR, Wasnich RD, Recker R, Cauley JA, Chestnut CH 3d, Ensrud KE, Burdeska A, Mills T; Oral Ibandronate Study Group. Oral daily ibandronate prevents bone loss in early postmenopausal women without osteoporosis. J Bone Miner Res 2004 Jan;19(1):11-8.

McDonnell DP. Mining the complexities of the estrogen signaling pathways for novel therapeutics. Endocrinology. 2003 Oct;144(10):4237-40.

Mehta NM, Malootian A, Gilligan JP. Calcitonin for osteoporosis and bone pain. Curr Pharm Des. 2003;9(32):2659-76.

Meunier PJ, Slosman DO, Delmas PD, Sebert JL, Brandi ML, Albanese C, Lorenc R, Pors-Nielsen S, de Vernejoul MC, Roces A, et al. Strontium ranelate: Dose-dependent effects in established postmenopausal vertebral osteoporosis—a 2-year randomized placebo controlled trial. J Clin Endocrinol Metab 2002 May;87(5):2060-6.

Meunier PJ, Roux C, Seeman E, Ortolani S, Badurski JE, Spector TD, Cannata J, Balogh A, Lemmel EM, Pors-Nielsen S, et al. The effects of strontium ranelate on the risk of vertebral fracture in women with postmenopausal osteoporosis. N Engl J Med 2004 Jan 29;350(5):459-68.

Morris AH, Zuckerman JD; AAOS Council of Health Policy and Practice, USA. American Academy of Orthopaedic Surgeons. National Consensus Conference on Improving the Continuum of Care for Patients with Hip Fracture. J Bone Joint Surg 2002 Apr;84A(4):670-4.

Morris CA, Cheng H, Cabral D, Solomon DH. Predictors of screening and treatment of osteoporosis: A structured review of the literature. Endocrinologist. 2004 Mar/Apr;14(2):70-75.

Mundy G. Metastasis to bone: Causes, consequences and therapeutic opportunities. Nat Rev Cancer 2002 Aug;2(8):584-93.

Neer RM, Arnaud CD, Zanchetta JR, Prince R, Gaich GA, Reginster JY, Hodsman AB, Eriksen EF, Ish-Shalom S, Genant HK, et al. Effect of parathyroid hormone (1-34) on fractures and bone mineral density in postmenopausal women with osteoporosis. N Engl J Med 2001 May 10;344(19):1434-41.

Onyia JE, Galvin RJ, Ma YL, Halladay DL, Miles RR, Yang X, Fuson T, Cin RL, Zeng QQ, Chandrasekhar S, et al. Novel and selective small molecule stimulators of osteoprotegerin expression inhibit bone resorption. J Pharmacol Exp Ther 2004 Apr;309(1):369-79.

Orwoll ES. Osteoporosis in men. Endocrinol Metab Clin North Am. 1998 Jun;27(2):349-67.

Orwoll E, Ettinger M, Weiss S, Miller P, Kendler D, Graham J, Adami S, Weber K, Lorenc R, Pietschmann P, Vandormael K, Lombardi A. Alendronate for the treatment of osteoporosis in men. N Engl J Med 2000 Aug 31;343(9):604-10.

Pal B. Questionnaire survey of advice given to patients with fractures. BMJ 1999 Feb 20;318(7182):500-1.

Parker CR, Blackwell PJ, Fairbairn KJ, Hosking DJ. Alendronate in the treatment of primary hyperparathyroid-related osteoporosis: A 2-year study. J Clin Endocrinol Metab 2002 Oct;87(10):4482-9.

Pettifor JM. Nutritional and drug-induced rickets and osteomalacia. In: Favus MJ, editor. Primer on the metabolic bone diseases and disorders of mineral metabolism. 5th ed. Washington, DC: American Society for Bone and Mineral Research; 2003. p. 399-407.

Pfeifer M, Begerow B, Minne HW. Effects of a new spinal orthosis on posture, trunk strength, and quality of life in women with postmenopausal osteoporosis: A randomized trial. Am J Phys Med Rehabil 2004 Mar;83(3):177-86.

Powles TJ, Hickish T, Kanis JA, Tidy A, Ashley S. Effect of tamoxifen on bone mineral density measured by dual-energy X-ray absorptiometry in healthy premenopausal and postmenopausal women. J Clin Oncol 1996 Jan;14(1):78-84.

Prestwood KM, Kenny AM, Kleppinger A, Kulldorff M. Ultralow-dose micronized 17$-estradiol and bone density and bone metabolism in older women: a randomized controlled trial. JAMA 2003 Aug 27;290(8):1042-8.Rauch F, Plotkin H, Travers R, Zeitlin L, Glorieux FH. Osteogenesis imperfecta types I, III, and IV: effect of pamidronate therapy on bone and mineral metabolism. J Clin Endocrinol Metab 2003 Mar;88(3):986-92.

Recker RR, Weinstein RS, Chestnut CH 3d, Schimmer RC, Mahoney P, Hughes C, Bonvoisin B, Meunier PJ. Histomorphometric evaluation of daily and intermittent oral ibandronate in women with postmenopausal osteoporosis: Results from the BONE study. Osteoporos Int 2004 Mar;15(3):231-7.

Reid DM, Hughes RA, Laan RF, Sacco-Gibson NA, Wenderoth DH, Adami S, Eusebio RA, Devogelaer JP. Efficacy and safety of daily risedronate in the treatment of corticosteroid-induced osteoporosis in men and women: A randomized trial. J Bone Miner Res 2000 Jun;15(6):1006-13.

Reid IR, Brown JP, Burckhardt P, Horowitz Z, Richardson P, Trechsel U, Widmer A, Devogelaer JP, Kaufman JM, Jaeger P, et al. Intravenous zoledronic acid in postmenopausal women with low bone mineral density. N Engl J Med 2002 Feb 28;346(9):653-61.

Riggs BL, Khosla S, Melton LJ 3rd. Sex steroids and the construction and conservation of the adult skeleton. Endocr Rev. 2002 Jun;23(3):279-302.

Ringe JD, Dorst A, Faber H, Ibach K. Alendronate treatment of established primary osteoporosis in men: 3-year results of a prospective, comparative, two-arm study. Rheumatol Int 2004 Mar;24(2):110-3.

Rittmaster RS, Bolognese M, Ettinger MP, Hanley DA, Hodsman AB, Kendler DL, Rosen CJ. Enhancement of bone mass in osteoporotic women with parathyroid hormone followed by alendronate. J Clin Endocrinol Metab 2000 Jun;85(6):2129-34.

Rosen CJ, Rackoff PJ. Emerging anabolic treatments for osteoporosis. Rheum Dis Clin North Am 2001 Feb;27(1):215-33.

Rossouw JE, Anderson GL, Prentice RL, LaCroix AZ, Kooperberg C, Stefanick ML, Jackson RD, Beresford SA, Howard BV, Johnson KC. Risks and benefits of estrogen plus progestin in healthy postmenopausal women: Principal results from the Women's Health Initiative randomized controlled trial. JAMA 2002 Jul 17;288(3):321-33.

Rubin C, Recker R, Cullen D, Ryaby J, McCabe J, Mcleod K. Prevention of postmenopausal bone loss by a low-magnitude, high-frequency mechanical stimuli: A clinical trial assessing compliance, efficacy, and safety. J Bone Miner Res 2004 Mar;19(3):343-51.

Rubin MR, Lee KH, McMahon DJ, Silverberg SJ. Raloxifene lowers serum calcium and markers of bone turnover in postmenopausal women with primary hyperparathyroidism. J Clin Endocrinol Metab 2003 Mar;88(3):1174-8.

Saag KG, Emkey R, Schnitzer TJ, Brown JP, Hawkins F, Goemaere S, Thamsborg G, Liberman UA, Delmas PD, Malice MP, et al. Alendronate for the prevention and treatment of glucocorticoid-induced osteoporosis. Glucocorticoid-Induced Osteoporosis Intervention Study Group. N Engl J Med 1998 Jul 30;339(5):292-9.

Schurch MA, Rizzoli R, Slosman D, Vadas L, Vergnaud P, Bonjour JP. Protein supplements increase serum insulin-like growth factor-I levels and attenuate proximal femur bone loss in patients with recent hip fracture. A randomized, double-blind, placebo-controlled trial. Ann Intern Med 1998 Mary 15;128(10):801-9.

Shane E, Addesso V, Namerow PB, McMahon DJ, Lo SH, Staron RB, Zucker M, Pardi S, Maybaum S, Mancini D. Alendronate versus calcitriol for the prevention of bone loss after cardiac transplantation. N Engl J Med 2004 Feb 19;350(8):767-76.

Shumaker SA, Legault C, Rapp SR, Thal L, Wallace RB, Ockene JK, Hendrix SL, Jones BN 3rd, Assaf AR, Jackson RD, et al. Estrogen plus progestin and the incidence of dementia and mild cognitive impairment in postmenopausal women: The Women's

Health Initiative Memory Study: a randomized controlled trial. JAMA. 2003 May 28;289(20):2651-62.

Shumaker SA, Legault C, Kuller L, Rapp SR, Thal L, Lane DS, Fillit H, Stefanick ML, Hendrix SL, Lewis CE, et al. Conjugated equine estrogens and incidence of probable dementia and mild cognitive impairment in postmenopausal women. The Women's Health Initiative Memory Study. JAMA 2004 Jun 23;291(24):2947-58.

Silverberg SJ, Gartenberg F, Jacobs TP, Shane E, Siris E, Staron RB, McMahon DJ, Bilezikian JP. Increased bone mineral density after parathyroidectomy in primary hyperparathyroidism. J Clin Endocrinol Metab 1995 Mar;80(3):729-34.

Silverberg SJ, Bone HG 3d, Marriott TB, Locker FG, Thys-Jacobs S, Dziem G, Kaatz S, Sanguinetti ES, Bilezikian JP. Short term inhibition of parathyroid hormone secretion by a calcium receptor agonist in primary hyperparathyroidism. N Engl J Med 1997 Nov 20;337(21):1506-10.

Silverberg SJ, Shane E, Jacobs TP, Siris E, Bilezikian JP. A 10-year prospective study of primary hyperparathyroidism with or without parathyroid surgery. N Engl J Med 1999 Oct 21;341(17):1249-55.

Silverman SL. Calcitonin. Endocrinol Metab Clin North Am. 2003 Mar;32(1):273-84.

Sinaki M, Itoi E, Wahner HW, Wollan P, Gelzcer R, Mullan BP, Collins DA, Hodgson SF. Stronger back muscles reduce the incidence of vertebral fractures: a prospective 10-year follow-up of postmenopausal women. Bone 2002 Jun;30(6):836-41.

Smith MD, Ross W, Ahern MJ. Missing a therapeutic window of opportunity: An audit of patients attending a tertiary teaching hospital with potentially osteoporotic hip and wrist fractures. J Rheum 2001 Nov;28(11):2504-8.

Solomon DH, Levin E, Helfgott SM. Patterns of medication use before and after bone densitometry: Factors associated with appropriate treatment. J Rheumatol 2000 Jun;27(6):1496-500.

Solomon DH, Finkelstein JS, Katz JN, Mogun H, Avorn J. Underuse of osteoporosis medications in elderly patients with fractures. Amer J Med 2003 Oct 1;115(5):398-400.

Sorensen OH, Crawford GM, Mulder H, Hosking DJ, Gennari C, Mellstrom D, Pack S, Wenderoth D, Cooper C, Reginster JY. Long-term efficacy of risedronate: A 5-year placebo-controlled clinical experience. Bone 2003 Feb;32(2):120-6.

Teng M, Wolf M, Lowrie E, Ofsthun N, Lazarus JM, Thadhani R. Survival of patients undergoing hemodialysis with paricalcitol or calcitriol therapy. N Engl J Med 2003 Jul 31;349(5):446-56.

Todd CJ, Freeman CJ, Camilleri-Ferrante C, Palmer CR, Hyder A, Laxton CE, Parker MJ, Payne BV, Rushton N. Differences in mortality after fracture of hip: The East Anglian audit. BMJ 1995 Apr 8;310(6984):904-8.

Tonino RP, Meunier PJ, Emkey R, Rodriguez-Portales JA, Menkes CJ, Wasnich RD, Bone HG, Santora AC, Wu M, Desai R, et al. Skeletal benefits of alendronate: 7 year treatment of postmenopausal osteoporotic women. Phase III Osteoporosis Treatment Study Group. J Clin Endocrinol Metab 2000 Sep;85(9):3109 15.

[a]Torgerson DJ, Bell-Syer SE. Hormone replacement therapy and prevention of nonvertebral fractures: A meta-analysis of randomized trials. JAMA 2001 Jun 13;285(22):2891-7.

[b]Torgerson DJ, Bell-Syer SE. Hormone replacement therapy and prevention of vertebral fractures: A meta-analysis of randomised trials. BMC Musculoskelet Disord 2001;2(1):7-10.

Udelsman R. Surgery in primary hyperparathyroidism: The patient without previous neck surgery. J Bone Miner Res 2002 Nov;17 Suppl 2:N126-32.

U.S. Department of Health and Human Services. Physical activity and health: A report of the Surgeon General. Atlanta (GA): U.S. Department of Health and Human Services, Centers for Disease Control and Prevention, National Center for Chronic Disease Prevention and Health Promotion, President's Council on Physical Fitness and Sports, 1996. 300p.

van Staa TP, Leufkens HG, Abenhaim L, Zhang B, Cooper C. Use of oral corticosteroids and risk of fractures. J Bone Miner Res 2000 Jun;15(6):993-1000.

Verschueren SM, Roelants M, Delecluse C, Swinnen S, Vanderschueren D, Boonen S. Effect of 6-month whole body vibration training on hip density, muscle strength, and postural control in postmenopausal women: A randomized controlled pilot study. J Bone Miner Res 2004 Mar;19(3):352-9.

Vestergaard P, Mosekilde L. Parathyroid surgery is associated with a decreased risk of hip and upper arm fractures in primary hyperparathyroidism: A controlled cohort study. J Intern Med 2004 Jan;255(1):108-14.

Ward K, Alsop C, Caulton J, Rubin C, Adams J, Mughal Z. Low magnitude mechanical loading is osteogenic in children with disabling conditions. J Bone Miner Res 2004 Mar;19(3):360-9.

Watts NB, Harris ST, Genant HK, Wasnich RD, Miller PD, Jackson RD, Licata AA, Ross P, Woodson GC 3d, Yanover MJ, et al. Intermittent cyclical etidronate treatment of postmenopausal osteoporosis. N Engl J Med 1990 Jul 12;323(2):73-9.

Wells G, Tugwell P, Shea B, Guyatt G, Peterson J, Zytaruk N, Robinson V, Henry D, O'Connell D, Cranney A; Osteoporosis Methodology Group and the Osteoporosis Research Advisory Group. Meta-analyses of therapies for postmenopausal osteoporosis. V. Meta-analysis of the efficacy of hormone replacement therapy in treating and preventing osteoporosis in postmenopausal women. Endocr Rev 2002 Aug;23(4):529-39.

Writing Group for the PEPI. Effects of hormone therapy on bone mineral density: Results from the Postmenopausal Estrogen/Progestin Interventions (PEPI) Trial. JAMA 1996 Nov 6;276(17):1389-96.

Yates J, Barrett-Connor E, Barlas S, Chen YT, Miller PD, Siris ES. Rapid loss of hip fracture protection after estrogen cessation: evidence from the National Osteoporosis Risk Assessment. Obstet Gynecol 2004 Mar;103(3):440-6.

Zuckerman JD, Skovron ML, Koval KJ, Aharonoff G, Frankel VH Postoperative complications and mortality associated with operative delay in older patients who have a fracture of the hip. J Bone Joint Surg Am 1995 Oct;77(10):1551-6.

Zuckerman JD. Hip fracture. N Engl J Med 1996 Jun 6;334(23):1519-25.

Chapter 10: Key Messages

- Individuals have a critical role to play in promoting their own bone health. All health care professionals, especially primary care providers, have the opportunity and responsibility to assist them in this task by promoting awareness of factors that influence bone health; identifying patients at risk of bone disease; and providing lifestyle and therapeutic interventions to prevent bone loss and fractures.

- Nurse practitioners, nurse midwives, and physician assistants can contribute significantly to the provision of bone health care. They can educate patients on nutrition and physical activity recommendations, ensure proper screening, and monitor compliance with treatment. Physical therapists, occupational therapists, pharmacists, and dietitians can play valuable roles in helping patients achieve maximal physical function and bone accrual.

- Childhood is an excellent time to initiate counseling aimed at encouraging appropriate nutrition and physical activities and discouraging the adoption of behaviors that negatively affect bone health.

- All young and middle-aged adults should be encouraged to adopt lifestyles that help prevent bone loss and promote overall health and the prevention of chronic disease. Young and middle-aged adult patients who have medical conditions or who are taking medications associated with bone loss should be considered for bone density testing and drug therapy.

- For older adults and the elderly, recommended levels of both calcium and vitamin D increase. Older adults should engage in regular physical activity, and many can follow the recommendations for younger adults. Weight-supporting activities may be more appropriate in older adults with compromised bone health, although with proper supervision and training they can safely engage in resistance exercises as well.

- Risk factors for bone loss and fracture should be assessed in all older women. In addition, all women aged 65 and older should undergo bone density testing as recommended by the U.S. Preventive Services Task Force and the National Osteoporosis Foundation. Bone density testing should be considered in men with fragility fractures; those on therapies that may cause bone loss, notably glucocorticoids or androgen deprivation; and men with multiple risk factors.

- Pharmacologic therapy should be considered in individuals who have osteoporosis. Individuals with low bone mass and multiple risk factors should also be considered for therapy. Selection of a therapeutic agent can be tailored to the severity of the patient's bone loss and other co-morbid conditions.

- Fall prevention strategies should also be discussed with every osteoporosis patient, and hip protectors should be considered for the frail elderly and patients at high risk for falling.

- A person of any age (especially an elderly individual) who represents a challenging clinical situation may benefit from a referral to an endocrinologist, rheumatologist, or other specialist in osteoporosis management.

Chapter 10

PUTTING IT ALL TOGETHER FOR THE BUSY HEALTH CARE PROFESSIONAL

As noted throughout this report, individuals have a critically important role to play in building and maintaining strong, healthy bones throughout life. All health care professionals, especially primary care providers, have the opportunity and responsibility to assist individuals in achieving this goal by promoting awareness of factors that influence bone health, identifying patients at risk of bone disease, and providing lifestyle and therapeutic interventions to prevent bone loss and fractures. Even though most osteoporotic fractures occur in older individuals, the risks of incurring such fractures are largely determined much earlier in life—both by the level of peak bone mass achieved during childhood and adolescence and by subsequent lifestyle choices and medical events of adulthood. As discussed earlier in this report, health care professionals could do a better job in preventing, identifying, and treating bone disease; osteoporosis remains underdiagnosed and undertreated. Since osteoporosis is a common disorder that can be diagnosed and treated in the primary care setting, much of the responsibility for promoting awareness, diagnosis, prevention, and treatment of osteoporosis falls on health care professionals who provide primary care. For example, pediatricians and other primary care providers for children and adolescents should

focus on maximizing bone accrual as discussed below in the section on infancy through adolescence. Primary care and other providers for adults can also help their patients maintain skeletal health by focusing on germane areas within their respective specialties. For example, obstetrics and gynecology providers should include recommendations for skeletal health in their discussions of nutrition and physical activity during family planning, lactation, pregnancy, and menopause, as discussed in the section on young and middle adulthood. Internists and specialists such as rheumatologists, gastroenterologists, oncologists, pulmonologists, dermatologists, and urologists should maximize lifestyle interventions and manage patients on pharmacotherapies, including oral glucocorticoids and gonadal hormone suppression therapies, that can cause bone loss, as discussed in the section on older adults and the elderly. Geriatricians, internists, emergency department physicians, and orthopedists have a unique opportunity to ensure that patients who present with fractures receive intensive interventions designed to maximize recovery and prevent future fractures. Certain health care professionals, such as nurse practitioners, nurse midwives, and physician assistants, can contribute significantly to the care of many patients and can educate patients on nutrition and lifestyle recommendations, ensure proper screening, and monitor compliance with treatment. Other health care professionals such as physical therapists, occupational therapists, pharmacists, dentists, optometrists, and dietitians can play valuable roles in helping patients achieve maximal physical function and bone accrual. For example, pharmacists can advise patients concerning calcium and vitamin D supplementation, the best way to take medications, and any potential drug interactions. Optometrists can help by ensuring that the vision of older patients is adequately corrected, which should decrease the risk of potentially debilitating falls. For their part, dentists may be able to detect bone loss in the jaw, which could lead to further investigation of the potential for osteoporosis.

Fortunately, recommendations related to bone health also promote overall health and therefore fit in well with other preventive recommendations. This chapter is devoted to identifying ways that health care professionals can incorporate recommendations focused on bone health into the advice they are already providing patients, and to offering practical advice on how providers can assist patients in implementing these recommendations into their lives. These recommendations are based largely on the evidence related to the maintenance of bone health, the diagnosis of bone disease, and the prevention and treatment of fractures outlined in Chapters 6, 7, 8, and 9, and therefore references are not included in this chapter except in cases where material has not previously been referenced.

Children and Adolescents

The period from infancy through adolescence is critical for building bones and developing healthful bone habits that help an individual to maintain a robust skeleton throughout life. As noted in Chapter 2, most individuals reach their "peak bone mass" during this time, which is determined by genetic factors and lifestyle choices (e.g., nutrition, physical activity) made by children with the influence of their parents during the first 18 years of life. The first 2 years of life and early adolescence are particularly important for future bone health, as they are characterized by rapid bone accumulation. Health care professionals who are involved in the health maintenance of infants, children, and adolescents have an opportunity to positively influence bone health for the rest of their patient's lives. While bone disease is quite rare in children and adolescents, health care professionals also need to be aware of the warning signs of potential problems that could be caused by genetic factors, lifestyle choices, certain diseases, or use of certain medications.

Nutrition

Achieving recommended levels of intake for calcium, vitamin D, and other nutrients during infancy, childhood, and adolescence is critical to maintaining healthy bones throughout life. (See Table 10-1 for a listing of the dietary calcium and vitamin D requirements for infants, children, and adolescents.) What follows is a more detailed discussion of how health care professionals can assist their patients in achieving these levels.

Calcium

Adequate calcium intake is critical for infants, children, and adolescents, as discussed below.

Infants: Nutrition is important to bone health even before birth. The largest influx of calcium into the fetal skeleton occurs during the last trimester of human pregnancy. Most newborns will receive adequate levels of calcium from their mothers during full-term pregnancies, and from breast milk, formula, and/or solid foods during the first year of life. Infants who are born prematurely "miss out" on some calcium before they are born and will likely have lower bone mass at birth than will a full-term infant. While breast feeding provides important advantages to premature infants, it may not provide for all of their needs. As a result, health care professionals should encourage parents of premature infants who are being breast fed to use supplements that provide added nutrients, particularly calcium, vitamin D, phosphorus, and protein (Schanler 2001). Health care professionals should advise the parents of premature infants who are not being breast fed about the importance of using infant formulas that are designed to provide calcium and phosphorus intakes similar to those that occur in utero during the last trimester of normal human pregnancy. Even when premature infants use such formulas, it can take up to 5 years for their bone mass to catch up with that of full-term newborns.

Table 10–1. Summary Recommendations for Bone Health

	Calcium (mg/day)	Vitamin D (IU/day)	Physical Activity	Bone Density Testing	Patients at Increased Risk
Infants					
0–6 Months	210	200	Interactive play	As clinically indicated in high risk patients.	Frequent fractures, anorexia, amenorrhea, chronic hepatic, renal, gastrointestinal, autoimmune disease. Medications in Table 10–2.
6–12 Months	270				
Children and Adolescents					
1–3 years	500	200	Moderate to vigorous activity at least 60 minutes per day. Emphasize weight bearing activity.	As clinically indicated in high risk patients.	
4–8 years	800				
9–18 years	1300				
Adults					
18–50 years	1000	200	Moderate activity at least 30 minutes per day, on most, preferably all, days of the week. Emphasize weight bearing activity. Fall prevention programs, modified for the frail elderly and spine fracture patients.	As clinically indicated in high risk patients.	
51–70 years	1200	400		Bone density testing by DXA in all women over age 65; consider in women under age 65 with risk factors. No consensus on men.	Individuals with risk factors in Table 10–4.
>70 years	1200	600			

Childhood: As shown in Table 10-1, children between 1 and 3 years old should get 500 mg per day of calcium, and those between 4 and 8 years old should consume 800 mg per day. Milk and foods derived from milk (e.g., cheese, yogurt) serve as the major food sources for calcium throughout childhood and adolescence. Any type of milk (whole, lowfat, or nonfat) provides the same level of calcium, but low-fat milk is the best choice for children over age 2. Additional sources include foodstuffs supplemented with calcium, such as fruit juices, fortified soy beverage, breads, and other breakfast foods, which can help to boost overall dietary calcium intake levels towards the recommended values. Since foods that contain calcium also have many other important nutrients, health care professionals should encourage parents and their children to strive for recommended levels of calcium intake through diet alone.

Adolescence: The second most rapid gains in bone mass occur with the onset of puberty, which also marks the time that calcium intake needs become greatest. As shown in Table 10-1, children 9 to 18 years old should consume 1,300 mg per day of calcium. Puberty is also the time that ethnic and gender differences in bone mass are first seen. As noted in Chapter 3, bone mass tends to be higher in African-Americans than in Caucasians, and higher in males than in females. Girls and boys experience their most rapid rate of bone growth during puberty, and by the end of puberty they have almost achieved peak mass. Hence the teenage years are especially critical to maximizing skeletal growth. Girls and, to a greater extent, boys also accumulate bone mass during and after puberty, with some additional mass being gained even in the third decade of life. Finally, it is worth noting that a delayed onset of puberty is associated with a reduction in peak bone mass attainment.

Few adolescents consume recommended levels of dietary calcium shown in Table 10-1. As indicated in Figure 6-4 based on data from the National Health and Nutrition Examination Surveys (NHANES), children up to age 9 consume the recommended amount of calcium. Consumption begins to decline slightly just as the calcium requirement to sustain pubertal growth goes up. Health care professionals should inquire specifically about calcium intake during check-ups. It is useful to remember that while fluid milk consumption decreases as children progress to adolescents, both children and adolescents consume mixed foods such as pizza that contain considerable amounts of calcium through cheese. Calcium intake in children and adolescents can be enhanced by incorporating fruit-flavored yogurt, milk-based puddings and shakes, cheese (including low-fat cheese products), and fortified foods such as orange juice into family meals, snacks, and packed school lunches. It is important to recognize that even in the context of obesity and other chronic disease prevention, low-fat and nonfat, calcium-rich dairy foods can be emphasized as a way to promote bone health without having a negative impact on efforts to manage weight. Calcium supplements may be used for those individuals who would otherwise have a chronic, sub-optimal intake of calcium and are unable to meet the requirement for calcium through diet alone. Interactive nutrition, physical activity, and bone health information geared toward girls and adolescents can be found on two Centers for Disease Control and Prevention (CDC) Web sites related to the *Powerful Bones, Powerful Girls campaign*: http://www.cdc.gov/powerfulbones/index2.html and http:www.cdc.gov/powerfulbones/parents.

Vitamin D

As with calcium, adequate levels of vitamin D are critical to forming and maintaining healthy bones throughout infancy, childhood, and adolescence. Full-term infants who are fed human breast milk appear to mineralize the skeleton similarly to infants fed commercial formulas, including soy-based formulas for infants with an intolerance to cow's milk. However, infants who are exclusively breastfed and who have limited exposure to sunlight are at increased risk of developing vitamin D deficiency. Severe vitamin D deficiency can lead to rickets. The American Academy of Pediatrics has suggested that all infants who are exclusively breastfed receive 200 IU (international units) of vitamin D daily to lessen the likelihood of developing rickets.

Vitamin D requirements during childhood are 200 IU daily, which is the amount contained in two glasses of fortified milk or in most children's multi-vitamins. There are also rare cases of rickets in children who have congenital disorders of vitamin D or phosphorus metabolism and health care professionals should be alert to this possibility. (See Chapter 3 for more details.) These bone diseases may not respond to vitamin D but can be treated by other means.

Protein, Salt, and Phosphorus

There has been some concern that the high intakes of protein, salt, and phosphorus that occur in children and adolescents who eat high-calorie, low-nutrient foods and drink soda can impair bone growth and mineralization. This may be true if these intakes are at the expense of calcium-rich foods, but studies in adolescents have shown that intake of the recommended levels of calcium intake can compensate for high levels of protein, salt, and phosphorus (Fitzpatrick and Heaney 2003).

Physical Activity

Bone mass may be increased in childhood by impact-bearing exercise or physical activity. Thus, health care professionals should emphasize the importance of physical activity at every visit and should encourage healthy children to be active everyday. At a minimum, they should engage in at least 60 minutes of moderate to vigorous physical activity on most days, preferably daily. Unfortunately, many children and adolescents do not get enough physical activity. Health care professionals should inquire about physical activity at each visit and urge children and adolescents to engage in physical activity for at least an hour a day. Health care professionals can also help promote the importance of physical education in the schools by speaking out in the community.

Other Lifestyle Factors

Childhood is an excellent time to initiate counseling aimed at discouraging the adoption of behaviors that may negatively affect bone health, including smoking and alcohol consumption. Such counseling should be continued throughout adolescence, at which time the dangers of anabolic steroids (which can increase the risk of osteoporosis) should also be discussed.

Risk Factor Assessment, Bone Density Testing, and Specialty Referral

The vast majority of children and adolescents will have healthy bone development, and the health care professional's goal is to encourage and support these young individuals and their parents to make the proper lifestyle choices (adequate nutrition and physical activity) to promote both bone health and overall health status. However, health care professionals should be alert to medical conditions and medications that place children and adolescents at risk for poor bone health.

In young individuals, skeletal disorders may present as children who fail to maintain their natural growth curve. While this can be due to any of a variety of factors, metabolic bone disease should be considered as part of a full workup.

Eating disorders such as anorexia and bulimia are uncommon, but can be extremely debilitating. General practitioners may observe changes in weight and appearance, as well as a history of delayed onset or cessation of menstrual periods. Individuals suspected of having eating disorders such as anorexia or bulimia should immediately be referred to an appropriate specialist or an eating disorders clinic.

All young females should be queried about onset and regularity of their menstrual periods. Regular menses signal an intact gonadal axis and adequate estrogen exposure. If menses have stopped after menarche for any reason investigation is warranted. Prolonged periods of amenorrhea have very serious and long-term consequences on bone health. In fact, the cessation of periods in a young, healthy woman should serve as a red flag, as it can lead to a high risk of immediate stress fractures as well as an increased long-term risk of osteoporosis and osteoporotic fractures. Its most common cause in young healthy women is participation in a very strenuous athletic activity like cross-country running or activities that are both strenuous and emphasize low-body weight, such as gymnastics or ballet. The absence of menstrual periods might be the only sign that these individuals need attention. The first step is to increase nutritional intake with calorie-dense foods (e.g., nuts, cheese) as part of an otherwise balanced diet. If the periods do not return within a couple of months, these individuals should be encouraged to curtail their athletic activity. To ensure that the activities are curtailed, health care professionals should make the adolescent, parents, and, if necessary, coaches and trainers aware of the short- and long-term consequences of amenorrhea to bone health.

Health care professionals should investigate the causes surrounding any fracture, including the level of trauma involved. Most fractures will be the result of common injuries (e.g., due to sports), but the potential for child abuse should also be considered. On the other hand, some of these children may have osteogenesis imperfecta, and it is also important to make this diagnosis and therefore avoid wrongful accusations of abuse. Health care professionals should also evaluate the potential for bone-related disorders, especially in children or adolescents who experience multiple fractures. Fractures are not uncommon during the early stage of puberty, which is a period (as discussed in Chapter 6) of rapid remodeling where the mineralization of newly formed bone lags behind the increase in the size of the bones. Nevertheless, any fractures in teenagers should be reported to their primary care providers, who should view it as a signal to further assess risk factors such as family and personal history to determine if additional steps are warranted. In some cases, especially fractures in infants, referral to a pediatric specialist who deals with metabolic bone disease (often an endocrinologist, nephrologist, or rheumatologist) will be necessary.

Children and adolescents taking certain medications or with certain diseases that are known to negatively affect bone health should also be carefully evaluated by a specialist. See Table 10-2 for a list of these diseases and medications. One group that is at particularly high risk of bone disease is the survivors of childhood cancer (Kaste 2004). In rare cases children may suffer from primary diseases that affect the bone due to genetic anomalies or from metabolic disorders that affect the processes that regulate systemic mineral homeostasis for calcium or phosphorus (Table 10-2). Health care professionals who suspect these problems because of poor growth, skeletal deformities, or unexplained fractures should refer the child to a specialist in pediatric bone disorders.

Bone density testing is not appropriate for healthy children and must be interpreted with caution even in at-risk children, since it is an imperfect approach to assessing bone before peak bone mass is achieved. If dual x-ray absorptiometry (DXA) is used, bone density should be expressed in Z-scores rather than the T-scores used for adults. T-scores compare individuals to peak bone mass (which does not occur until the third decade of life), while Z-scores provide an age-matched comparison. Comparing children or adolescents to adult peak bone mass rather than age-specific bone mass will inappropriately underestimate their bone density. The measurement of bone density in children is further complicated by the lack of a large, uniform reference database for pediatric patients and by the fact that bone age and chronologic age may not match in children with chronic diseases. The bones of these children are more similar to those of younger children, and thus their bone density may be lower.

Adults

Nutrition

The recommended diet for optimal bone health is consistent with diets recommended for the prevention of other diseases. Therefore, health care providers have opportunities at many patient encounters to establish and reinforce nutritional recommendations that benefit bone and overall health. There are many very common conditions such as hypertension, diabetes, and weight management for which nutritional counseling is vital, providing health care professionals with an excellent opportunity to also incorporate recommendations for bone health.

Table 10-2. Representative Disorders of the Pediatric Skeleton: Developmental Disorders of Bone and Cartilage

Developmental Disorders of Bone and Cartilage
• Osteogenesis Imperfecta • Chondrodysplasia
Metabolic Bone Diseases [primary]
• Idiopathic Juvenile Osteoporosis • Fibrous Dysplasia • Hypophosphatasia(s)
Metabolic Bone Diseases [secondary]
• Hypophosphatemic Vitamin D Resistant Rickets • Vitamin D Dependent Rickets Type I or Type II • Anorexia Nervosa • Celiac Disease • Cystic Fibrosis • Gaucher's Disease • Immobilization • Malignancy • Muscular Dystrophies • Organ (Bone Marrow, Renal) Transplantation
Medications That Can Cause Disorders
• Antiepileptic Medications • Oral Glucocorticoids • Gonadal Hormone Suppression After Puberty • Immunosuppressive Agents (Cancer Chemotherapy)

Calcium

Calcium intake should be 1,000 mg per day during early and middle adulthood. A quick assessment of calcium intake can be made by estimating that a diet without dairy products contains approximately 250–300 mg per day of calcium (Weinberg et al. 2004). Calcium intake from dairy products, calcium-fortified foods, and supplements can be added to this baseline to obtain a rapid, reasonable estimate of the total daily intake. See Chapter 7 for a quick assessment tool that patients can use.

Common food sources of calcium have the added benefit of providing additional nutrients as well. Significant food sources of calcium include dairy products, calcium-set tofu, canned fishes with bones, and other calcium-fortified foods (see table 10-3). Some individuals with lactose intolerance can consume lactose-reduced milk, live culture yogurt, fortified soy beverage, tofu, and hard cheeses. For maximum calcium nutrition, health care professionals should encourage consumption of low-oxalate vegetables such as broccoli, kale, mustard greens, and turnip greens, as oxalates can impair calcium absorption. Vegetarians and vegans can consume tofu brands that are set with calcium (this type of tofu can be identified by checking the label), vegetables with calcium, almonds, and calcium-fortified foods and beverages, such as fortified orange juice and fortified soy beverage. Fortunately, the array of calcium-fortified foods is expanding, providing consumers with a wide variety of options for achieving adequate calcium intake. A table of calcium-containing foods, organized by calcium content per serving, can be found in Table 10-3.

To assist individuals in determining how much calcium they are getting from the food they consume, food labels express calcium content as a percentage of 1,000 mg—in other words, an item with 20 percent of the daily recommended

amount of calcium contains 200 mg of calcium. The calcium content of foods, including fresh fruits and vegetables, can be found on the USDA National Nutrient Database Web site at http://www.nal.usda.gov/fnic/cgi-bin/nut_search.pl.

Calcium supplements can be critical for those persons who cannot meet calcium requirements through food alone. In the absence of gastrointestinal disease, all major forms of calcium supplements are absorbed equally well when taken with meals. The citrated salts may be more readily absorbed in individuals with gastrointestinal disease or decreased stomach acid production. Since different types of supplements may contain different amounts of elemental calcium, it is important to check the label and to determine the exact amount of calcium in the supplement, in order to achieve the targeted level of calcium intake. Patients should be encouraged to check supplement labels to ensure that their calcium supplement meets United States Pharmacopoeia lead standards. Some calcium supplements may contain other nutrients such as vitamin D or vitamin K. This should be discussed with individuals on warfarin therapy who need calcium supplements, since their response to therapy may be altered by high vitamin K intake. Finally, calcium supplements should be ingested no less than 4 hours before or after taking iron or thyroid medications, since calcium may decrease the absorption of these other medications.

The efficiency of calcium absorption from supplements is greatest when calcium is taken in doses of 500 mg or less. In other words, calcium intake, be it through food and/or supplements, should be spread throughout the day, and the daily requirement should not be consumed at a single setting.

Finally, it is important to emphasize to patients that the upper tolerable level for calcium

Table 10–3. Calcium Containing Foods By Calcium Content Per Serving with 100 mg

Food	Serving size	Calcium, mg
>400 mg		
Tofu, regular with calcium sulfate	½ cup	434
Tofu, firm with calcium sulfate	½ cup	860
Fortified cereal	¾ cup	varies by brand
300–400 mg		
Whole milk	1 cup	291
Milkshake	8 oz.	300
Lowfat yogurt	8 oz.	300
Fortified orange juice	1 cup	300
Fortified soy milk	1 cup	300
Fortified rice milk	1 cup	300
Skim, 1%, or 2% milk	1 cup	321
Fortified cereal	¾ cup	varies by brand
Fortified oatmeal	1 pkt	350
200–300 mg		
Cheddar, monterey or provolone cheese	1 oz.	206
Soybeans, roasted	1 cup	237
Spinach (cooked)	1 cup	245
Mixed cheese dish	1 cup	250
Fortified energy bar	1	250
Soybeans (cooked)	1 cup	261
Swiss cheese	1 oz.	272
Plain yogurt	8 oz	274
100–200 mg		
Pizza	1 slice	100
Fortified waffles	2	100
Fortified butter or margarine	1 Tbsp.	100
Sherbet	1 cup	103
Mustard greens (cooked), Bok Choy	1 cup	104
Spaghetti, lasagna	1 cup	125
Cottage cheese	1 cup	138
Baked beans	1 cup	142
Dandelion greens or turnip greens (cooked)	1 cup	147
Ice cream	1 cup	151
Frozen yogurt or pudding	½ cup	152
American, Feta, or Mozzarella cheese	1 oz.	174
Soybeans, boiled	1 cup	175

Source: USDA 2002.

intake recommended by the Institute of Medicine is 2,500 mg per day. In some cases, this limit should be even lower, since some individuals who are susceptible can become hypercalciuric with calcium intakes as low as 1,500 mg per day. Health care professionals should ask their patients if they regularly take antacids, since many of them may not know that common antacids contain high levels of calcium. As a result, those individuals who take antacids regularly may be consuming calcium at the higher-than-recommended levels.

Vitamin D

The following recommendations for adequate intake do not take into account vitamin D that is absorbed from the sun, since it is difficult for an individual to determine how much vitamin D he or she gets from exposure to sunshine. Young and middle-aged adults should consume about 200 IU per day of vitamin D, although intakes of up to about 1,000 IU per day are generally considered safe. Much higher intakes can be toxic for healthy individuals, although physicians may prescribe higher dosages for individuals with a vitamin D deficiency. Primary food sources of vitamin D are limited to fortified milk (100 IU per cup), egg yolk (25 IU per yolk), fortified cereals, and fish oils. Sunlight exposure contributes variably to circulating and active vitamin D formation, depending on age, race, clothing, and latitude. Sunscreen with an SPF above eight will block the ultraviolet B radiation that stimulates vitamin D production; the extent to which this can lead to vitamin D deficiency is not well defined. However, particularly in northern climates and among older individuals, vitamin D deficiency is becoming recognized as very common. Health care professionals should educate individuals about recommended levels and sources of vitamin D and encourage adequate intake

through food sources, supplements, and appropriate amounts of sun exposure. Physicians should consider measuring the circulating form of vitamin D in the blood—25-hydroxy vitamin D—in individuals who have any of the following characteristics: low dietary intake of vitamin D, inadequate exposure to the sun, signs of poor absorption of vitamin D, or the presence of a gastrointestinal disorder that might decrease their vitamin D supply. Individuals found to be vitamin D deficient by a physician may be given pharmacologic doses of vitamin D to replenish stores and maximize bone mineralization (Pettifor 2003).

Protein

Adequate dietary protein is important for bone health. In short-term studies, low protein intakes have been shown to result in decreased calcium absorption, while protein supplementation after hip fracture has been shown to speed healing and decrease mortality. However, increasing protein intake also increases urine calcium excretion. The long-term effect of both high and low protein diets on skeletal health has yet to be determined. Following the current dietary guidelines for servings of protein-containing foods such as meat, poultry, beans, and dairy products does not present any problems for calcium and bone health. These guidelines can be achieved by consuming 2–3 servings of meat or beans and 2–3 servings of milk and cheese per day. Higher intakes may be necessary in individuals with a history of low protein intake and those who are recovering from fracture in order to bring protein levels back to normal (as long as they also are getting sufficient levels of calcium intake). Important sources of protein include low-fat dairy products, which also provide calcium, phosphorous, and other important nutrients. Most vegetables provide fiber and minerals in addition to small amounts of protein, while soy protein sources such as tempeh, soybeans, and full-fat tofu provide isoflavones (plant compounds with estrogenic effects), which have been shown to increase bone density in some short-term clinical trials (long-term studies are ongoing). Nutritional supplements containing protein are available for those who cannot get enough protein from diet.

Other Nutrients

Sodium chloride intake increases urine calcium excretion, and excessive intake of salt may increase bone resorption in postmenopausal women, although this effect may be offset by adequate calcium intake. However, bone health is yet another reason to maximize the intake of fresh, unprocessed foods and achieve the Institute of Medicine recommendation for an intake of no more than 2,400 mg per day of sodium. Individuals can reduce their intake by avoiding canned, jarred, cured, and processed foods in home cooking. Individuals can reduce their intake of salt by carefully checking the labels of processed foods used in the home and choosing fresh fruits, vegetables, and meats without sauces and dressings when eating away from home. Caffeine consumption leads to a small decrease in calcium absorption; carbonated beverages do not appear to significantly affect calcium excretion independent of caffeine. As long as adequate levels of calcium intake are maintained, however, both carbonated and caffeinated beverages can be consumed in moderation.

Many other minerals such as phosphorus, magnesium, copper, and boron also contribute to bone health to varying degrees. Adequate amounts of these elements can generally be consumed by focusing on an overall healthful diet that includes an adequate intake of lean protein, abundant consumption of fruits and vegetables, and appropriate intake of calcium and vitamin D

along with moderate consumption of sodium and caffeine. (See Table 7-5 for more details.)

Physical Activity

Physical activity should be promoted throughout adulthood, as appropriate to the physical capabilities of the individual. Physical activity not only promotes bone health, but it also helps to optimize weight control, metabolic parameters, muscle strength, and cardiovascular fitness. Programs that have demonstrated skeletal benefits have all included impact activities or resistance-training exercises, including walking, jumping, jogging, running, soccer, racquet sports, weight lifting, dancing, hiking, and stair climbing. To promote bone and overall health, adult patients should be encouraged to accomplish at least 30 minutes per day of moderate intensity physical activity on most, preferably all, days of the week. Some strength or resistance training can be particularly beneficial to bone health. Engaging in longer periods of moderate activity and/or increasing the intensity of activity (i.e., at least 20 minutes of vigorous intensity activity) are the best ways to promote cardiovascular health.

Initiating and maintaining a program is a significant challenge for sedentary patients. Patients should be encouraged to engage in even small amounts of daily activity, since these activities may have some health benefits. Some individuals may find it easier to start with manageable goals that incorporate physical activity into their daily activities, such as parking farther from their destination or using the stairs instead of the elevator. Long-term compliance with physical activity routines may be enhanced by enlisting the support of family members or friends, advocating moderate intensity that is within the person's capabilities, devising programs that individuals can accomplish at home, offering flexibility in activity choices, and providing feedback and incentives. Participating in a physical activity that the individual enjoys, such as gardening, a walk with a friend, or a community exercise or dance class, also helps maintain compliance. Individuals should be encouraged to find an activity they like enough to continue and to be ready to try a different program if they lose interest in the current one.

Patient education materials, including pamphlets and videos with specific exercises and instructions for moving safely and maintaining optimal posture, can be obtained from the National Institute on Aging at http://www.niapublications.org or from the National Osteoporosis Foundation at http://www.nof.org.

Other Lifestyle Measures

Excessive alcohol and tobacco use increases the risk for fracture. Thus, patients should be encouraged to quit smoking and to limit alcohol intake to moderate use, not only to optimize bone health, but also for their overall health and well-being. In addition, general safety measures to reduce the risk of trauma, such as consistent use of seatbelts, should be advised.

Pregnancy and Lactation

While the data are somewhat limited, it appears that there is a transient decrease in bone density during pregnancy and lactation, but the healthy mother's skeleton rapidly recovers after lactation is completed. Thus, there does not appear to be a long-term detrimental effect of pregnancy and lactation on bone health. Pregnant and lactating women should follow their obstetrician's recommendations for optimal nutrition and physical activity. The current recommended intakes during pregnancy and lactation are 1,000 mg per day of calcium and 200 IU per day for vitamin D. A higher intake of 1,300 mg per day of calcium is recommended for women under age 18.

Risk Factor Assessment and Bone Density Testing

All young and middle-aged adults should be encouraged to adopt lifestyles that help to prevent bone loss and to promote overall health and the prevention of chronic disease. Bone density testing of asymptomatic young and middle-aged adults without significant risk factors is not recommended. Although the radiation exposure of testing is very low, this exam should not be performed on women who may be pregnant.

Young and middle-aged adult patients with medical conditions associated with bone loss, such as hyperthyroidism, hyperparathyroidism, hypogonadism (either endogenous or medically induced), malabsorptive syndromes or eating disorders, significantly impaired mobility, or chronic renal or hepatic failure, warrant special attention. In addition to being strongly encouraged to adopt appropriate nutrition and lifestyle choices, they should also be considered for bone density testing and pharmacologic therapy. A bone density test should be performed on patients requiring medications that can result in bone loss, such as oral glucocorticoids, anticonvulsants, immuno-suppressants (cyclosporine A, tacrolimus, methotrexate), and heparin for more than a month. Since bone loss can occur rapidly after the initiation of glucocorticoid therapy, health care professionals should consider bone density testing prior to the start of such therapy; patients with low bone density should be considered for concurrent antiresorptive therapy.

In addition, younger patients with conditions that increase fracture risk should be encouraged to adhere to maximal nutrition and lifestyle measures aimed at preventing bone disease. Specific therapy such as antiresorptive drugs should also be considered in those with significantly low bone mass based on a bone density test.

Interpretation of bone density exams in this age group should focus on the T-score values, even though specific T-score thresholds for the diagnosis and treatment of osteoporosis have not been established for younger individuals. T-scores can be interpreted for patients by explaining that the T-score compares their bone density to the average maximum lifetime bone density (peak bone mass) in young adults. Patients should be advised that a positive T-score means that their bone density is above the average for a young adult around age 30, while a negative number means their bone density is below that of the average 30-year-old. The World Health Organization (WHO) has established definitions of normal (T-score above -1), low bone mass/osteopenia (T-score between –1 and –2.5), and osteoporosis (T-score less than –2.5) based on epidemiologic data. However, it should be remembered that the risk of bone fracture increases continuously as bone density decreases. In other words, there are no precipitous changes in fracture risk associated with these "break" points. The relationship between T-scores and fracture risk has been conducted primarily in postmenopausal women; data in younger individuals are limited. It should also be remembered that the WHO diagnostic definitions were derived from DXA data and therefore should not be applied to other bone density testing modalities.

Treatment and Monitoring Therapy

With the exception of glucocorticoid-induced osteoporosis, there have been few trials of osteoporosis medications in young and middle-aged adults. Therapy in this age group should focus on maximizing nutrition and lifestyle modifications and addressing any underlying medical conditions such as hypogonadism that can lead to low bone mass. Comorbid conditions that may affect bone should be treated; for example, care should be taken to ensure serum thyroid stimulating hormone (TSH) remains in the normal range in individuals with hypothyroidism who are on L-thyroxine therapy. Young and middle-aged adults who have osteoporosis even after non-pharmacologic therapies have been employed should be considered for anti-resorptive therapy, options for which are discussed in Chapter 9.

For individuals who have received bone density testing prior to menopause, additional bone density exams should be conducted only if the results could prompt a change in therapeutic plan. Early postmenopausal women with normal or marginally low bone density do not need repeat bone density scanning for at least 3–5 years, unless an intervening medical condition that could accelerate bone loss develops. Individuals on anti-resorptive therapy may benefit from a follow-up DXA scan. However, due to the variability of densitometry measurements, at least 18 to 24 months should elapse between scans to ensure that any changes are large enough to be clearly detected. Since there is variability between DXA scans even with rigorous quality assurance and careful technique, care should be taken not to alter treatment regimens in response to small changes in bone density values. While they can be significant in research trials, changes in hip or spine bone density of 4 percent or less are at the detection limits of office-based densitometry and should be interpreted cautiously in the clinical setting. Osteoporotic patients who cannot readily see signs that therapy is working or failing often do not take their prescription drugs appropriately (i.e., adherence is poor) and/or they do not stick with their drug regimen over time (i.e., persistence is poor). A recent study of osteoporotic patients showed that monitoring by a nurse, with or without the use of a biochemical marker of bone resorption, could improve both adherence to and persistence with therapy over time. Moreover, better adherence was found to be associated with better outcomes (Clowes et al. 2004).

Specialty Referrals

Specialists can assist primary care providers with additional expertise in those young and middle-aged adults who represent challenging situations, including individuals for whom the etiology of low bone mass is unknown, those who require an evaluation for secondary causes of bone loss, those being considered for long-term antiresorptive therapy, and those who either do not tolerate or do not respond to therapy. These patients may benefit from a referral to an endocrinologist, rheumatologist, or other specialist in osteoporosis management. Referrals to dietitians and physical therapists can also be helpful in implementing nutrition and physical activity programs, particularly for those individuals with significant dietary and mobility limitations.

A broad approach to assessing bone health, preventing bone disease, and managing osteoporosis in adults is illustrated in Figure 10-1.

Older Adults

Nutrition

The nutrition guidance outlined for young and middle-aged adults also applies to older individuals and the elderly. Specific additional recommendations pertinent to this age group are discussed below.

Calcium and Vitamin D

Calcium and vitamin D absorption decreases with aging, and older individuals with limited mobility tend to receive less sunlight, leading to rates of vitamin D deficiency (as measured by serologic testing) of up to 57 percent in this population (Thomas et al. 1998). As a result, recommended levels of both calcium and vitamin D

increase in this population. Total calcium intake should be 1,200 mg per day after age 50. Older individuals should be educated in how to read labels for calcium content, since calcium is expressed as a percent of 1,000 mg on labels (the recommended level for younger adults). Since the calcium intake goal for older adults is greater than 1000 mg per day, these individuals actually need to consume more than 100 percent of the level recommended on food labels. Since older persons may suffer constipation as a side effect of calcium supplements, health care professionals should emphasize food sources of calcium and also recommend increasing fluid and fiber intake. Inability to secrete acid in the stomach (achlorhydria) may limit the absorption of calcium carbonate salts; citrated salts may be absorbed better in these patients, but carbonate salts will still be absorbed if taken with meals.

Individuals between the ages of 51 and 70 should consume 400 IU per day of vitamin D, while those over age 70 should get 600 IU per day. Since it may be difficult for older individuals to achieve these levels of intake through food alone, many individuals will require multi-vitamins or specific vitamin D supplements. Individuals who have low vitamin D dietary intake and/or low sun exposure should have their vitamin D level measured. Persons found to have vitamin D deficiency should receive pharmacologic doses of vitamin D.

Other nutrients

Recommendations for other nutrients for older adults are the same as those for younger adults. In addition, protein supplementation has been shown to speed healing and reduce mortality in older individuals suffering hip fractures. These patients should have a nutritional evaluation during post-fracture rehabilitation.

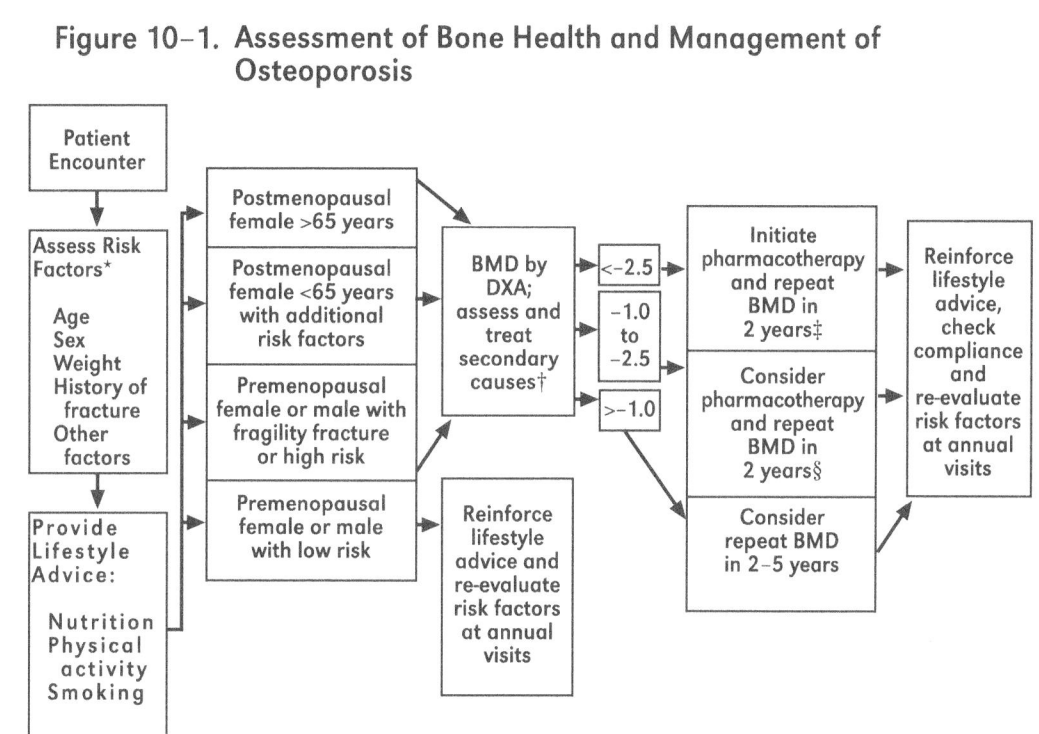

Figure 10–1. Assessment of Bone Health and Management of Osteoporosis

Note: This flow chart outlines a broad approach to assessing bone health and preventing bone disease, determining who should have bone density measurements, and deciding on pharmacologic treatment for osteoporosis. More details on each of these topics can be found in Chapters 6, 7, 8, and 9. The flow chart does not include the use of biochemical markers of bone turnover, which, as discussed in Chapter 8, is a promising approach to assessing early response to or subsequent compliance with pharmacotherapy. This flow chart is based on the assumption that health care providers will see their patients annually, and will briefly evaluate risk factors, assess compliance to lifestyle and nutritional advice, and review medications at each visit. Because there are often no symptoms in individuals whose bone health is declining, this annual "bone check-up" by health care providers is essential.

Footnotes:
* There is no clear-cut definition of "high" and "low" risk at the present time, although the presence of multiple factors that contribute to bone loss (e.g., a family history of osteoporosis, low body weight, and endocrine, musculoskeletal, or nutritional disorders) should be considered an indication of high risk. The analysis of risk factors should include not only those that affect bone fragility, but also those that contribute to the risk of falling.

† If DXA of the spine and hip are not available, peripheral measurements may be used to assess risk, but the T-score cut-offs for treatment have not been established. It is important to evaluate possible secondary causes of bone loss as well as other skeletal disorders in all patients, but particularly in those who are being considered for pharmacotherapy. In most patients pharmacotherapy and treatment for secondary causes can be initiated at the same time.

‡ A generalized approach to pharmacotherapy is outlined in Chapter 9. But it is likely that the development of new drugs and the acquisition of new data on currently available drugs will lead to changes in treatment in the near future.

§ Individuals with low bone density or osteopenia (defined as BMDs between –1.0 and –2.5) are clearly at increased risk of fracture. The decision to recommend pharmacotherapy for these individuals will depend on many factors. Conservative therapy consisting of calcium, vitamin D, and exercise may be appropriate for young individuals with low BMD who have not had a fragility fracture.

Physical Activity

Older adults should maintain as high a functional status as possible and regularly engage in physical activity. Many older adults can follow the same recommendations for younger adults outlined above. Weight-supporting activities such as stationary bicycling, deep-water walking, and floor exercises may be more appropriate in older adults with compromised bone health although with proper supervision and training these individuals can safely engage in resistance exercises as well. Individualized programs devised by physical therapists or physiatrists can safely improve strength, mobility, and functional capacity in vulnerable older adults. Physical therapists can also train individuals in specific postural exercises to strengthen back extensor muscles, which may relieve pain and decrease development or progression of kyphosis.

Patients with spine fractures should avoid activities that flex the spine and increase pressure on compromised vertebral bodies. In addition, activities such as golf, bowling, tennis, and horseback riding place significant force on the spine and should be avoided in patients with compromised bone health. People with osteoporosis of the spine should avoid use of exercise machines that involve trunk rotation or forward bending, as these movements can cause a fracture in individuals with osteoporosis. Machines to avoid include abdominal exercisers, biceps, rowing, and cross-country ski machines, stationary bicycles with moving handlebars, or upper body ergometers.

Physical therapists play an important role in both fracture prevention and treatment. They can evaluate balance and the risks of falling and teach specific exercises and techniques to minimize that risk. Since nearly all hip fractures are associated with a fall, preventing falls in older individuals is fundamental to preventing fractures. Occupational therapists can evaluate the home environment and make modifications that minimize the risks of falling, including eliminating loose rugs; installing hand rails, shower chairs, and hand-held nozzles in the bathroom; installing bedside lamps, nightlights in hallways and bathrooms, and strips of contrasting tape on stair treads; and recommending the use of canes and walkers as appropriate as well as the avoidance of certain types of clothing, including long garments and trailing hems.

Patient education materials, including pamphlets and videos with specific exercises and instructions for exercise, moving safely, and maintaining optimal posture, can be obtained from the National Institute on Aging at http://www.niapublications.org/shopdisplay products.asp?id=17&cat=Exercise+for +Older+People or from the National Institutes of Health Osteoporosis and Related Bone Diseases~National Resource Center (http://www.osteo.org).

Risk Factor Assessment and Bone Density Testing

Risk factors for bone loss and fracture should be assessed in all women over 65. Commonly identified risk factors for fracture are listed in Table 10-4.

One of the best validated instruments to help identify patients at risk of low bone mineral density (BMD) (and thus in need of a DXA) is the three-item Osteoporosis Risk Assessment Instrument (ORAI). As shown in Table 10-5, ORAI uses age, weight, and current use of hormone therapy to identify women at risk for osteoporosis (Cadarette et al. 2000).

Another easy-to-use tool that many clinicians and their patients may find appealing is the Osteoporosis Self-Assessment Tool (OST). As shown in Figure 10-2, this tool combines age and weight in a simple nomogram. Assuming that

BMDs are performed on those with a score of less than two (the upper two sections of the chart), the OST tool identifies over 90 percent of women with osteoporosis—and 100 percent of those over age 65—as defined by WHO criteria (Cadarette et al. 2004). This finding not only helps to validate OST, but it also provides further evidence to support current guidelines recommending BMD testing in all women over age 65. However, as with other risk-assessment tools, OST has low specificity, as about 55 percent of the women identified by this tool as needing a BMD actually do not have osteoporosis (Cadarette et al. 2004). Since the OST index is easy to calculate, it may be the most useful available tool in clinical practice at this time.

As noted in Chapter 8, one risk factor that is not included in these screening instruments is height loss. Careful measurement of height can be useful both in assessing risk and in monitoring patients on therapy. A height loss of more than one inch should serve as a "red flag" for the potential of osteoporosis and/or spinal fractures.

Both the NOF and USPSTF recommend bone density testing for women age 65 and older. The USPSTF also recommends that bone density testing begin at age 60 for women who are at increased risk for osteoporotic fractures. Expert organizations differ, however, on when to conduct routine screening in women under age 60. The USPSTF has found evidence that screening women who are at lower risk for osteoporosis or fracture can identify additional individuals who may be eligible for treatment for osteoporosis. This evidence also suggests that such widespread screening would prevent a small number of fractures, since younger individuals with low BMD and no other risk factors are at low risk of fracture. The NOF guidelines recommend bone density testing in postmenopausal women under age 65 with risk factors for

---

Table 10-4. Risk Factors for Fracture

- Older age (>65 years)
- Fracture after age 45
- First-degree female relative with a fracture in adulthood
- Self report health as "fair" or "poor"
- Current tobacco use
- Weight less than 127 lbs.
- Menopause prior to age 45 years
- Amenorrhea
- Lifelong low calcium intake
- Excess alcohol consumption
- Poor vision despite correction
- Falls
- Minimal weight-bearing exercise
- Medical Conditions
    - ~ Hyperthyroidism
    - ~ Chronic lung disease
    - ~ Endometriosis
    - ~ Malignancy
    - ~ Chronic hepatic or renal
    - ~ disease
    - ~ Hyperparathryoidism
    - ~ Vitamin D deficiency
    - ~ Cushing's disease
    - ~ Multiple sclerosis
    - ~ Sarcoidosis
    - ~ Hemachromotosis
- Medications:
    - ~ Oral glucocorticoids
    - ~ Excess thyroxine replacement
    - ~ Antiepileptic medications
    - ~ Gonadal hormone suppression
    - ~ Immunosuppressive agents

---

osteoporosis. It should also be noted that the majority of the evidence upon which these guidelines are based was obtained in White women. There is no consensus regarding screening in men; however, bone density testing should be considered in men with fragility fractures, those on therapies that may cause bone loss, notably glucocorticoids or androgen deprivation, and men with multiple risk factors.

Table 10–5. Scoring System for Osteoporosis Risk Assessment Instrument (ORAI)

Variable	Score
Age, yr	
≥ 75	15
65–74	9
55–64	5
45–54	0
Weight, kg	
<60	9
60–69	3
≥ 70	0
Current estrogen use	
No	2
Yes	0

Women with a total score of 9 or greater would be selected for bone densitometry.

Note: The Osteoporosis Risk Assessment Instrument (ORAI) uses age, weight, and the use of estrogen as an aid to selecting postmenopausal patients for bone density testing. A score greater than 9 would indicate testing is warranted.

Source: Cadarette 2000. Development and validation of the Osteoporosis Risk Assessment Instrument to facilitate selection of women for bone densitometry —Reprinted from CMAJ 02–May–00: 162(9), Page(s) 1289–1294 by permission of the publisher. ©2000 Canadian Medical Association.

Measuring bone density at the hip by DXA is the best predictor of hip fracture. Some members of the original WHO working group recommended that the diagnosis of osteoporosis should be based only on the T-score obtained through DXA measurement at the hip (Kanis et al. 2000). These members indicated that while measurements at other sites and with other technologies may be useful for assessing risk of fracture, they should not be used for diagnosis of osteoporosis.

Bone density T-scores can be interpreted for older individuals in the same way they are for young and middle-aged adults. Although there are no data, many experts also evaluate the Z-scores in older individuals. The Z-score compares the patient's bone density to that expected for their age, rather than to peak bone mass. While this approach has not been validated, many experts will more strongly consider a laboratory evaluation of vitamin D levels and of potential secondary causes of osteoporosis in patients with Z-scores of –2 or less (meaning the patient's bone density is two standard deviations or more below that expected for their age). It is important to consider the possibility of secondary causes in all patients with osteoporosis, even those with Z-scores higher than -2. Laboratory evaluation for secondary causes should be guided by clinical judgment as well as findings from the patient's history and a physical examination. There are many different types of conditions and medications that can lead to secondary osteoporosis, as summarized in Tables 3-1 and 3-2 in Chapter 3.

Treatment and Monitoring Therapy

Pharmacologic therapy should be instituted in individuals who have osteoporosis, as defined by WHO criteria or the existence of fragility fractures. Individuals with low bone mass and multiple fracture risk factors should also be con-

Figure 10-2. Osteoporosis Self-Assessment Tool (OST) Chart

Body Weight lbs.	45–49	50–54	55–59	60–64	65–69	70–74	75–79	80–84	85–89	90–94	95–99	Body Weight lbs.
66–75	–3	–4	–5	–6	–7	–8	–9	–10	–11	–12	–13	66–75
76–87	–2	–3	–4	–5	–6	–7	–8	–9	–10	–11	–12	76–87
88–98	–1	–2	–3	–4	–5	–6	–7	–8	–9	–10	–11	88–98
99–109	0	–1	–2	–3	–4	–5	–6	–7	–8	–9	–10	99–109
110–120	1	0	–1	–2	–3	–4	–5	–6	–7	–8	–9	110–120
121–131	2	1	0	–1	–2	–3	–4	–5	–6	–7	–8	121–131
132–142	3	2	1	0	–1	–2	–3	–4	–5	–6	–7	132–142
143–153	4	3	2	1	0	–1	–2	–3	–4	–5	–6	143–153
154–164	5	4	3	2	1	0	–1	–2	–3	–4	–5	154–164
165–175	6	5	4	3	2	1	0	–1	–2	–3	–4	165–175
176–186	7	6	5	4	3	2	1	0	–1	–2	–3	176–186
187–197	8	7	6	5	4	3	2	1	0	–1	–2	187–197
198–208	9	8	7	6	5	4	3	2	1	0	–1	198–208
209–219	10	9	8	7	6	5	4	3	2	1	0	209–219
220–230	11	10	9	8	7	6	5	4	3	2	1	220–230

AGE (years)

Note: The OST Chart uses age and weight as a decision assistance tool for postmenopausal women. The heavy lines divide high, medium, and low risk. Patients with a score of less than two (those with medium and high risk, in the unshaded area of the chart) would be recommended for bone density. This figure refers to postmenopausal White women. Cut points may be different for women of other races or for men.

Source: Cadarette 2004.

sidered for therapy (in addition to emphasizing appropriate lifestyle and nutritional intake). The FDA has approved several anti-resorptive therapies (bisphosphonates, selective estrogen receptor modulators, estrogen, and calcitonin) as well as a single anabolic agent, teriparatide (PTH), which is currently available only as a daily injection. Selection of therapeutic agent can be tailored to the severity of the patient's bone loss and other comorbid conditions. The risks and benefits of these agents, as determined by clinical trials, are discussed in Chapter 9. Finally, fall prevention strategies should be discussed with every osteoporosis patient, and hip protectors should be considered for the frail elderly and patients at high risk for falling.

Combinations of antiresorptive agents have been tested for their impact on bone density, and results suggest that this approach produces modestly greater increases in BMD than do single agents used alone. There are no data, however, on the efficacy of combination therapy in reducing the risk of fracture. In addition, using bisphosphonates in conjunction with teriparatide provides no added benefit over use of each agent individually.

As with younger individuals, follow-up bone density exams should be conducted only when the results could prompt a change in therapeutic plan. Older individuals with normal or minimally low bone density likely do not need to repeat bone density scanning for at least 3–5 years, unless an accelerated rate of bone loss is suspected that might lower their bone density to a level at which treatment would be considered. As with younger and middle-aged adults, individuals on anti-resorptive therapy may benefit from a follow up DXA scan at least 18 to 24 months after the initial scan.

The utility of markers of bone resorption in monitoring response to therapy shows promise but has not been firmly established. Some experts use marker measurements in the evaluation of patients with an apparent lack of response to antiresorptive therapy, but this approach has not been validated. Much work continues to determine the clinical utility of using markers of bone activity. A complete discussion can be found in Chapter 8.

Non-bone medication use should be evaluated as part of the treatment plan for elderly individuals with low bone density. Medications associated with dizziness, low blood pressure, falls in blood pressure upon standing (orthostasis), and sedation can increase the risk of falling, and their use should be minimized or avoided. In addition, alcohol use should be reviewed, as it may cause older individuals to become unsteady and susceptible to falls.

Follow-up for Fractures

There is significant morbidity and mortality following fractures in older individuals. In addition, these individuals are at very high risk for future fractures. Thus, health care providers should aggressively intervene to maximize bone health, minimize morbidity, and prevent future fractures in these patients. All nutrition and lifestyle modifications should be strongly encouraged, specific osteoporotic pharmacologic therapy should be instituted, and appropriate rehabilitation should be achieved. Identifying and intervening in patients with osteoporotic fractures presents an exceptional opportunity to dramatically reduce the consequences of this disease. Yet, as noted in Chapter 9, a significant number of fracture patients do not receive optimal long-term care focused on bone health. All health care providers involved in the care of fracture patients must dedicate themselves to ensuring not only adequate treatment for the acute fracture, but also aggressive implementation of all therapeutic and rehabilitative measures to prevent further fractures. Specific post-fracture treatment recommendations are found in Chapter 9.

Specialty Referrals

Osteoporosis is often diagnosed and treated in the primary care setting. However, as with younger individuals, older persons and the elderly with particularly challenging clinical situations can benefit from a referral to an endocrinologist, rheumatologist, or other specialist in osteoporosis management. For example, such referrals may be appropriate in cases where secondary osteoporosis is suspected, therapy is not tolerated, bone density declines, or a fragility fracture occurs during treatment.

Physical therapists and occupational therapists provide vital assistance in the management of older patients with osteoporosis by working with them to increase strength, balance, and physical activity and to reduce the risk of falls. Referrals to physical and occupational therapists should be strongly considered for all osteoporotic individuals at risk for falls and/or with limited exercise capacity. Older individuals at risk for fracture should also be referred to an eye care professional, who should perform refraction, cataract removal, and/or glaucoma therapy as appropriate, as such treatments maximize visual acuity and minimize the risk of falls.

Elderly individuals with vertebral fractures, particularly those with persistent pain, may benefit from referral to an orthopedist and to a physical therapist, who can fit them for a back brace that helps to reduce kyphosis.

Strategies to Maximize Adherence

Long-term adherence, defined as the percentage of prescribed medication taken, and persistence, defined as the percentage of individuals who take a medication for the prescribed period of time, are poor with any therapy, with rates for both being around 50 percent (Clowes

et al. 2004). It is not known, moreover, whether certain strategies, such as feedback to patients on the results of repeat bone density testing or increased use of biochemical markers of bone turnover, can improve long-term compliance with osteoporosis therapies. In fact, while measurement of bone resorption markers has been advocated to improve compliance to therapy, monitoring by a nurse without such measurements has been found to be equally effective in improving compliance (Clowes et al. 2004). This study suggests that the key to maximizing adherence to any therapy is for health care professionals to follow up with patients to ensure that they are taking their medications appropriately.

Specific follow-up strategies that have been shown to improve adherence to other types of medical regimens should be utilized in patients with osteoporosis as well. These include counseling about the importance of the planned treatment regimen, enlisting the support of the patient's social network, sending reminders about follow-up appointments, recognizing adherence efforts, simplifying and organizing the treatment regimen, addressing patient concerns about side effects, and maintaining an encouraging provider-patient relationship. Many of these approaches are time and labor intensive; non-physician health care professionals can be invaluable resources in making the most of these strategies in a busy practice. Patient education materials on many aspects of osteoporosis are available free on-line from the National Institutes of Health Osteoporosis and Related Bone Diseases~National Resource Center (http://www.osteo.org).

Key Questions for Future Research

Research questions related to the prevention, diagnosis, and treatment of bone disease are provided at the end of Chapters 6, 8, 9, and 11.

References

Cadarette SM, Jaglal SB, Kreiger N, McIsaac WJ, Darlington GA, Tu JV. Development and validation of the osteoporosis risk assessment instrument to facilitate selection of women for bone densitometry. CMAJ 2000 May 2;162(9):1289-94.

Cadarette SM, McIsaac WJ, Hawker GA, Jaakkimainen L, Culbert A, Zarifa G, Ola E, Jaglal SB. The validity of decision rules for selecting women with primary osteoporosis for bone mineral density testing. Osteoporos Int 2004 Jan 17.

Clowes, JA, Peel NF, Eastell R. The impact of monitoring on adherence and persistence with antiresorptive treatment for postmenopausal osteoporosis: A randomized controlled trial. J Clin Endocrinol Metab 2004 Mar; 89(3):1117-23.

Fitzpatrick L, Heaney RP. Got soda? J Bone Miner Res 2003 Sep;18(9):1570-2.

Kanis JA, Gluer CC. An update on the diagnosis and assessment of osteoporosis with densitometry. Committee of Scientific Advisors, International Osteoporosis Foundation. Osteoporos Int. 2000;11(3):192-202.

Kaste SC. Bone-mineral density deficits from childhood cancer and its therapy: A review of at-risk patient cohorts and available imaging methods. Pediatr Radiol 2004 Feb 12.

Pettifor JM. Nutritional and drug-induced rickets and osteomalacia. In: Favus MJ, editor. Primer on the metabolic bone diseases and disorders of mineral metabolism. 5th ed. Washington, DC: American Society for Bone and Mineral Research; 2003. p. 399-407.

Schanler RJ. The use of human milk for premature infants. Pediatr Clin North Am. 2001 Feb;48(1):207-19.

Thomas MK, Lloyd-Jones DM, Thadhani RI, Shaw AC, Deraska DJ, Kitch BT, Vamvakas EC, Dick IM, Prince RL, Finkelstein JS. Hypovitaminosis D in medical inpatients. N Engl J Med. 1998 Mar 19;338(12):777-83.

U.S. Department of Agriculture, Agricultural Research Service. Nutrient Data Laboratory [homepage on the Internet]. 2002. USDA Nutrient Database for Standard Reference, Release 15. Available from: http://www.nal.usda.gov/fnic/foodcomp/search/.

Weinberg LG, Berner LA, Groves JE. Nutrient contributions of dairy foods in the United States, Continuing Survey of Food Intakes by Individuals, 1994-1996, 1998. J Am Diet Assoc. 2004 Jun;104(6):895-902.

Part Five

WHAT CAN HEALTH SYSTEMS AND POPULATION-BASED APPROACHES DO TO PROMOTE BONE HEALTH?

This part of the report examines how health systems and population-based approaches can promote bone health.

Chapter 11 looks at the key systems-level issues and decisions that affect bone health care, including evidence-based medicine, clinical practice guidelines, training and education of health care professionals, quality assurance and quality improvement techniques, coverage policies, and disparities in prevention and treatment. It also evaluates the key roles of various stakeholders in promoting a more systems-based approach to bone health care, including individual clinicians; medical groups; health plans and other insurers; hospitals and rehabilitation facilities; public health departments; and other stakeholders, such as academic medical centers and public and private employers.

Chapter 12 describes the various potential components of population-based approaches to promoting bone health at the local, State, and Federal levels and reviews the evidence supporting their use. One of the key messages of this chapter is that well-crafted population-based interventions should be highly effective in improving bone health as well as other aspects of health. To illustrate this point, the chapter includes seven detailed profiles of innovative and/or effective population-based programs, each of which was selected to illustrate an important concept in population-based health.

Chapter 11: Key Messages

- Individual organizations—even very small ones—can apply a "systems-based" approach to clinical care and other services by putting into place any of a variety of formal policies and processes.
- There are four distinct systems-based activities that collectively encompass the overall goal of improving the bone health status of Americans:
  - ~ Identifying and developing intervention strategies for various risk levels of the population.
  - ~ Educating and raising awareness among clinicians and the public about bone disease.
  - ~ Ensuring that individuals receive appropriate preventive, diagnostic, and treatment services based upon their level of risk.
  - ~ Monitoring and evaluating bone health outcomes within populations and the community.
- The most important role for individual clinicians in promoting a systems-based approach to bone health is to educate themselves and their patients about prevention, assessment, diagnosis, and treatment.
- Medical groups have the opportunity to implement a systems-based approach as well. For example, they can dedicate staff to certain important tasks; use bench-marking data or academic detailing to promote quality improvement; or implement evidence-based care paths and computerized reminder systems that promote the provision of timely and appropriate care. Some groups may be able to develop specialized osteoporosis clinics or disease management programs.

- Hospitals and rehabilitation facilities can go beyond their traditional role of simply treating bone-related problems or symptoms by developing strategies for improving overall bone health and preventing future falls.
- Skilled nursing homes can institute measures to prevent falls and fractures; to assure that residents receive appropriate amounts of calcium and vitamin D; and to include activities that strengthen bones in their daily regimens.
- Health plans and insurers can get involved in managing bone health by assessing and monitoring provider performance; engaging in quality improvement programs; and/or implementing pay-for-performance initiatives.
- The public health system and other government agencies can play a vitally important role in promoting a systems-based approach to bone health, including:
  - ~ Promote awareness among consumers and clinicians of bone health and disease.
  - ~ Improve linkages between health care organizations, community-based organizations, and the public health system.
  - ~ Train health professionals to promote bone health and recognize and treat bone disease.
  - ~ Develop strategies to promote bone health and appropriate treatment.
  - ~ Monitor and evaluate activities within a community and the Nation as a whole.
- Other institutions, organizations, and agencies can facilitate a systems-based approach to bone health through research, education, and purchasing policies.

Chapter 11

SYSTEMS-BASED APPROACHES TO BONE HEALTH

Overview

The health care system in the United States is not a system *per se*. Rather, it is a collection of independent enterprises, some small and some large, that provide or pay for various aspects of health care. Despite the fragmented nature of this system, individual organizations—even very small ones—can apply a "systems-based" or "systematic" approach to providing clinical care and other services in order to function most effectively. Under this approach, health care organizations and other facilitators (such as employers and other purchasers) put into place any of a variety of formal policies and processes that are designed to ensure that individual consumers receive timely and appropriate preventive, diagnostic, and treatment measures to promote bone health. The nature of these measures is tailored to the underlying risk of bone disease.

For example, an individual clinician's office can create a simple protocol or flow sheet to ensure that a consistent approach is taken to a specific health issue, such as administering preventive care. Larger organizations can make use of more complicated systems such as computerized reminders and triggers based on clinical indicators and/or prescribing patterns.

Systems-based approaches to the prevention and treatment of osteoporosis can be exceptionally valuable both in improving the management of osteoporosis care and in reducing adverse outcomes from poor bone health. This type of approach can help to overcome the problems created by poor communication and a lack of collaboration among the various components of the health care system (e.g., government, communities, provider organizations, health plans, employers, the media, academics). Fragmentation makes the system ill equipped to serve the chronically ill and to provide population-based care (IOM 2002). It also means that those who finance care may not receive the benefits of such care. With increasing job turnover, employees commonly change insurers, even while remaining with the same health care provider. As a result, employers and insurers may have little incentive to cover expensive preventive services (e.g., drug therapy to prevent future osteoporotic fractures) that may not pay dividends until the patient is covered by a different plan or by Medicare.

This chapter lays out four distinct systems-based activities that collectively encompass the overall goals of the larger health system within the United States for improving the bone health status of Americans. The four activities are as follows:

1. Identifying the various risk levels of the population being served and developing an intervention strategy for individuals

Population-Based Risk Stratification: A Prerequisite to a Systems-Based Approach

There is one overriding principle that governs systems-based approaches to osteoporosis and bone health—that is, to focus on populations. A population-based approach considers the health of a group of persons (as defined by factors such as age, gender, geography, or risk factors) who may have diverse needs rather than the patient who has individual needs. Good population-based interventions also accommodate individual needs. The overall goal is to ensure that all persons receive the care they need, especially those at high risk of debilitating and costly fractures. To that end, two tasks must be accomplished. The first is to categorize the population being served into subgroups defined by their underlying risk of bone disease, falls, and fractures. The second is to define appropriate preventive, assessment, and therapeutic strategies for each subgroup based on the best available evidence. These steps should be taken by each of the various components of the health system, be it an individual provider assessing risks among his or her patients, a medical group assessing risks among its patient population, a health plan evaluating the risks of its enrollees, an academic health center educating providers, or a public health department surveying risks in the community at large. When implemented well, risk-stratification and population-based approaches provide ample opportunity for decision-making by providers. For more information on risk stratification, please see Chapter 8.

in each category of risk, with a particular focus on high-risk individuals.

2. Educating and raising awareness among clinicians and the public at large about the risks of bone disease, as well as the best ways to prevent, diagnose, and treat it in the various risk categories identified above.

3. Ensuring that individuals receive appropriate prevention, diagnostic, and treatment services based upon their level of risk.

4. Monitoring and evaluating bone health outcomes within specific populations and the community to identify problem areas and assess the impact of strategies and interventions for improving bone health.

The chapter is organized around each of the individual entities that make up the overall system—individual clinicians, medical groups, health plans/insurers, public health, and other facilitators of bone health, such as public (e.g., Medicare and Medicaid) and private purchasers (e.g., employers) and academic medical centers. Separate sections describe each of their respective roles and responsibilities within each of the activities listed previously. The individual organizations within the overall system need to collaborate and coordinate their activities. To facilitate this type of collaboration, Table 11-1 summarizes the potential participants in a broad set of major interventions and activities designed to promote bone health. It is important to remember, however, that the distinctions between the various levels are somewhat arbitrary. For example, a staff-model health maintenance organization (HMO) includes both a medical group and health plan. Thus, while the strategies discussed within the chapter will appear where they are most commonly employed, it is perfectly conceivable that other stakeholders can and should consider their use as well.

Table 11–1. Health Systems Interventions for Osteoporosis and Bone Health That Can Be Provided at Different Organizational Levels

Intervention/Activity	Individual Clinician	Medical Group	Hospital or Post-Acute Facility	Health Plan or Insurer	Government and Public Health Department	Voluntary Health Organizations and Professional Associations	Academic Institution	Health Care Purchaser	Industry
Promoting bone healthy lifestyles (nutrition, physical activity, no smoking)	■	■	■	■	■	■	■	■	■
Awareness campaigns	■	■	■	■	■	■	■	■	■
Guidelines/evidence-based reports	■	■	■	■	■	■			
Continuing education	■	■	■	■	■	■	■		
Sponsored programs (e.g., education, exercise, fall prevention)		■	■	■	■	■	■	■	■
Behavioral approaches (e.g., computerized reminders, chart flags, structured notes)	■	■	■	■					
Specialization of staff		■	■						
Benchmarking		■	■	■					
Academic detailing		■	■	■	■				
Quality improvement projects		■	■	■	■		■	■	
Patient registries		■	■	■		■			
Specialized clinics		■		■					
Disease management programs		■		■				■	■
Community-based targeted screening programs		■		■	■	■		■	■
Pre-discharge assessment/protocols			■						
Standing orders			■						
Testing (e.g., BMD) requirements prior to prescription authorization				■					
Performance reporting				■				■	■
Training of health care professionals					■	■	■		
Developing research agenda, conducting research					■	■	■		
Monitoring and surveillance					■	■			
Insurance coverage for desired management				■	■			■	■
Policy interventions (e.g. regulations, tax credits, urban planning, standards for densitometry)					■	■	■		

Finally, examples of systems-based approaches to osteoporosis and bone health are provided whenever possible. Since such approaches are still rare in bone health, examples of successful systems approaches to other lifelong or chronic health issues are also included. They contain valuable lessons that may potentially be relevant to bone health.

Systems-Based Approaches for Various Stakeholders

While all components of the health system should engage in risk stratification, the roles and responsibilities for different types of organizations will vary when it comes to implementing systems-based approaches. This section discusses each of the key stakeholders, including individual clinicians, medical groups, insurers, public health departments, and other facilitators.

Systems-Based Approaches for Individual Clinicians

Perhaps the most important roles for the individual clinician in promoting a systems-based approach to bone health relate to 1) educating themselves and their patients about bone health prevention, treatment, and assessment, and 2) putting into place systems to ensure that patients receive appropriate services based on their risks and needs.

Unfortunately, however, clinicians may not always fulfill these roles. Evidence-based interventions (i.e., those whose effectiveness has been demonstrated) are often not used on those who need them. For example, a recent large-scale study of older patients who had suffered hip or forearm fractures found that roughly four out of five did not fill a prescription for an osteoporosis medication in the 6 months after the fracture (Solomon et al. 2003). Moreover, most individuals who did fill a prescription were already on a medication before the fracture,

meaning that the net number of individuals initiating drug therapy was quite small. The same study also found that certain groups, including men, non-Whites, and those with other medical conditions, are less likely than White women to receive treatment for osteoporosis. There are also certain characteristics of health care providers that can predict their rates of diagnosis and treatment of osteoporosis (Morris 2004), such as gender, specialty, and years since medical school. However, there are no studies on the effectiveness of programs to increase awareness in improving diagnosis and therapy. Two recent large studies conducted in managed care settings generated similar findings, with only a minority of post-menopausal women who had sustained a fracture receiving pharmacologic treatment following the fracture (Feldstein et al. 2003b, Andrade et al. 2003). These studies highlight the important role for physicians in both prescribing the appropriate therapy and in encouraging patients to comply.

Evidence alone, even when compelling, is frequently insufficient to change provider practice patterns. To overcome the barriers to change, it might make sense to consider adoption of a comprehensive model for accelerating the diffusion of innovations. One such approach, known as the Rodgers Diffusion model, provides insight into both the limitations of current behavioral change techniques and potential strategies for accelerating diffusion of evidence-based innovations (Rodgers 1995). This model lays out five stages to the process of deciding when and how to use a new innovation: 1) knowledge; 2) persuasion; 3) decision; 4) implementation; and 5) confirmation.

Knowledge

There are two aspects to the knowledge stage. The first is the need for consumers to be aware of the importance of the health issue. While individual clinicians can help in educating their patients, this public awareness role is best played by medical groups, health plans/insurers, public health departments and other government agencies, and potentially other facilitators, such as medical societies. It is important to remember, however, that these awareness campaigns are not the only sources of information for individual consumers. They also receive information from the media (e.g., newspapers, magazines, television program-ming) and pharmaceutical companies (e.g., via direct-to-consumer advertising). For more information on public awareness campaigns, see the section on the role of public health.

The second aspect of the knowledge stage relates to making sure that clinicians are aware of the evidence related to best practices for bone health. Individual clinicians can employ a variety of systems-based approaches to ensure their own awareness of up-to-date information on best practices. Among these systems are practice guidelines and evidence-based medicine reports that synthesize findings from multiple studies and sources. These reports and guidelines have been issued by government agencies (e.g., the U.S. Preventive Services Task Force [USPSTF], a panel of experts with representation from the non-Federal sector that is housed at the Agency for Health Care Research and Quality [AHRQ]) and by professional and public societies (e.g., American Association of Clinical Endocrinology, the National Osteoporosis Foundation). The National Guideline Clearinghouse (NGC) serves as a comprehensive source for credible guidelines related to bone disease and other diseases. Sponsored by AHRQ in partnership with the American Medical Association and America's Health Insurance Plans, NGC includes 71 general and specific guidelines related to osteoporosis and bone health.

Since the evidence base is often not sufficiently developed to allow the crafting of comprehensive guidelines, supplemental information based on expert opinion is often added, thus leading to variations across guidelines. This lack of complete evidence also means that guidelines often do not answer all clinical questions of interest, including the applicability of the guideline to important subpopulations (e.g., minorities, older persons) or the role of comorbidities. In addition, guidelines and evidence-based reports often fail to incorporate patient preferences, although this is changing. In spite of their limitations, guidelines and evidence-based reports should be seriously considered by individual clinicians, since they attempt to provide the best recommendations for what clinicians should do. See Chapter 8 for more on risk assessment guidelines and Chapter 9 for more on treatment guidelines.

In addition, as discussed in Chapters 8 and 10, individual clinicians should also consider the use of risk assessment tools such as the Osteoporosis Risk Assessment Instrument (ORAI) and the Osteoporosis Self-Assessment Tool (OST). These tools, which are based on risk factors that have been demonstrated to be associated with osteoporosis, are helpful in identifying individuals who are at risk of bone disease and/or fracture and who therefore might benefit from further assessment and/or treatment.

Persuasion

Just because guidelines and evidence-based reports exist, there is no guarantee that clinicians will read and absorb them. Even if they do, the evidence suggests that they may not change their behavior by implementing the recommended practices. In fact, the gap between evidence-based care and the actual care provided in the community (the "knowledge-practice gap") is well recognized as a barrier to quality care (Reuben 2002).

Several steps are needed, therefore, to ensure that individual clinicians become aware of and act on the evidence. One common strategy is the use of professional education to disseminate guidelines and evolving research, including presentations at meetings and other common continuing medical education (CME) activities.

However, these techniques have generally been ineffective in changing provider behavior on their own (Grimshaw et al. 2001, Grol and Grimshaw 2003). In fact, it has proven remarkably difficult to convince clinicians to implement evidence-based changes for improving care within clinical settings. Many factors related to knowledge, attitudes, and behaviors contribute to this inertia. These barriers have been well described (Cabana et al. 1999) and are listed below:

- Lack of awareness or familiarity with the guidelines
- Disagreement with specific guidelines or guidelines in general
- Doubt that following the guideline will lead to desired outcomes
- An inability to overcome existing practice habits
- Patient factors, such as preferences
- Environmental factors, such as lack of time or resources

The disappointing results from CME and guidelines has led to the use of other approaches for persuading providers, including academic detailing (described in the next section) and opinion leaders. These techniques have long been used by the pharmaceutical industry in marketing new products to prescribers. They also fit within the model described earlier, which relies on respected peers to assist with persuasion.

Decision and Implementation

Even after clinicians become convinced of the merits of adopting an evidence-based practice, they still may need help in deciding when and how to implement it on a daily basis. For that reason, a variety of systems-based approaches have been developed to assist individual physicians in practicing evidence-based medicine. One common approach is computerized reminder systems, which have been used in a variety of settings, including hospitals (Dexter et al. 2001). These systems are commonly employed to promote use of preventive services such as influenza immunizations (Gaglani et al. 2001) and to support adherence to clinical protocols (Demakis et al. 2000). The same kind of approach can be taken in bone health. For example, a recent study demonstrated the usefulness of sending e-mail messages to primary care providers of patients who had recently suffered an osteoporotic fracture but had not yet received a bone mineral density (BMD) test; 51 percent of the patients of doctors who received the e-mail message were given a BMD test or a medication for osteoporosis, compared to just 6 percent in a usual care group (Feldstein et al. 2003a). A less technologically sophisticated but similar approach involves the use of chart flags (Melville et al. 1993), which alert physicians on the paper chart when they should consider a particular evidence-based course of action for a patient. Flow diagrams or algorithms represent similar approaches that have been used to determine who needs testing (e.g., mammography) and how often they need it (Melville et al. 1993).

Confirmation

All of these steps outlined above are not enough to result in lasting behavior change (Rodgers 1995), unless the clinicians who change behavior receive confirmation after the fact that they made a wise decision in doing so. For example, clinicians who agree to try using a pre-visit questionnaire will need to see that it has achieved its intended results (and not caused any unanticipated problems, such as negatively affecting office work flow) before the change will be permanent. Without this confirmation step, innovations tend to be dropped after a period of time.

Summary

The best approach for individual clinicians is to adopt a comprehensive behavior-change plan that targets the different barriers to change with distinct strategies aimed at each (Grol and Grimshaw 2003). One example of a multi-component strategy aimed at individual physicians was developed during the intervention phase of the Assessing Care of Vulnerable Elders (ACOVE) project ([a]Reuben et al. 2003). This intervention is aimed at changing practice behaviors related to the care of three geriatric conditions (falls, cognitive impairment, and urinary incontinence) through the following:

- Use of medical record prompts via structured visit notes
- Delegation of some tasks to office staff to encourage performance of essential care processes by clinicians
- Patient education, including encouraging the patient to play an active role in follow-up, which may also be quite influential in changing physician behavior (Maly et al. 1996)

Finally, it is important to remember that individual clinicians not only need to change their own behavior, but they also need to encourage their patients to do the same. To that end, clinicians should constantly be advising their patients about appropriate lifestyle changes related to bone health, as discussed in Chapter 10. In addition, clinicians should provide their patients with information on resources that can assist them in changing behavior. For example, ACOVE provides information to patients about community-based resources, such as exercise programs that reduce the risk of falls. (See Chapter 6 for more information.) These programs are particularly valuable for high-risk individuals. Unfortunately, the quality and availability of community-based programs and resources varies considerably within and across geographic areas. Most clinicians do not currently have readily available information for their patients about community-based programs and resources, including where they are located and how to access them. This represents an area where public health departments and clinicians could collaborate.

An Example of a Systems-Based Approach

An action plan for the prevention of osteoporotic fractures in the European Community provides an interesting example of a systems-based approach (Compston 2004). In 2002, the European Union Osteoporosis Consultation Panel was formed to develop an action plan to implement recommendations for the prevention of osteoporotic fractures. Six action steps were developed to achieve the stated goal of reducing the social and economic burden of osteoporotic fractures by 2005: 1) awareness campaigns targeted at potentially high-risk individuals, e.g. postmenopausal women; 2) preventive lifestyle strategies, including the development of government-backed health education programs and policies and the harmonization of public health policies; 3) evidence-based guidelines, including developing guidelines in member States, making existing guidelines more accessible, and providing government endorsement and financial support to these efforts; 4) evidence-based fracture care and fall prevention programs, along with multidisciplinary approaches to rehabilitation; 5) economic data and analysis, including the identification of resource needs (particularly bone densitometry systems) and the analysis of the cost-effectiveness of interventions; and 6) the European fracture database, including a survey of existing data, development of data collection methods, and economic modeling and planning of health care resources.

Systems-Based Approaches for Medical Groups

Medical groups should be able to employ all of the approaches available to individual clinicians. In addition, because of their larger size, medical groups have the opportunity to implement a greater degree of systematization. For example, office staff can be assigned to perform a small number of targeted functions (e.g., checking visual acuity as a component of an evaluation of the risk of falls), thereby reducing the burden on clinicians and allowing staff to develop expertise in specific tasks. Group practices also have an additional tool available to them to promote behavior change—benchmarking, a process that allows physicians to compare their performance with that of others or with a "gold standard." Benchmarking can also allow an individual clinician to track his or her performance over time. When complemented with other quality improvement techniques, benchmarking has been shown to improve performance in managing conditions such as diabetes (Kiefe et al. 2001). It is important to note that individual clinicians who are members of independent practice associations (IPAs) may also have access to benchmarking data through the IPA's central office.

Larger group practices can also employ other formal quality improvement techniques based on measurement of processes (Nelson et al. 1998) and outcomes, with the goal of reducing variations in care delivery and improving overall outcomes. For example, medical groups can employ rapid-cycle improvement techniques such as the "Plan, Do, Study, Act" (PDSA) cycle. The PDSA cycle begins with clinicians planning and conducting small-scale, local tests of change in their own offices and in the health care organizations in which they work. After studying the results, clinicians and health care organizations can then apply relevant systems-based improvements to everyday practice. In many cases, PDSA cycles are often more appropriate and informative in facilitating systems-based improvement than are formal studies with experimental designs (such as randomized trials) or the implementation of changes without evaluative measurement (Berwick 1998). The Institute for Health Care Improvement has been successful using the PDSA approach in the areas of diabetes and depression.

Medical groups also have the ability to create registries of patients with specific disorders so that evidence-based interventions can be delivered systematically to the population in need. These registries also allow the monitoring of patients' responses to these interventions. For example, medical groups have used registries to ensure that patients with diabetes receive glycosylated hemoglobin testing and eye care referrals. Within bone health, a registry of patients with higher-than-average risk for osteoporotic fractures could help to identify those who are not taking medications to improve bone health. Similarly, a registry of those who have fallen or are at high risk of falling could facilitate preventive measures such as environmental modifications (e.g., installation of grab bars, hand rails, raised toilet seats) and/or referrals to a fall prevention program. The registry could also be used to monitor those who have fallen and/or those who have a fear of falling to determine whether progress in addressing these problems has been made.

Medical groups can also implement systematic education efforts aimed at physicians and other health professionals, such as academic detailing (Siegel et al. 2003, Solomon et al. 2001). Academic detailing involves having trained professionals advise individual providers in one-on-one sessions about how to follow evidence-based practice guidelines in a specific area, such as appropriate use of a diagnostic test (e.g., dual x-ray absorptiometry [DXA]) or of pharmacologic therapies. Some groups may even serve enough patients to sponsor education classes, Internet resources, and exercise programs.

Very large groups may be able to develop specialized clinics for caring for specific disorders, such as osteoporosis. These clinics can be a practical approach to ensuring that the quality of care for the disorder is uniform throughout the group. They can also allow for the concentration of expensive resources such as bone densitometers in a few locations. These clinics may also allow personnel to develop in-depth expertise in caring for patients with conditions such as osteoporosis. For example, nurse practitioners have gained such expertise in treating patients with heart failure (Crowther 2003) and diabetes (Litaker et al. 2003). Although experience with osteoporosis clinics has been limited, a nurse practitioner-led Fracture Liaison Clinic in Glasgow was successful in increasing the frequency of BMD testing and treatment in fracture patients as compared to historical controls. The clinic identifies patients who have suffered one or more fractures in emergency departments and then follows up with their health care providers to encourage BMD testing and treatment (McLellan and Fraser 2002).

Specialized clinics can also refer patients with osteoporosis and those at risk of falling to therapists and community-based exercise programs with expertise in addressing their specific needs (as discussed earlier, individual clinicians can do this as well). The optimal staffing, referral criteria, and volume of patients needed to justify an osteoporosis clinic are unknown. In particular, innovative, effective strategies for using nurses, nurse practitioners, physician assistants, physical therapists, and other health professionals to promote bone health need to be identified.

Large medical groups may have enough patients with bone disease to justify the development of their own disease management programs. (Smaller groups and individual clinicians may be able to refer patients to programs run by health plans, if they exist.) In disease management programs, persons identified as having specific medical conditions are followed more intensely. The goals are to improve health outcomes and reduce costs by preventing declines in health status that lead to the need for costly medical care, including hospitalizations and emergency department visits. Disease management programs tend to be utilized primarily for conditions associated with frequent hospitalizations and high expenditures, such as heart failure (Rich et al. 1995), diabetes, and asthma (Legoretta et al. 2000). These programs also tend to be relevant for conditions that require intensive monitoring and frequent changes in regimens (e.g., diuretics for congestive heart failure, insulin doses for patients with diabetes). As they require considerable human resources (e.g., frequent telephone calls and visits), the typical disease management programs are likely to be too expensive for a disease like osteoporosis, which does not demand frequent adjustment of medication schedules. A possible exception, however, is disease management for those who have had prior falls or are at high risk for falling. In fact, some fall prevention programs look very similar to disease management programs (Tinetti 1986), and it can be argued that the high risk of fracture among persons who have already fallen or who have multiple risk factors for falls merits the intensive monitoring and resources associated with disease management programs.

As an example, Kaiser Permanente Northwest (with 450,000 members in Oregon and Washington) is instituting a comprehensive program to manage osteoporosis after fractures and to prevent falls. The program is based on a pilot study, described earlier in this chapter, which demonstrated the effectiveness of sending e-mail reminder notices to the physicians of patients suffering recent fractures (Feldstein et al. 2003a). The e-mail reminders include recommendations on BMD testing and osteoporosis treatment. If a patient is identified as being at risk of falling, clinicians can enter an order for a low- or high-risk referral into Kaiser's electronic medical record. For those patients identified as being at low risk for a fall, Kaiser's health education department sends educational information about osteoporosis and fall prevention along with a referral to a community-based exercise program. Those at high risk for a fall also receive educational materials and a referral to an exercise program, and they are also referred to an outpatient falls prevention program run by the physical therapy department. This 8-week program provides a complete assessment of the risk of falling along with muscle strengthening, balance, and gait-training programs. This regional, population-based program is provided through a physician assistant in Kaiser's Department of Endocrinology with oversight by an endocrinologist.

Finally, large group practices and vertically integrated health systems can consider taking a more population-based approach. For example, large group practices may implement community-based screening for osteoporosis. Such approaches have been employed successfully in increasing mammography screening for breast cancer (Reuben et al. 2002).

Systems-Based Approaches for Hospitals and Post-Acute Rehabilitation Facilities

The consequences of poor bone health and osteoporosis frequently lead to admission to hospitals and post-acute rehabilitation facilities. Osteoporotic fractures of the hip, pelvis, and spine (if symptoms are severe) frequently require hospitalization for surgery or symptom control. A systems-based approach to osteoporosis requires more than just treating the immediate problems or symptoms; rather, it should include efforts to both improve bone health and prevent future falls. Similar approaches have been employed in managing coronary artery disease (Fonarow et al. 2001) to ensure that patients in the hospital after a heart attack are discharged on appropriate medications that reduce the risk of future heart attacks. For osteoporosis, this type of approach would entail patient education about nutrition, orders for pharmacologic therapy, referrals for physical therapy or exercise programs, and social services (if needed).

A large group of hospitalized patients may not yet have been diagnosed with osteoporosis, but their admitting diagnosis (e.g., falls, syncope, gait instability, failure to thrive) may nonetheless serve as a "red flag" about a high future risk of fracture. A systems-based approach to caring for these patients could involve putting into place a process for identifying these individuals at admission and then conducting BMD tests prior to discharge to determine if they are osteoporotic or osteopenic. However, the current diagnosis-related group (DRG) reimbursement system for fee-for-service Medicare discourages the performance of screening tests during the hospital stay, since reimbursement is the same whether or not these tests are performed. Furthermore, scheduling additional tests such as BMD during the hospitalization may delay discharge. At a minimum, however, clinical risk factors for osteoporotic fractures should be assessed using standardized protocols during the hospital stay or at discharge, unless such action is precluded by the patient's acute illness.

Many patients who suffer fractures or falls, as well as those with gait and balance disorders, are discharged to skilled nursing facilities to receive additional rehabilitation. These patients typically do not qualify for Medicare reimbursement in an acute inpatient rehabilitation facility. (Under current Medicare guidelines, patients must need at least 3 hours per day of a combination of different types of rehabilitation, such as physical therapy, occupational therapy, and speech therapy, to qualify for reimbursement.) Similar to hospitalized patients, a systems-based approach to skilled nursing facility residents who suffer fractures would consider them as candidates for specific bone and fall prevention interventions. Those who are at high risk of falling but who have not fractured should be considered candidates for rehabilitation to reduce this risk. However, the assessment and treatment of frail patients can be challenging. Although BMD testing may not be available in many nursing homes, many of the patients have already suffered fractures and testing is therefore unlikely to provide additional, useful information. The goal for these individuals should be the prevention of new fractures. Since the frail elderly are especially prone to falling, residential settings such as nursing homes should take advantage of the opportunity for social group exercise activities that reduce the risk of falling by building muscle strength and improving balance. In addition, medication administration can be challenging in the frail elderly who live in nursing homes and in the community, since many of these individuals are cognitively impaired and therefore may have trouble with compliance. In these situations, long-acting medications, including those that could be administered once a year intravenously (e.g., intravenous bisphosphonates are currently under development) or by injection (e.g., vitamin D) hold great promise, as do drinks fortified with calcium and the use of hip protectors in those most prone to falling.

In addition, other systems-based approaches to improving bone health in the nursing home are possible. For example, a nursing home could implement a policy of "standing" orders for vitamin D and calcium supplementation (in those who can tolerate it) that are followed unless the clinical provider specifically rejects the order. Similar "standing" orders are common for laxatives and for mild pain medications (e.g., acetaminophen). Another possibility would be "standing" orders for hip protectors for all residents at risk of falling (Lauritzen et al.1993). (See Chapter 9 for more details on hip protectors.)

Systems-Based Approaches for Health Plans and Insurers

The role of health plans and insurers in systems-based approaches to medical conditions varies considerably from plan to plan and insurer to insurer. It depends in large part on the degree to which health plans and insurers hold their contracted medical groups accountable for management of specific diseases, including the processes of care. To date, most health plans and insurers have played a limited role in promoting optimal care for patients with bone disease. Some of these organizations might have limited incentives to invest today in preventive services and programs that likely will not yield financial and/or clinical benefits for many years (perhaps when those who receive the services have changed health plans or are covered by Medicare). Nonetheless, there are ways in which all health plans and insurers affect bone health—that is, coverage policies that directly affect the provision of services, procedures, and medications used to promote bone health and to prevent, diagnose, and treat bone disease. In addition, at least some plans and insurers are getting more intimately involved in a systems-based approach to bone health and disease. These plans are assessing and monitoring performance, engaging in quality improvement programs, and/or implementing pay-for-performance initiatives that reward high-quality, evidence-based care. The rest of this section covers these various leverage points for plans and insurers—that is, coverage, performance measurement, quality improvement, and pay-for-performance.

Medicare and Private Sector Coverage

The Medicare program tends to set the standard with respect to coverage policies for testing and treatment within the area of bone health. In other words, most private insurers tend to follow Medicare's lead.

Coverage of Tests for Screening and Monitoring. Under a provision of the Balanced Budget Act of 1997 (P.L. 105-33), Medicare is required to cover BMD testing every 2 years for people at risk of developing osteoporosis or under treatment for osteoporosis (USDHHS 1998). This law is applicable to individuals enrolled in Medicare fee-for-service and Medicare + Choice plans. Under this law, BMD testing is defined as radiologic, radioisotopic, or other procedures approved by the FDA for the purpose of identifying bone mass, detecting bone loss, and interpreting bone quality. Although many different testing modes and devices have been approved by the FDA and are covered by Medicare and some private payers, it is important to remember that not all of these tests have been shown to have a strong predictive relationship with fracture risk (see Chapter 8 for a more detailed discussion). The most thoroughly investigated tool is DXA, which measures bone density at the most likely sites of fracture, the hip and spine. Since DXA is expensive and not available everywhere, ultrasound of the heel can be used as an initial screening tool, to be followed by a DXA test in those identified as having low bone density. Individuals with the following characteristics are considered at risk and eligible for Medicare coverage of BMD testing:

- Women who are estrogen deficient as defined by their physicians and who are at risk for osteoporosis
- Individuals with vertebral abnormalities, osteoporosis, or spine fracture determined by x-ray
- Individuals with primary hyperparathyroidism
- Individuals being monitored to assess the response to or efficacy of an FDA-approved osteoporosis drug therapy
- Individuals receiving or expecting to receive glucocorticoid therapy, equivalent to ≥ 7.5 mg of prednisone per day, for more than 3 months

Men and minority (especially Black) women who present with these risk factors are often not recognized as being in need of BMD testing. White women are known to have a higher risk of fracture, but it is important to remember that individuals in other racial and ethnic groups need to be tested and, if appropriate, treated if they exhibit the risk factors cited above or have suffered a fragility fracture at any site.

Policies for coverage of BMD testing by private health plans generally follow the eligibility criteria for Medicare, though individual plans vary in their coverage. For example, BlueCross of California considers all women age 65 and older as eligible regardless of additional risk factors (BlueCross of California 2002). Likewise the specific tests to assess BMD that are covered may vary from plan to plan.

Coverage of Pharmacologic Treatment. The Medicare Modernization Act (MMA) was signed into law in 2003 and provides beneficiaries with access to some level of coverage for drugs that treat bone disorders. In addition, Medicare beneficiaries enrolled in Medicare Advantage (formerly Medicare + Choice) plans with pharmacy benefits typically have some level of coverage for medications related to bone health. Neither traditional Medicare or Medicare Advantage beneficiaries have coverage for nutritional supplements, such as calcium and vitamin D. Most private health plans do cover estrogen and at least one of the bisphosphonates. Coverage for selective estrogen receptor modulators (raloxifene), calcitonin, and parathyroid hormone varies among different plans.

Coverage of Non-Pharmacologic Treatment. Physical therapy is covered under Medicare Part B for certain diagnoses related to falls. Medicare does not cover physical therapy for individuals solely on the basis of being at high risk of falling. Effective September 1, 2003, there is a combined $1,590 annual limit on Medicare coverage of outpatient physical therapy and therapy for speech-language pathology. Private health plans have variable coverage for physical therapy.

Coverage for vertebroplasty and kyphoplasty under Medicare Part B varies from state to state. These procedures are generally covered for painful spine fractures that have not responded to conventional therapy. The coverage policies of private health plans for these procedures is limited, due largely to the lack of solid evidence on their effectiveness. For example, BlueCross and BlueShield of Montana will consider coverage of vertebroplasty and kyphoplasty on an individual basis for patients who have failed to respond to standard non-surgical treatment (BlueCross BlueShield of Montana 2003). Aetna considers kyphoplasty to restore bone height lost due to painful osteoporotic fractures to be an experimental/investigational intervention and consequently does not cover this procedure (Aetna 2003).

Performance Assessment

In addition to coverage policies, health plans and insurers are uniquely positioned to employ a systems-based approach to improving bone health through the use of performance assessment. Health plans can use their data about diagnoses and utilization of services to assess whether indicated preventive measures and treatment are provided to their members, whether such measures and treatments work, and whether members are satisfied with the care that they receive. To date, plan-driven programs to improve quality have largely focused on the assessment and reporting of performance for preventive services and selected chronic diseases. Osteoporosis has not been a target of performance assessment, although it may become a target condition in 2004 with the introduction of a performance measure for osteoporosis by the National Committee for Quality Assurance (NCQA).

NCQA is a nonprofit health care oversight organization that accredits managed care plans and has produced a widely used quality reporting system called the Health Plan Employer Data and Information Set (HEDIS). HEDIS measures were initially designed to provide information to large purchasers about the quality

New HEDIS Performance Measure for Osteoporosis

A new HEDIS performance measure related to osteoporosis goes into effect in 2004. The measure will evaluate how well a health plan does in diagnosing and treating osteoporosis in elderly women who suffer a fracture. The measure is defined as: "The percentage of women age 67 or older who suffer a fracture who receive either a BMD test or prescription treatment for osteoporosis with 6 months of the date of the fracture." The new HEDIS measure will evaluate the care of women age 67 or older on Medicare who are enrolled in a managed care plan.

of care delivered to their employees. More recently, the audience for HEDIS results has broadened, and they are often reported in consumer-oriented report cards. Since HEDIS has standard measures and uniform data reporting requirements, comparisons can be made between various health plans.

With the planned implementation of a performance measure for osteoporosis in 2004, health plans and insurers will have an opportunity to assess performance and promote quality care for osteoporosis. The measure reports the percentage of women age 67 or older who suffer a fracture who receive either a BMD test or prescription treatment for osteoporosis within 6 months of the date of the fracture.

A complementary approach to the HEDIS measures has been the development of quality indicators (e.g., those developed in the Assessing Care of the Vulnerable Elderly [ACOVE] project) that can be used to identify deficiencies in care provided (Wenger

and Shekelle 2001, Shekelle et al. 2001). While guidelines exist that can assist in determining appropriate services for other populations, ACOVE spells out seven evidence-based quality indicators that specifically apply to elderly individuals (i.e., those over age 75) at high risk of functional decline due to osteoporosis (Table 11-2). Some are based on chart review of documented care and others on data obtained in interviews with elderly individuals (Grossman and MacLean 2001, RAND 2004).

Quality Improvement Initiatives

Health plans and insurers that sponsor performance measurement can and often do supplement these activities with other programs designed promote use of evidence-based medicine. While osteoporosis has generally not been a major focus of such activities, existing quality improvement programs could be adapted to osteoporosis. For example, like some medical groups, health plans have implemented disease management programs targeting high-cost, common diseases such as diabetes, heart failure, and asthma. Given the high cost of osteoporotic fractures both in terms of health (Tosteson et al. 2001, OTA 1994) and dollars (Max et al.2002), disease management programs for osteoporosis might be beneficial for both plans and patients, especially if individuals who have already sustained (or are at high risk for) osteoporotic fractures are targeted. In fact, some osteoporosis disease management programs have been implemented (although the details of most of these are considered proprietary). For example, one osteoporosis disease management program implemented by the BlueShield of Northeastern New York contains components aimed at both members and providers. Among the member-centered interventions were mailings, education days at local pharmacies, and newsletter articles

Table 11-2. ACOVE-2 Quality Indicators for the Management of Osteoporosis in Vulnerable Elders

Indicator Purpose	Process Measure
Quality Indicator 1 Prevention	ALL female persons age 75 or older should be counseled at least once regarding intake of dietary calcium and vitamin D and weight-bearing exercise.
Quality Indicator 2 Smoking Cessation	ALL female persons age 75 or older who smoke should be counseled annually about smoking cessation.
Quality Indicator 3 Pharmacologic Preventive Therapy	EVERY female person age 75 or older should be counseled about risk for osteoporosis and the potential need for pharmacologic prevention of osteoporosis at least once.
Quality Indicator 4 Identifying Secondary Osteoporosis	IF a person age 75 or older has a new diagnosis of osteoporosis, THEN during the initial evaluation period an underlying cause of osteoporosis should be sought by checking medication use and current alcohol use.
Quality Indicator 5 Calcium and Vitamin D for Osteoporosis	IF a person age 75 or older has osteoporosis, THEN calcium and vitamin D supplements should be recommended at least once.
Quality Indicator 6 Calcium and Vitamin D With Corticosteroid Use	IF a person age 75 or older is taking corticosteroids for more than 1 month, THEN the patient should be offered calcium and vitamin D.
Quality Indicator 7 Treatment of Osteoporosis	IF a person age 75 or older is newly diagnosed with osteoporosis, THEN the patient should be offered treatment with hormone replacement therapy, SERMs, bisphosphonates, or calcitonin within 3 months of diagnosis.*

* *Note:* Estrogen is listed as an option, with the Women's Health Initiative finding that it is effective for the prevention of hip fractures. Potential increases in risk of cardiovascular disease may make it a less favorable choice.

Source: RAND 2004.

that were all focused on osteoporosis. These were supplemented with infomercials on a local cable channel and posters developed for placement in local clinicians' offices. To support providers in providing evidence-based osteoporosis care, the plan developed guidelines and encouraged adherence to them by sending notices and placing stickers on the patient's chart alerting providers when patients had been contacted about osteoporosis. In addition, providers were given information about compliance issues related to specific patients. For example, providers were notified if a patient did not fill his or her prescription for osteoporosis drugs at least 80 percent of the time. Finally, the plan initiated a requirement that BMD be measured before the approval of new prescriptions for osteoporosis drugs. The program appears to be working; during its first year BMD usage doubled and medication compliance rates increased by almost 60 percent (Paccione 2003).

Despite this anecdotal evidence of success, disease management for osteoporosis has not yet been adequately evaluated to determine its cost-effectiveness. It may be possible for osteoporosis disease management programs to be integrated into similar types of programs for other chronic diseases, such as heart disease or diabetes.

Pay-for-Performance Initiatives

Reimbursement policies represent one of the most innovative ways that health plans and insurers can promote quality and quality improvement. In fact, the National Health Care Purchasing Institute, through an initiative of the Robert Wood Johnson Foundation, identified 11 potential provider incentive models for improving quality of care (Bailit 2002). Several plans have recently started to tie reimbursement to performance within specific conditions. However, it is important to recognize that clinical performance is typically not the only parameter assessed when determining the level of the incentive payment. Other factors that may be considered include patient satisfaction, availability of providers (e.g., office hours that are favorable to the patient), and use of educational services.

One example of such an approach comes from California, where a coalition of health plans and physician groups has initiated, "Pay for Performance". This statewide program will pay physician groups extra if they can document strong performance in caring for patients with certain diseases (Integrated Health Care Association 2003). Participants include Aetna, BlueCross of California, BlueShield of California, CIGNA Health Care of California,

Health Net, and PacifiCare, each of which has agreed to use common performance measures for asthma, coronary artery disease, and diabetes. These plans have also agreed to implement "significant" financial incentives based on performance, although the size of the incentive and the distribution methodology for the payments will be determined independently by each plan. The first payments to medical groups under this plan will be in 2004 based on 2003 performance data.

Systems-Based Approaches for Government and Public Health Agencies

Federal, State, and local governments, including the public health system, can play vitally important roles within many of the four core activities described earlier. In fact, a recent Institute of Medicine (IOM) report made a number of general recommendations on the appropriate role of governments and public health agencies that are applicable to bone health and osteoporosis (IOM 2002). Among these were urging local health departments to support community-led, joint efforts between the corporate community and public health agencies to strengthen health promotion and disease and injury prevention programs for employees and their communities, along with a call for increased collaboration between public health officials and local and national entertainment media to facilitate the communication of accurate information about diseases and medical and health issues.

As the IOM report suggests, perhaps the most important role for public health agencies is to promote awareness among consumers and clinicians of the importance of bone health, and of the best methods for preventing, assessing, and treating bone disease. While the lack of a cohesive health care system creates challenges for the prevention and treatment of bone disease, the public health system can help overcome these problems by mobilizing to increase awareness.

A better informed and more concerned public can facilitate adherence to recommended care management practices by influencing provider behavior (Maly et al. 1996) and policy changes.

To that end, public health agencies may sponsor broad-based and targeted public awareness campaigns, with messages tailored to different population subgroups. For example, for younger persons, the emphasis may be on nutrition (e.g., calcium intake), lifestyle choices (e.g., smoking avoidance and cessation), and physical activity to build peak bone-mass. In contrast, for older persons who have already suffered an osteoporotic fracture, the message may focus on whether they are receiving appropriate medications and fall prevention measures. The choice of venues should vary based upon the message. Younger persons might best be reached through the Internet, advertising on evening television and billboards, and/or in magazines oriented at youth. In contrast, the elderly might best be reached through daytime television programs, magazines, and senior centers. Of course, other stakeholders within the overall health system, including health plans/ insurers, large medical groups, and professional associations can assist with these awareness campaigns, while individual clinicians can reinforce the campaign's messages during their interactions with consumers.

Public health agencies may also want to consider supplementing their awareness activities with broad-based and/or targeted screening programs, provided either independently or in collaboration with health care delivery systems. Similar types of programs have been conducted in other areas, including nationwide programs promoting vaccinations for influenza and polio and local screening programs for disorders like hypertension and hypercholesterolemia.

Another potential role for public health and government is to improve the linkages between health care organizations, community-based organizations, and the public health system. At present the lack of such linkages makes it difficult to provide consumers—especially those with multiple, chronic health conditions—with a full range of beneficial services. While public health agencies do not typically provide the continuity of care that is required for management of chronic conditions like osteoporosis, they may be able to play a vital role in bridging the gap between health care organizations, community-based and educational resources, and other complementary services in various aspects of bone health, including fall prevention and BMD screening. For example, public health agencies could partner with community-based organizations to provide consumers with an assessment of their risk of bone disease (possibly including BMD screening). Consumers could take this information to their health care provider (a referral could be provided, if necessary), who could then work with the individual to determine the appropriate course of action. Some individuals may need a referral to a specialist or an osteoporosis clinic, while others can continue to have their bone health managed by their primary care provider. By educating consumers and engaging the health system in this manner, public health can play a critical role in helping to ensure that consumers receive appropriate, evidence-based care.

Yet another area for public health is in helping to train health care professionals to be more skilled at promoting bone health and in recognizing and treating bone disease. Public health agencies can work with health professional associations to co-sponsor conferences and seminars and can work with academic institutions in the development and promotion of curricula.

Policy-making represents another strategy that governmental agencies at the local, State, and Federal level can use to promote bone health and appropriate treatment of bone disease. They can use policies to promote bone health and to encourage the prevention, timely diagnosis, and early, appropriate treatment of bone disease and fractures. For example, regulations could require the installation of grab bars in the showers of all retirement communities. Financial incentives such as tax credits could promote the widespread availability of fitness centers that provide exercise classes to seniors at risk for falling. Local urban planning policies can also promote bone health by developing public spaces that minimize the risk of falling and that offer opportunities for outdoor exercise. Finally, governmental agencies can also set quality control standards for assessing BMD tests and certification standards for densitometer operators.

A final, vitally important role for public health is in monitoring and surveillance activities. These activities relate not only to monitoring compliance with regulations, but also to implementing ongoing surveillance methods to monitor and assess trends in the following:

- The prevalence of bone disease and fractures in the community
- The degree to which individuals engage in bone-healthy behaviors
- The degree to which community-wide and institution-specific interventions are influencing consumer and clinician behavior and having an impact on bone health outcomes

Other Facilitators

Individual clinicians, medical groups, health care delivery systems, insurers, and public health departments are the primary drivers of systems-based approaches to improving bone health and reducing the consequences of osteoporosis. Other institutions, organizations, and agencies can facilitate these efforts through research, education, and purchasing policies and power. Diverse entities such as voluntary health organizations and professional associations, academic institutions, health care purchasers, and industry (including pharmaceutical and technology companies) are all stakeholders in the system. While they have rarely collaborated in developing approaches to health care problems such as osteoporosis, a cohesive approach could provide substantial momentum towards optimization of bone health on a large scale.

The Role of Voluntary Health Organizations and Professional Associations

Voluntary health organizations (or advocacy groups) and professional associations play important roles in any systems-based approach to bone health. They are able to reach the public and providers with critical information quickly and often with fewer constraints than can government organizations.

One of the most important roles for voluntary organizations is to raise public awareness about specific health problems such as bone disease. By including individuals who have personally been touched by bone disease, these organizations are uniquely positioned to provide important guidance to other sectors of the health system regarding the real-life impact of bone disease on individuals, families, and communities.

Lacking the label of government and being composed of persons from the community, voluntary health organizations also can be quite effective in persuading local residents—their peers—to adopt the lifestyle changes necessary to prevent the onset or progression of bone and other diseases. For some diseases, the absence of the government label has also made it possible for voluntary health organizations to develop registries of affected individuals, thereby improving access to information and other resources related to the treatment of the disease.

Professional associations also play a critical role in promoting a systems-based approach to bone health. They are key facilitators in the training of professionals needed to address public health problems such as bone health. They also promote changes in the curricula of professional schools and provide continuing education to practicing bone health professionals. These associations can also be instrumental in the development of evidence-based prevention and treatment guidelines and standards of care for bone health. These guidelines help to ensure that individuals who have or are at risk of getting bone disease can benefit from the best practices related to prevention, assessment, diagnosis, and treatment.

The Role of Academic Institutions

Academic institutions can be critical facilitators through their two core missions of education and research. Typically, health professions education has focused more on teaching the clinical aspects of care than on the delivery or systems aspects. With respect to osteoporosis and bone health, various professionals are essential for promoting bone health, including physicians, nurses, physician assistants, dietitians, physical and occupational therapists, social workers, dentists, ophthal-mologists, optometrists, and pharmacists. While the amount of training each professional student receives in bone health and osteoporosis has not been quantified systematically, discipline-specific curricula could be created. For example, some schools have created "bone curricula" that teach basic science and clinical aspects related to bone health and bone diseases such as osteoporosis, osteomalacia, and bone tumors. Teaching tools such as CD-

ROMs, standardized patient case studies, and videotapes have been created to help teach this material. Equally important is the development of professional skills to become effective members of a health care team that focuses on improving bone health and preventing adverse outcomes. For example, trainees from different disciplines (e.g., medical students and residents, nurse practitioners, physician assistants) could be given the opportunity to rotate through osteoporosis clinics. Although a variety of models for interdisciplinary team training have been implemented, organizational challenges ([b]Reuben et al. 2003) and discipline-specific barriers to such cross-discipline training (Reuben et al. 2004) may impede these efforts. Finally, academic institutions may also serve an important educational role for the general public by teaching lifestyles that promote bone health in primary and secondary schools and colleges. Schools must begin to play a role in promoting and supporting good dietary habits and regular physical activity, beginning in childhood.

The second role of academia is to advance research on bone health. To date, such research has focused primarily on clinical issues, but some academic institutions have active research programs on health care delivery. While many of these have focused on preventive measures (e.g., cancer screening, smoking cessation), a few have attempted to improve bone health.

The Role of Health Care Purchasers

Health care purchasers have begun to use their power both individually and collectively to influence health care delivery. For example, the Leapfrog Group, a coalition of major employers around the country, has attempted to change health care delivery by encouraging adoption of computerized physician order entry (CPOE) systems, referral of patients to specialized, high-volume centers for some surgical procedures, and minimum requirements for physician staffing in intensive care units (Leapfrog Group 2003). If successful, these types of efforts by purchasers may be very influential in promoting evidence-based care, and thus may represent a potential top-down approach to ensuring that good bone health care is provided. As mentioned previously, the Federal and State governments in their roles as purchasers can also influence bone health and osteoporosis care by coverage and other purchasing-related decisions. It is important to remember that the role of purchasers in promoting better bone health will likely continue to be limited in a financing environment where those that pay for prevention, assessment, and treatment today frequently do not realize the benefits of such investments, which tend to materialize over the long term.

The Role of Industry

The pharmaceutical and medical device industries have been important facilitators in reducing the consequences of poor bone health through the development and promotion of drugs, devices, and other technologies. In fact, these companies are critical sources of information for providers and the public on the use of pharmaceutical agents to prevent and treat bone disease. This information needs to be combined with a more comprehensive approach to promoting bone health, including appropriate diet and physical activity.

In addition, there are other, independent companies that focus on disease management that can promote bone health by contracting with health plans, insurers, and other organizations to provide evidence-based care, just as they are doing now for conditions such as heart failure and diabetes. As mentioned previously, however, it is not clear to what extent these companies focus on osteoporosis today or what type of services they provide.

Special Populations

Several populations deserve special attention by all components of the health care system because they face barriers in accessing care and/or limitations in medical knowledge that may prevent them from receiving good care. These populations include the uninsured and underinsured, the poor, minority populations, men, nursing home residents, frail elderly persons, and rural or other remote populations.

The Uninsured

Thanks largely to government programs such as Medicare and to commercial insurance, the vast majority of persons who are at risk of poor bone health and osteoporosis have or are eligible for health care coverage. In fact, most persons lacking insurance in the United States are working age-adults and children who, in the absence of medical conditions and medications that interfere with good bone health, are at low risk of short-term adverse bone health outcomes. Nevertheless, children and adults without access to health care may not receive important information about behaviors that promote peak bone mass (e.g., appropriate diet and levels of physical activity, avoidance of smoking). Those uninsured individuals who are at high risk of bone disease represent a particularly vulnerable population, since all of their costs for medical care and pharmacotherapy must be borne out of their own pockets or through uncompensated care mechanisms. In many cases these individuals fail to access preventive care services and to obtain early diagnosis and treatments, waiting instead until their health deteriorates to the point that they face an urgent or emergent situation.

The Underinsured

A potentially bigger problem than the uninsured is the far larger number of Americans with health insurance coverage who are "underinsured." These individuals often face problems in getting access to appropriate services to promote bone health and to treat osteoporosis. Medications designed to treat or prevent bone loss can be expensive and the costs can be highly variable. For example, in June 2004, costs ranged from $25 per month for persons who only receive conjugated equine estrogens, to $64 per month for bisphosphonates, to $502 per month for those receiving teriparatide (Drugstore.com 2004). Of course, the new Medicare drug benefit will provide some level of coverage to beneficiaries. However, hip protectors, which cost only $50–$100 and may prevent fractures in frail elderly persons (Kannus et al. 2000, Parker et al. 2001), are not covered by Medicare, while coverage for important environmental modifications such as grab bars, railings, and raised toilet seats is inconsistent. Items considered to be durable medical equipment (e.g., raised toilet seats) are covered under Part B Medicare, but home modifications (e.g., installation of grab bars) are not. Some of these modifications may be provided, typically on a sliding scale basis, by programs sponsored by the Administration on Aging.

Minority Groups

Along with the uninsured and underinsured, people of color also need special consideration with respect to bone health and osteoporosis. As noted in earlier chapters, the definition of osteoporosis and assessments of fracture risk from BMD test results are based upon standards developed for Whites. Minority groups that have different average body and bone size, such as Asians and Blacks, present some challenges for the assessment of bone health by standard bone density tests. Blacks have higher bone density and a lower risk of fracture than do Whites of the same age. Nevertheless, the presence of strong risk factors such as a previous fracture or the use of glucocorticoid drugs, especially when combined with low body weight and/or older age, should be a signal for immediate attention to the potential need for intervention. In other words, while a person's race may suggest a lower average risk of fracture, it by no means indicates that there is no risk.

The bone density of Asians is similar to that of Whites after accounting for a smaller average body and bone size (Finkelstein et al. 2002). Nevertheless, standard bone density assessment does not compensate for these differences, and thus it is important to evaluate family and personal history of fracture and other risk factors in Asians (and small Whites) before determining if they are at high enough risk to warrant the initiation of treatment.

With respect to prevention and treatment of bone disease in minorities, there is no indication that pharmacologic interventions act differently or less effectively in minority populations. Blacks and Asians are more prone to lactose intolerance than are other groups, and thus they may be at greater risk of consuming inadequate levels of calcium and vitamin D. Thus, it is important to promote alternative sources of calcium and vitamin D in those who are lactose intolerant. (See Chapter 7 for more details.)

Another issue facing people of color is timely access to all health care services. The goal of better bone health for all Americans cannot be reached without significant improvements in preventive services, screening, diagnosis, and treatment, as well as significant changes in individual behaviors. This goal will not become a reality for people of color unless there are major improvements in their ability to access care on a timely basis. These minority populations are at the highest risk for poor health, yet they rely on an unorganized patchwork of providers for services that are necessary to prevent illness and maintain health. Emergency facilities are a major source of care for people of color, and their dependence on these often overcrowded facilities continues to grow (IOM 2002). These facilities are ill equipped to provide or even facilitate the coordinated, ongoing preventive and treatment services that people of color need to maintain bone health and overall health and well-being.

People of color not only have difficulty in accessing care, but there are also concerns about the quality of those services that they do receive. A recent study by the Institute of Medicine concluded that people of color tend to receive lower quality health care than does the majority population, even after accounting for access-related factors (Smedley et al. 2003). These disparities are consistent across a wide range of services, including those critical to bone health. A recent study found that few Black women (11.5 percent) had been screened for osteoporosis despite the presence of important risk factors for low bone density; the study also found that the prevalence of low bone density among these Black women was substantial (Wilkins and Goldfeder 2004). Overcoming these disparities will require specific strategies and programs geared towards bringing improvements in bone health to minority populations.

Men

Men represent another population of concern, since far less is known about the epidemiology, risk factors, and treatment of osteoporosis in males. As noted in Chapter 4, men account for roughly 20 percent of all hip fractures. It is unclear whether the diagnostic criteria for osteoporosis in women should be applied to men. While aging is associated with bone loss in men, the pattern of loss does not appear to be the same as that experienced by women for several years after menopause. (See Chapter 3 for more details.) The National Osteoporosis Foundation recommends BMD testing for men who present with fractures or are receiving treatment with a GNRH agonist for prostate cancer, as well as for all individuals who have primary hyperparathyroidism or are on long-term glucocorticoid treatment (NOF 2003). For more details on the evidence related to BMD in men, see Chapter 8. With respect to therapy, bisphosphonate and PTH treatments are effective in men (Finkelstein et al. 2003, Orwoll et al. 2000). The use of testosterone for bone and muscle loss in elderly men has been debated due to the possible increased risk of prostate cancer (Liverman and Blazer 2004). At this time, testosterone would not be considered a first-line treatment to prevent fractures.

The Frail Elderly

As with men, the knowledge base for how best to manage frail elderly persons with osteoporosis is not fully developed. As discussed earlier, the frail elderly living in nursing homes and retirement communities can benefit greatly from group-based exercise programs that reduce the risk of falling by improving muscle strength and balance. These supervised programs help to reduce some of the barriers to getting frail individuals to become more physically active, including lack of knowledge about what types of activities are safe and effective and the fear of falling or becoming injured while exercising. As noted earlier, the frail elderly also stand to benefit from the development of long-acting medications that make compliance problems less of an issue.

Populations in Underserved Rural and Inner City Areas

Individuals living in areas that lack health care resources, including rural areas and inner cities, represent another special population to be considered. Although many of the therapeutic options for promoting bone health are accessible nationwide, some communities may lack bone densitometry services and/or specialists with expertise in osteoporosis. Furthermore, newly developed procedures are not available in every community.

Conclusions

Major advances in bone health have been made over the past decade. The knowledge base needed for clinical decision-making has grown substantially, resulting in a much better understanding of the risk factors for poor bone health outcomes and strategies and interventions for reducing that risk. Measurement of bone density has become more widely available as the hardware for BMD testing has become less expensive. New, well-tolerated drugs have been introduced that are effective in increasing BMD and preventing fractures. Fall prevention programs have been developed and demonstrated to be effective, as described in Chapters 6 and 7. For those individuals who are at extremely high risk of fracture, rigorously tested hip protectors can significantly reduce the risk of fracture from a fall. Some payment decisions (e.g., Medicare's decision to cover BMD testing) have facilitated identification of those who need specific treatment to help prevent fracture. Finally, there has been increased public awareness of the importance of bone health and the potential consequences of osteoporosis.

In the context of these advances, systems-based approaches offer the potential to make substantial improvements in bone health and to reduce the adverse outcomes of bone disease. Historically, a number of barriers have prevented the widespread application of such approaches. These barriers include the lack of a comprehensive evidence base to guide decision making on osteoporosis and bone health, the fragmented nature of the delivery system, a financing and payment system that does not always create the proper incentives for the promotion of bone health, a workforce that has not historically been trained to engage in a cross-disciplinary, systems-based approach to care, and the lack of a strong push for improvement from outside facilitators, such as purchasers.

Fortunately, some of these barriers are being broken down. Further progress is possible through changes in policy, financing, organizational management, and education. Such changes are critically important to improving the bone health of Americans. As the evidence base continues to grow, a piecemeal approach to translating research findings into practice will no longer suffice. On the contrary, to benefit the largest numbers of individuals, it will be essential to utilize systems-based approaches that promote use of evidence-base bone health care for a broad spectrum of Americans, including the special populations discussed earlier in this chapter.

Key Questions for Future Research

Many systems-based approaches have been found to be effective in promoting certain aspects of health, but few have been specifically tested in bone health. Key research questions in this area are listed below:

- What are the most effective methods for increasing consumer and health care provider awareness of the need for improving bone health? Do these methods need to vary depending upon the racial and ethnic make-up of the target population? If so, how? How do these differ by age group and treatment goals (e.g., preventive versus therapeutic)?

- What are the most cost-effective methods for stratifying the population according to risk of bone disease? What role can measures of bone density and of fall risk play in the risk-stratification process?

- What are the optimal diagnostic and therapeutic approaches for special populations (e.g., men, racial and ethnic minorities, nursing home residents) for whom the evidence base is lacking?

- What are the optimal clinical, educational, and social rehabilitation programs for persons who have sustained hip or painful vertebral fractures?

- Which provider incentives and quality improvement techniques are most effective in changing current patterns of care for osteoporosis and bone health to be consistent with commonly accepted guidelines?

- What systems changes (e.g., computer-

ized reminders, registries, standing orders) can be broadly implemented in various settings to guide osteoporosis and bone health care in a manner that is consistent with commonly accepted guidelines?

- What are the best measures for assessing the quality of comprehensive osteoporosis care?

- Is the use of specialized osteoporosis clinics a more cost effective way to improve bone health than attempting to improve practice patterns among primary care physicians?

- How can health care providers and systems effectively link with community-based organizations to reduce the risk of falling?

- How can the public health system be most effectively engaged as a partner in improving bone health?

- How effective are fall prevention clinics in reducing the risk of future falls?

- What screening tools are most appropriate for provider organizations to use in primary care settings?

- How is screening and treatment for osteoporosis best integrated into management of other chronic diseases?

References

Aetna U.S. Health care [home page on the Internet]. Hartford (CT): Aetna, Inc.; 2003 May 16 [cited 2003 Aug 28]. Clinical Policy Bulletins: Treatment of Back Pain: Invasive Procedures. Available from: http://www.aetna.com/cpb/data/CPBA0016.html.

Andrade SE, Majumdar SR, Chan A, Buist DS, Go AS, Goodman M, Smith DH, Platt R, Gurwitz JH. Low frequency of treatment of osteoporosis among postmenopausal women following a fracture. Arch Intern Med 2003 Sep 22;163(17):2052-7.

Bailit Health Purchasing, LLC. Provider Incentive Models for Improving the Quality of Care [monograph on the Internet]. Washington (DC): National Health Care Purchasing Institute; 2002 Mar [cited 2003 Aug 28]. Available from: http://www.nhcpi.net/pdf/models.pdf.

Berwick DM. Developing and testing changes in delivery of care. Ann Intern Med 1998 Apr 15;128(8):651-6.

Black D, Nevitt M, Cummings SR. Bone densitometry and spine films. In: Cummings SR, Cosman F, Jamal SA, editors. Osteoporosis: An evidence-based guide to prevention and management. Philadelphia (PA): American College of Physicians; 2002. p. 29-58.

BlueCross BlueShield of Montana [home page on the Internet]. Montana: BlueCross BlueShield Association; c2003 [cited 2003 Aug 28]. Percutaneous vertebroplasty and kyphoplasty. Available from: http://mt1-bcbs.bcbsmt.com/bsd/MedicalPolicy.nsf/0/0f9b7d7482acb31d87256be300568e3f?Open Document.

BlueCross of California [home page on Internet]. Bone Mineral Density Measurement. California: BlueCross Association February 2002 [cited 2003 Aug 28]. Available from: http://medpolicy.bluecrossca.com/policies/medicine/bone_min.htm.

Cabana MD, Rand CS, Powe NR, Wu AW, Wilson MH, Abboud PA, Rubin HR. Why don't physicians follow clinical practice guidelines? A framework for improvement. JAMA. 1999 Oct 20;282(15):1458-65.

Compston J. Action Plan for the prevention of osteoporotic fractures in the European Community. Osteoporos Int. 2004 Apr;15(4):259-62.

Crowther M. Optimal management of outpatients with heart failure using advanced practice nurses in a hospital-based heart failure center. J Am Acad Nurse Pract 2003 Jun;15(6):260-5

Demakis JG, Beauchamp C, Cull WL, Denwood R, Eisen SA, Lofgren R, Nichol K, Woolliscroft J, Henderson WG. Improving residents' compliance with standards of ambulatory care: Results from the VA Cooperative Study on Computerized Reminders. JAMA 2000 Sep 20;284(11):1411-6.

Dexter PR, Perkins S, Overhage JM, Maharry K, Kohler RB, McDonald CJ. A computerized reminder system to increase the use of preventive care for hospitalized patients. N Engl J Med 2001 Sep 27;345(13):965-70.

Drugstore.com [homepage on Internet] [cited 2004 Jun 22]. Available from: http://www.drugstore.com.

[a]Feldstein AC, Elmer PJ, Smith DH, Aickin M, Herson MK, Orwoll ES, Chen C, Swain MC. Results of a randomized controlled trial to improve the management of osteoporosis after fracture. Presented at: 26th Annual Meeting of the American Society for Bone and Mineral Research; 2003 Sep 19-23; Minneapolis, MN.

[b]Feldstein A, Elmer PJ, Orwoll E, Herson M, Hillier T. Bone mineral density measure-

ment and treatment for osteoporosis in older individuals with fractures: A gap in evidence-based practice guideline implementation. Arch Intern Med 2003 Oct 13;163(18):2165-72.

Finkelstein JS, Lee ML, Sowers M, Ettinger B, Neer RM, Kelsey JL, Cauley JA, Huang MH, Greendale GA. Ethnic variation in bone density in premenopausal and early perimenopausal women: Effects of anthropometric and lifestyle factors. J Clin Endocrinol Metab 2002 Jul;87(7):3057-67.

Finkelstein JS, Hayes A, Hunzelman JL, Wyland JJ, Lee H, Neer RM. The effects of parathryroid hormone, alendronate, or both in men with osteoporosis. N Engl J Med 2003 Sep 25;349(13):1216-26.

Fonarow GC, Gawlinski A, Moughrabi S, Tillisch JH. Improved treatment of coronary heart disease by implementation of a Cardiac Hospitalization Atherosclerosis Management Program (CHAMP). Am J Cardiol 2001 Apr 1;87(7):819-22.

Gaglani M, Riggs M, Kamenicky C, Glezen WP. A computerized reminder strategy is effective for annual influenza immunization of children with asthma or reactive airway disease. Pediatr Infect Dis J 2001 Dec;20(12):1155-60.

Grimshaw JM, Shirran L, Thomas R, Mowatt G, Fraser C, Bero L, Grilli R, Harvey E, Oxman A, O'Brien MA. Changing provider behavior: An overview of systematic reviews of interventions. Med Care 2001 Aug;39(8 Suppl 2):II2-45.

Grol R, Grimshaw J. From best evidence to best practice: Effective implementation of change in patients' care. Lancet 2003 Oct 11;362(9391):1225-30.

Grossman JM, MacLean CH. Quality indicators for the management of osteoporosis in vulnerable elders. Ann Intern Med 2001 Oct 16;135(8 Pt 2):722-30.

Institute of Medicine. The future of the public's health in the 21st century. Washington (DC): National Academy Press; 2002.

Integrated Health Care Association [homepage on the Internet] Walnut Creek (CA): Integrated Health Care Association [cited 2003 Aug 28]. History of IHA's Pay for Performance Available from: http://www.iha.org/payfprfd.htm.

Kannus P, Parkkari J, Niemi S, Pasanen M, Palvanen M, Jarvinen M, Vuori I. Prevention of hip fracture in elderly people with use of a hip protector. N Engl J Med 2000 Nov 23;343(21):1506-13.

Kiefe CI, Allison JJ, Williams OD, Person SD, Weaver MT, Weissman NW. Improving quality improvement using achievable benchmarks for physician feedback: A randomized controlled trial. JAMA 2001 Jun 13;285(22):2871-9.

Lauritzen JB, Petersen MM, Lund B. Effect of external hip protectors on hip fractures. Lancet 1993 Jan 2;341(8836):11-3.

The Leapfrog Group for Patient Safety [homepage on the Internet]. Washington (DC): AcademyHealth; c2003 [cited 2003 Aug 28]. Available from: http://www.leapfroggroup.org.

Legorreta AP, Leung KM, Berkbigler D, Evans R, Liu X. Outcomes of a population-based asthma management program: Quality of life, absenteeism, and utilization. Ann Allergy Asthma Immunol 2000 Jul;85(1):28-34.

Litaker D, Mion L, Planavsky L, Kippes C, Mehta N, Frolkis J. Physician - nurse practitioner teams in chronic disease management: The impact on costs, clinical effectiveness, and patients' perception of care. J Interprof Care 2003 Aug;17(3):223-37.

Liverman CT, Blazer DG, eds. Testosterone and

aging: Clinical research directions. Committee on assessing the need for clinical trials of testosterone replacement therapy, Board on Health Sciences Policy, Institute of Medicine. Washington (DC): The National Academies Press; 2004. 240 p.

Maly RC, Abrahamse AF, Hirsch SH, Frank JC, Reuben DB. What influences physician practice behavior? An interview study of physicians receiving consultative geriatric assessment recommendations. Arch Fam Med 1996 Sep;5(8):448-54.

Max W, Sinnot P, Kao C, Sung HY, Rice DP. The burden of osteoporosis in California, 1998. Osteoporos Int 2002;13(6):493-500.

McLellan AR, Fraser MA. 28 month audit of the efficacy of the fracture liaison service in offering secondary prevention for patients with osteoporotic fractures. Available at http://www.asbmr.org/pages/pass1.htm or from JointandBone.org Rheumawire Oct 2, 2002.

Melville SK, Luckmann R, Coghlin J, Gann P. Office systems for promoting screening mammography. A survey of primary care practices. J Fam Pract 1993 Dec;37(6):569-74.

Morris CA, Cheng H, Cabral D, Solomon D. Predictors of screening and treatment of osteoporosis: a structured review of the literature. The Endocrinologist. IN PRESS.

North American Menopause Society. Management of postmenopausal osteoporosis: position statement of the North American Menopause Society. Menopause 2002 Mar-Apr;9(2):84-101.

National Osteoporosis Foundation. Physician's guide to prevention and treatment of osteoporosis. Washington (DC): National Osteoporosis Foundation; 2003. 37 p.

Nelson EC, Splaine ME, Batalden PB, Plume SK. Building measurement and data collection into medical practice. Ann Intern Med 1998 Mar 15;128(6):460-6.

Office of Technology Assessment, U.S. Congress. Hip Fracture Outcomes in People Age 50 and Over-Background Paper. Washington, DC: US Government Printing Office; July 1994. OTA-BP-H-120.

Orwoll E, Ettinger M, Weiss S, et al. Alendronate for the treatment of osteoporosis in men. N Engl J Med. 2000; 343:604-610.

Paccione PA (BlueShield of Northeastern New York, Albany, NY). Personal communication. August 2003.

Parker MJ, Gillespie LD, Gillespie WJ. Hip protectors for preventing hip fractures in the elderly. Nurs Times. 2001 Jun 28-Jul 4;97(26):41.

RAND Health [homepage on the Internet]. Santa Monica (CA): RAND Corporation; c2004 [cited 2004 June 18]. Assessing Care of Vulnerable Elders. Available from http://www.rand.org/health/tools/vulnerable.elderly.html.

Reuben DB. Organizational interventions to improve health outcomes of older persons. Med Care 2002 May;40(5):416-28.

Reuben DB, Bassett LW, Hirsch SH, Jackson CA, Bastani R. A randomized clinical trial to assess the benefit of offering on-site mobile mammography in addition to health education for older women. Am J Roentgenol 2002 Dec;179(16):1509-14.

[a]Reuben DB, Roth C, Kamberg C, Wenger NS. Restructuring primary care practices to manage geriatric syndromes: the ACOVE-2 intervention. J Am Geriatr Soc 2003 Dec;51(12):1787-93.

[b]Reuben DB, Yee MN, Cole K, Waite M, Nichols L, Benjamin BA, Zellman G, Frank

JC. Organizational issues in establishing geriatrics interdisciplinary team training. Gerontol Geriatr Educ. 2004;24(2):13-34.

Reuben DB, Levy-Storms L, Yee MN, Lee M, Cole K, Waite M, Nichols L, Frank JC. Disciplinary Split: A Threat to Geriatrics Interdisciplinary Team Training. J Am Geriatr Soc 2004 Jun;52(6):1000-6.

Rich MW, Beckham V, Wittenberg C, Levin CL, Freidland KE, Carney RM. A multidisciplinary intervention to prevent the readmission of elderly patients with congestive heart failure. N Engl J Med 1995 Nov 2;333(18):1190-5.

Rodgers, E.M. Diffusion of innovations. 4th ed. New York: Free Press; 1995.

Shekelle PG, MacLean CH, Morton SC, Wenger NS. Assessing care of vulnerable elders: Methods for developing quality indicators. Ann Intern Med 2001 Oct 16;135(8 Pt 2):647-52.

Siegel D, Lopez J, Meier J, Goldstein MK, Lee S, Brazill BJ, Matalka MS. Academic detailing to improve antihypertensive prescribing patterns. Am J Hypertens 2003 Jun; 16(6):508-11.

Smedley, Brian D.; Stith, Adrienne Y.; Nelson, Alan R. editors. Unequal treatment: Confronting racial and ethnic disparities in health care. Committee on Understanding and Eliminating Racial and Ethnic Disparities in Health Care, Board on Health Sciences Policy. Institute of Medicine. Washington (DC): National Academies Press; 2003. 764 p.

Solomon DH, Van Houten L, Glynn RJ, Baden L, Curtis K, Schrager H, Avorn J. Academic detailing to improve use of broad-spectrum antibiotics at an academic medical center. Arch Intern Med 2001 Aug 13-27;161(15):1897-902.

Solomon DH, Finkelstein JS, Katz JN, Mogun H, Avorn J. Underuse of osteoporosis medications in elderly patients with fractures. Amer J Med 2003 Oct 1;115(5):398-400.

Tinetti ME, Williams TF, Mayewski R. Fall risk index for elderly patients based on number of chronic disabilities. Am J Med. 1986 Mar;80(3):429-34.

Tosteson AN, Gabriel SE, Grove MR, Moncur MM, Kneeland TS, and Melton LJ 3d. Impact of hip and vertebral fractures on quality-adjusted life years. Osteoporos Int 2001 Dec;12(12):1042-9.

U.S. Department of Health and Human Services, Health Care Financing Administration. Medicare program; Medicare coverage of and payment for bone mass measurements. Fed Regist 1998 Jun 28;63(121):34320-8.

Wenger NS, Shekelle PG. Assessing care of vulnerable elders: ACOVE project overview. Ann Intern Med 2001 Oct 16;135(8 Pt 2):642-6.

Wilkins CH, Goldfeder JS. Osteoporosis screening is unjustifiably low in older African-American women. J Natl Med Assoc. 2004 Apr;96(4):461-7.

Chapter 12: Key Messages

- Population-based interventions are targeted toward promoting the overall health status of the community by preventing disease, injury, disability, and premature death. A population-based health intervention should include the following: assessment, health promotion, disease prevention, monitoring of services, and evaluation. Some methods include public education programs, community projects, and media interventions.

- Bone health is particularly amenable to population- and community-based interventions, for several reasons.
  - ~ Bone loss and fractures affect a large portion of the population and can be prevented during all stages of life.
  - ~ There is a widespread lack of knowledge about prevention among providers and the public.
  - ~ State and local governments have an incentive to promote this approach, since the costs of caring for bone disease are frequently borne by government and the benefits from population-based interventions extend to other areas of health.
  - ~ Well-crafted population-based interventions have been shown to be effective in improving bone health and other aspects of health, including increases in physical activity and decreases in smoking within a target population.

- Communication is an essential tool in many population-based health interven-

tions. Public sector (social marketing, mass media campaigns) and private sector (direct-to-consumer advertising) approaches can be used to reach target populations.

- This chapter includes seven case examples of successful and/or innovative interventions that can serve as building blocks for future population-based approaches to bone health:
  - ~ Any campaign should be based upon credible evidence and be evaluated on a continuing basis to ensure that objectives are being met and/or that corrective action can be taken.
  - ~ A number of evidence-based tools are available for developing interventions.
  - ~ Basic education about bone health is an important component.
  - ~ Building local partnerships is critical to success. Health care providers; education, environmental, and housing agencies; organizations serving the aged; churches, synagogues, and other religious organizations; and other groups can help to build a comprehensive strategy for maximizing the bone health of community residents.
  - ~ Useful prevention messages are available for every age group, although age should not be the only variable affecting the design of interventions.
  - ~ Health policy and environmental changes are important tools in health promotion.

Chapter 12

POPULATION-BASED APPROACHES TO PROMOTE BONE HEALTH

This chapter defines and provides examples of population-based interventions for promoting bone health that are tailored to different populations, addresses evidence regarding their effectiveness, and identifies some key aspects of successful programs.

Definition of Population-Based Interventions

In contrast to clinical services provided to individual patients in an effort to improve their health status, population-based interventions are targeted toward populations to promote the overall health status of the community by preventing disease, injury, disability, and premature death. A population-based health intervention should include the following: assessment, health promotion, disease prevention, monitoring of services, and evaluation. Some methods to accomplish these goals include public education programs, community projects, and media interventions. Some programs involve combinations of these approaches.

Most of these interventions are tailored to reach a subset of a population although some may be targeted towards the population at large. Populations and subsets may be defined by geography, culture, race and ethnicity, socioeconomic status, age, or other characteristics. Many of these characteristics relate to the health of the described population (Keller et al. 2002).

Bone health is a topic particularly amenable to population-based interventions, for a variety of reasons. Bone loss and fractures affect a large portion of the population, and they can be prevented during all stages of life. As discussed elsewhere in this report, there appears to be a widespread lack of knowledge about prevention approaches among both health providers and the general population. Finally, State and local governments have an incentive to promote population-based bone health interventions, for several reasons. First, the complications of osteoporosis are easily observed, and the costs of caring for these complications are frequently borne by these governments. Second, such interventions, including promoting exercise and appropriate diet, provide many other health benefits to community residents as well.

The most effective population-based approaches in bone health often involve a combination of individual- and population-level initiatives. The story of the Elder Floridian Foundation in the text box below highlights the interplay of individual- and population-level interventions and the importance of reaching beyond traditional health practices to produce positive changes in the population's health.

Personal Perspective of a Volunteer With the Elder Floridians Foundation

As a teenager, I watched my grandmother and her sisters get shorter. After my grandmother broke her hip, I spent many weekends cleaning for my grandparents while my mother prepared meals for the upcoming week. Grandmother never fully recovered from her fracture and died within a year. I was not able to name the primary reason for my grandmother's death until much later.

I learned about osteoporosis by researching the disease and writing press releases and background papers as a volunteer for the Elder Floridians Foundation. These materials were used for a media campaign to support proposed Florida legislation that would mandate the diagnosis and treatment of osteoporosis. Learning that it is possible to keep bones healthy and prevent fractures was an incredible discovery. Although I felt strongly that all older women should have this information, I did not feel that it applied to me. After all, I was in my mid-40s and healthy.

During the Governor's kick-off news conference event, which involved bone density (DXA) tests for reporters and elected officials, I got a big surprise. Results of my own DXA indicated low bone density of the hip.

I was alarmed that more than a million women in Florida might be in a similar situation, and it became my mission to educate them about their risk for this disabling disease. The media campaign was successful. Legislation was passed that mandated insurance coverage for medically necessary diagnosis and treatment of osteoporosis for high-risk individuals.

It also resulted, however, in an unfunded mandate to create an education and awareness program in Florida. To fill this gap, the Elder Floridians Foundation launched *Project Osteoporosis: Be Smart, Be Dense, Know the Difference* in September 1997.

The goal of *Project Osteoporosis* is to alert Florida's citizens through community-based education programs to the vital need to prevent, diagnose, and treat osteoporosis. These programs consist of a risk assessment survey, an educational slide presentation, a question and answer opportunity with health care professionals, and a peripheral bone density scan of the forearm (pDXA). Women's organizations, civic and faith groups, universities, and professional associations are among the Foundation's grassroots partners. They enthusiastically host *Project Osteoporosis* programs in local communities and at regional and State conventions.

Project Osteoporosis has traveled to 53 of Florida's 67 counties, providing hundreds of thousands of screenings to many grateful Floridians. The program has also shown that osteoporosis happens to people from all walks of life. Many of the people touched by this campaign have already suffered the consequences of osteoporotic fractures. Here is the story of one woman who was meaningfully affected by *Project Osteoporosis*:

Lucy was in her early 70s, had lost 5 inches in height and was no longer capable of growing new bone. Unfortunately, she suffered three compression fractures before a physician recommended a bone density test and prescribed treatment. By this time, Lucy's bones had become so brittle that she had two more compression fractures of the spine after beginning treatment. She said two things that still have a tremendous impact on the volunteers who work for *Project Osteoporosis*: "Be sure to tell people about the pain" and "I wish I had known."

Evidence of the Effectiveness of Population-Based Interventions

There is every reason to believe that well-crafted, population-based interventions can be highly effective in improving bone health and other aspects of health. For example, in 1993, it was estimated that while 10 percent of early deaths in the United States could be prevented through medical treatment, 70 percent could be prevented through programs that reduce health risks such as tobacco, drug, and alcohol use; sedentary lifestyle; poor nutrition; violence and environmental factors (McGinnis and Foege 1993). Over the past two decades, a variety of public health and health care professionals and organizations have developed methods for conducting standardized reviews of the effectiveness of interventions, including population-based interventions. These standardized assessments of an entire body of evidence for a specific intervention are known as "systematic reviews." Systematic reviews have contributed to methods for translating evidence into recommendations for practice (Canadian Task Force on the Periodic Health Examination 1994, Preventive Services Task Force [U.S.] 1996, Briss et al. 2000, Fiore et al. 2000). These "evidence-based recommendations" provide a method for linking the strength of a recommendation to the availability and quality of supporting evidence.

The Guide to Community Preventive Services (the Community Guide) provides systematic reviews on the effectiveness of various population-based interventions for a variety of public health topics, and then translates the evidence of effectiveness into evidence-based recommendations (Truman et al. 2000, Zaza et al. 2000). To date, the Task Force on Community Preventive Services has published reviews and recommendations on population-based interventions for nine public health topics (Guide to Community Preventive Services 2003).

The Community Guide includes completed reviews of interventions on two topics directly related to improving bone health: increasing physical activity (Task Force on Community Preventive Services 2002) and reducing tobacco use and exposure to environmental tobacco smoke (Task Force on Community Preventive Services 2001). These reviews and recommendations provide an initial set of population-based intervention options for communities and health care systems, and illustrate the range of settings and strategies to consider when developing population-based approaches to promote bone health.

Population-Based Interventions To Increase Physical Activity

Regular physical activity is associated with improved health and reduced risk of overall mortality (Lee et al. 1995, Paffenbarger et al. 1993). Physical activity and fitness have many bone health benefits, including reduced risk of osteoporosis and fractures (Bonaiuti et al. 2002, Karlsson 2004) and fall-related injuries (Carter et al. 2001, Robertson et al. 2002).

The Task Force on Community Preventive Services selected and reviewed 11 interventions related to physical activity. Recommendations were based primarily on the demonstration of changes in physical activity behaviors or aerobic capacity. As shown in Table 12-1, the task force found sufficient or strong evidence on the effectiveness of six interventions (Task Force on Community Preventive Services 2002), including community-wide, multi-component information campaigns; point-of-decision prompts to encourage stair use; school-based physical education; social support interventions in the community; health-behavior change programs

Table 12–1. Recommendations from the Task Force on Community Preventive Services, 2001– Use of Selected Interventions to Increase Physical Activity (PA) Behaviors and Improve Physical Fitness

Intervention	Number of Qualifying Studies	Task Force Recommendation
Informational approaches to increasing physical activity		
Community-wide campaigns (multi-component intervention)	10	**Recommended** (strong evidence on effectiveness)
Mass media campaigns	3	**Insufficient evidence**
Point-of-decision prompts to encourage stair use	6	**Recommended** (sufficient evidence on effectiveness)
Classroom-based health education focused on information provision	10	**Insufficient evidence**
Behavioral and social approaches to increasing physical activity		
Individually adapted health behavior change programs	18	**Recommended** (strong evidence on effectiveness)
School-based physical education (PE)	13	**Recommended** (strong evidence on effectiveness)
Classroom-based health education focusing on encouragement to turn off the television	3	**Insufficient evidence**
College-age physical education/health education	2	**Insufficient evidence**
Social support interventions in community contexts	9	**Recommended** (strong evidence on effectiveness)
Social support interventions in families	11	**Insufficient evidence**
Environmental and policy approaches to increasing physical activity (additional reviews in progress)		
Creation of or enhanced access to places for physical activity	10	**Recommended** (strong evidence on effectiveness)
Point-of-decision prompts to encourage stair use		See above under Informational approaches

Source: CDC 2001.

adapted for individual needs; and environmentally enhanced access to places for physical activity.

Evidence was insufficient to assess the effectiveness of five interventions selected for review, meaning that there is not enough information to conclude whether these strategies are effective. These five interventions include the following: classroom-based health education focused on information provision (due to inconsistent results); family-based social support (inconsistent results); mass media campaigns when implemented alone (insufficient number of studies); college-based physical and health education (insufficient number of studies); and classroom-based health education focused on reducing television viewing and video game playing (insufficient evidence of an increase in physical activity). For a more detailed explanation of the evidence for these interventions as well as others that were evaluated, see http://www.thecommunityguide.org/pa/pa.pdf. Conclusions from the task force document the strength of the available evidence and demonstrate that a variety of community-based interventions lead directly to increases in physical activity within the targeted population. These increases should ultimately lead to bone-health benefits, given the direct link between regular physical activity and stronger, healthier bones. The recommendations identify and support a range of effective, population-based options for schools, businesses, health care systems, and communities to increase physical activity. Programs, planners, and decision-makers can review the information, identify the efforts most appropriate for their local circumstances (setting, goals, target population, and resources), and translate the selected recommendations into specific, actionable interventions.

Population-Based Interventions To Reduce Tobacco Use

Smoking can be detrimental to bones, and therefore tobacco prevention and control efforts can have a positive impact on bone health. More broadly, these programs provide an excellent model for understanding how to assess, translate, and apply evidence on the effectiveness of population-based interventions.

The Community Guide reports strong evidence-based conclusions on the effectiveness of population-based interventions in tobacco control (Task Force on Community Preventive Services 2001). Table 12-2 lists task force recommendations developed from 14 population-based interventions. These recommendations illustrate several important points.

First, policies themselves are effective interventions. The concept of policies as interventions is firmly established in tobacco prevention and control programs. Laws and/or ordinances related to clean indoor air and excise taxes on tobacco products have proven to be effective population-based policy interventions. (See the Michigan case study later in this chapter for an example of the use of State polices to improve bone health.) Second, health care systems can be important settings for population-based interventions. Policies and programs implemented by health care systems, or by large employers or other entities that purchase health care for large groups of people, can target both patients and providers. Evidence of the effectiveness of clinical interventions that were documented in previous reviews (U.S. Preventive Services Task Force 1996, Fiore et al. 2000) enabled the Task Force on Community Preventive Services to focus on interventions designed to motivate patients and/or providers to make greater use of such interventions. (See Chapter 11 for addi-

Table 12–2. Recommendations From the Task Force on Community Preventive Services, 2000—Selected Population-Based Interventions To Reduce Tobacco Use and Exposure to Secondhand Tobacco Smoke

Intervention	Number of Qualifying Studies	Task Force Recommendation
Strategies to reduce exposure to secondhand tobacco smoke		
Smoking bans and restrictions	10	**Recommended** (strong evidence on effectiveness)
Community-wide education to reduce exposure in the home	1	**Insufficient evidence**
Strategies to reduce the initiation of tobacco use		
Increasing the unit price of tobacco products	8	**Recommended** (strong evidence on effectiveness)
Mass media education campaigns when combined with additional interventions	12	**Recommended** (strong evidence on effectiveness)
Strategies to increase tobacco-use cessation		
Increasing the unit price of tobacco products	17	**Recommended** (strong evidence on effectiveness)
Mass media education campaigns when combined with additional interventions	15	**Recommended** (strong evidence on effectiveness)
Mass media education-smoking cessation series	9	**Insufficient evidence**
Mass media education-smoking cessation contests	1	**Insufficient evidence**
Telephone cessation support when combined with additional interventions	32	**Recommended** (strong evidence on effectiveness)
Health care provider reminder systems when combined with provider education with or without patient education	31	**Recommended** (strong evidence on effectiveness)
Health care provider reminder systems when implemented alone	7	**Recommended** (sufficient evidence on effectiveness)
Reducing patient out-of-pocket costs for effective cessation therapies	4	**Recommended** (sufficient evidence on effectiveness)
Health care provider education when implemented alone	16	**Insufficient evidence**
Health care provider feedback	3	**Insufficient evidence**

Source: CDC 2000.

tional discussion of the role of health systems in population health.)

Third, interventions are often implemented and evaluated in combination. Four of the 14 interventions reviewed in Table 12-2 consist of multiple components. In many cases, the independent effects of the various components of the interventions cannot be determined based on the available body of evidence. The Michigan example described later in this chapter illustrates the use of a combination of interventions to improve bone health.

The concept of a comprehensive population-based approach to address a public health problem has become essential to tobacco prevention and control programs (Centers for Disease Control and Prevention 1999). Comprehensive multi-component efforts acknowledge that reducing tobacco use requires a population-based change in attitudes as well as behaviors (National Cancer Institute 2000). Bone health advocates can benefit from examining the multifaceted programs used in community tobacco interventions.

Communication Tools for Population-Based Interventions

Communication is an essential tool in many population-based health interventions. Its role and effectiveness are described extensively in the Institute of Medicine report, "The Future of the Public's Health in the 21st Century" (Committee on Assuring the Health of the Public in the 21st Century 2003). Public sector (social marketing, mass media campaigns) and private sector (direct-to-consumer advertising) approaches can be used to communicate with target populations in order to improve health.

Social Marketing

Social marketing, which has been used since the 1970s, is based on the principles of commercial marketing. It involves the planning and implementation of an orchestrated marketing effort, usually involving multiple organizations and institutions, with the ultimate goal of generating behavior change. It is commonly described as being based on the "four Ps": product, price, place, and promotion. "Product" is the targeted behavior, which may be the initiation of a new behavior or the cessation of a current behavior. "Price" is the individual's perception of what may be lost or given up for the sake of behavior change. "Place" is where individuals have access to the products or services or where they engage in the desired behaviors. "Promotion" is communicating to target audiences about behavior change through a variety of ways, including media relations, personal selling, and special events (McKee 1992, Siegel and Donor 1998).

The development of effective social marketing campaigns requires extensive formative research, including qualitative and quantitative methods that are used throughout the process to understand the specific needs, desires, beliefs, and attitudes of the target audience (Andreason 1995). (For an example of formative research for social marketing purposes, see the description of the National Bone Health Campaign in this chapter.) Currently, the Robert Wood Johnson Foundation is sponsoring a Social Marketing Collaborative in its Turning Point program to develop social marketing resource guides for U.S. agencies and organizations (Social Marketing Collaborative 2002).

Direct-to-Consumer Advertising

Direct-to-consumer advertising (DTCA) has become a common way for pharmaceutical companies to market new products. In 1997, the Food and Drug Administration released guidelines on consumer-oriented drug marketing. Since then, DTCA has become a multibillion-dollar aspect

Learning From Other Campaigns: The National Cholesterol Education Program

Successful national educational campaigns for other diseases can serve as useful models for what might be achievable through coordinated efforts to improve bone health. One such model is the National Cholesterol Education Program (NCEP), launched in the fall of 1985 and modeled after another successful program—the National High Blood Pressure Education Program. NCEP was administered and coordinated by the NIH National Heart, Lung, and Blood Institute (NCEP 2003). More than 35 national medical, public health, and voluntary health organizations and Federal agencies served as active partners and members of the program's coordinating committee. The multidisciplinary partnership included researchers, clinicians, public health officials, and policy advocates at the national, State, and local levels. NCEP had a number of objectives. First, it attempted to keep health providers up to date on science-based clinical guidance. Second, it promoted awareness in the general population of the consequences of uncontrolled high blood cholesterol and urged individuals to "know your number" and what it means to you. The ultimate goal was to lower elevated cholesterol levels as a means of reducing heart attacks and heart attack deaths.

With input from its partners, the program developed television public service announcements, print ads and other media materials, public health information publications, and patient guides. It also produced physician kits and clinical guidelines.

In addition, the vast memberships and State chapters of its Coordinating Committee partners carried out many of their own initiatives via their far-reaching collective channels.

The impact has been significant. In 1983, only 35 percent of Americans said they had had their cholesterol checked. By 1995, that figure jumped to 75 percent. In other words, some 70–80 million Americans who were unaware of their blood cholesterol levels in 1983 took action to find out where they stood and what they needed to do to protect their hearts. Physicians became more aware of cholesterol detection and treatment as well, as core NCEP clinical guidelines are now firmly established in everyday practice. The average total cholesterol level of American adults has fallen significantly, and coronary heart disease mortality has continued to decline. These indicators show the considerable impact that cholesterol education has had (NCEP 2003).

Ten Lessons Learned From the National Cholesterol Education Program

The lessons learned from the NCEP are valuable for any national campaign being developed to improve health:

1. Establish a solid scientific base that can bring credibility and persuasion to effort.
2. Create a multidisciplinary and far-reaching partnership that includes interested organizations with State and local chapters.
3. Make sure partners and target audiences have input at the concept stage, not just the dissemination stage.

Ten Lessons Learned From the National Cholesterol Education Program (cont.)

4. Pursue collaboration with outside interests, such as industry, as appropriate opportunities arise.
5. Develop a comprehensive program plan that includes roles for all partners.
6. Reach a consensus on consistent key messages that can be repeated and reaffirmed by many partners through many channels and outlets.
7. To reach desired goals and objectives, make sure the effort has the type of long-term commitment in terms of leadership and funding from sponsoring organizations that is necessary to make it sustainable over the long term.
8. Both population and clinical approaches will be needed in order to change behavior at the personal, family, and community level, and choices between these two types of interventions should not be made.
9. Establish or acquire baseline data pertinent to established goals and objectives so progress, or lack thereof, can be measured and program direction can be altered as needed.
10. Build in a reassessment and renewal process to keep the effort vital and current.

Similarities Between Osteoporosis and Cholesterol

There are similarities in expression of the two risk factors, osteoporosis and elevated cholesterol, that suggest that a program comparable to the NCEP has the potential to be effective in improving bone health. These include:

1. The first symptom often can be a serious event (a fracture in one case, a heart attack in the other).
2. Osteoporosis is now and cholesterol was then underdetected, underdiagnosed, undertreated, and underappreciated.
3. Osteoporosis does and cholesterol did require a two-prong approach, e.g., lifestyle change and early detection and control.
4. The ability to assess, educate, and monitor each respective condition by knowing one's number, i.e. blood cholesterol level on one hand, T-score on the other.
5. There did exist with cholesterol and does exist with osteoporosis a tremendous need to increase awareness that these conditions are common with potentially serious consequences that can be prevented and/or treated.

of pharmaceutical marketing (Rosenthal et al. 2002). Theorists argue for and against its use, with debate usually centered on whether DTCA informs and empowers consumers or encourages them to seek inappropriate and expensive care. Several surveys have demonstrated that consumers are aware of DTCA and take action as a result of it (such as asking doctors about products) (Lyles 2002). Evidence of direct health benefits from DTCA, however, is limited (Weissman et al. 2003).

The mass media, including television programming, movies, radio, newspapers, and magazines, represents another communication tool for the promotion of bone health. Health campaigns for other causes, including those aimed at reducing cholesterol levels, smoking rates, and the incidence of sexually transmitted diseases, have been successful in having their messages and/or desired behaviors portrayed in the mass media. Specialty and niche media can be used to reach racial and ethnic groups. One common approach for television and cinema is to suggest story lines and/or character portrayals that reinforce the intended message to the target audience. Similar efforts could be made in bone health. An example of a promising effort in social marketing is the $VERB_{TM.}$ *It's what you do.* campaign, a national, multicultural, social marketing campaign initiated in 2002 by the Centers for Disease Control and Prevention (CDC) to encourage young people between 9 and 13 years old to be physically active every day. Telephone surveys of youth and their parents conducted before the launch of the campaign and a year later indicate a 34 percent increase in the number of times each week that 9- and 10-year-olds engage in physical activity during their free time. There are 8.6 million children in the United States in this age group (Potter et al. 2004).

Population-Based Interventions: Conclusions

Despite challenges in mobilizing populations to improve health by addressing risk behaviors, a number of population-based interventions have been found to be effective. Evidence reviews provide a concise summary of the evidence on effectiveness and help decision-makers and program planners to weigh intervention options for local applications. Evidence reviews do not replace the important steps of conducting local assessments and enlisting community participa-

tion. Interventions should be well matched to local conditions (settings, needs, goals, target populations, and resources) and carefully implemented and evaluated.

As the evidence on different approaches continues to grow, several recurring themes and strategies emerge. While innovative application of new theories, strategies, and interventions will remain important to improving bone health, evidence-based reviews of what is already being done can play a significant role in supporting population-based program planning and decision-making.

Program Examples

Many of the following examples of population-based interventions in the area of bone health represent evidence-based interventions that draw upon research findings that have been presented in previous chapters of this report. In other cases, the examples illustrate innovative approaches where the evidence base is not yet fully developed. As a result, formal evaluation results are not available for some programs. In these cases, other evidence of the program's impact have been highlighted, including data related to "process" outcomes, such as number of Web site "hits," or proxy measures for bone health, such as the percentage of program participants who increased their calcium intake. Regardless of the evidence base for the programs, they were chosen for inclusion in this report because they each illustrate one or more key concepts in population-based interventions, which are summarized at the end of the chapter. However, this chapter is not intended to provide a comprehensive review of all successful population-based bone health interventions. The included examples are illustrative of the vast array of innovative programs that exist throughout the country.

Primary Prevention Messages for Young Girls:

The *National Bone Health Campaign*

The *National Bone Health Campaign* illustrates both the need and the ability to use population-based approaches early in life in an effort to reduce the chance of developing bone disease later. It also illustrates how a specific audience (in this case, girls age 9–12) can be the target of a prevention program.

Background

The *National Bone Health Campaign* (NBHC) is a multiyear national campaign created in 1998 by congressional mandate. Managed in partnership by the Centers for Disease Control and Prevention CDC, the Office on Women's Health (OWH) of U.S. Department of Health and Human Services, and the National Osteoporosis Foundation, this campaign uses a social marketing approach to educate preadolescent girls, their parents, and other adult influencers about behaviors that will help to prevent low bone density, thereby reducing the risk of osteoporosis later in life.

Before the campaign's materials were developed, formative research was conducted to get a better understanding of how information about calcium consumption and physical activity would be most effectively conveyed to this age group, a subject that was poorly understood. Racial- and ethnic-specific focus groups were the primary method for this research, along with a baseline survey of parents and daughters. The results indicated that bone health was neither well understood by, nor considered to be important to, girls and their parents.

The research also found that girls and their parents wanted messages that offer information, motivate them to act, provide action steps, and address the environments in which desired behaviors occur (USDHHS 2001). Girls also want messages provided in a context of fun, power, and social interaction.

The Intervention

The overall goal of the campaign is to educate and encourage girls to establish lifelong healthy habits—particularly increased calcium consumption and physical activity—that build and maintain strong bones. In the short term, the campaign is striving to increase girls' and parents' knowledge about how calcium intake and physical activity relate to bone health. Over the long term, the focus will shift to building on this increased knowledge in order to change behaviors.

To reach these goals, the campaign developed six main messages: 1) bone health is an important part of fitness, strength, and power; 2) calcium-rich foods and regular physical activity build strong bones; 3) calcium can be obtained from a variety of tasty and easily accessible foods; 4) there are a variety of easy and fun ways to get physical activity every day; 5) being more physically active is fun, and provides energy, fitness, health, and social interaction; 6) good nutrition helps you stay fit and active. All campaign materials are designed to convey easy ways to consume 1,300 mg of calcium and to participate in weight-bearing physical activity every day. To appeal to the girls' desire for inner strength, all six messages are held together by the campaign tag line: *Powerful Bones. Powerful Girls.*™

The cornerstone of the campaign is a Web site that helps girls understand how calcium and weight-bearing physical activity can be a fun, important part of everyday life. The site's spokes-character, Carla (Figure 12-1), emphasizes the basics of a bone-healthy lifestyle. The site also includes interactive games and quizzes, recipes for tasty foods with calcium, and tips on ways to get weight-bearing physical activity (Centers for Disease Control and Prevention 2003).

The campaign also uses other channels to reach young girls, including paid advertisements in children and youth magazines (such as Nickelodeon, Sports Illustrated Kids, and Girls Life), radio advertisements (434 radio ads ran between July and December 2001), a radio media tour (which included 200 interviews), and print materials such as calendars with stickers, presentations, and fact sheets.

For parents, four main messages are consis-tently used in the campaign: 1) as part of your daughter's healthy development and future, it is vital to build strong bones early in her life; 2) foods with calcium are an essential part of a healthy, balanced diet; 3) your actions do make a difference, participating in your daughter's activities or sports programs actively or as an observer is a way to spend time with her and be part of her healthy lifestyle; and 4) creating an environment to facilitate your daughter's cal-cium consumption and physical activity is an easy way to ensure her health in the future. The four messages are distributed through tip sheets,

Figure 12–1. Powerful Bones. Powerful Girls. The National Bone Health Campaign

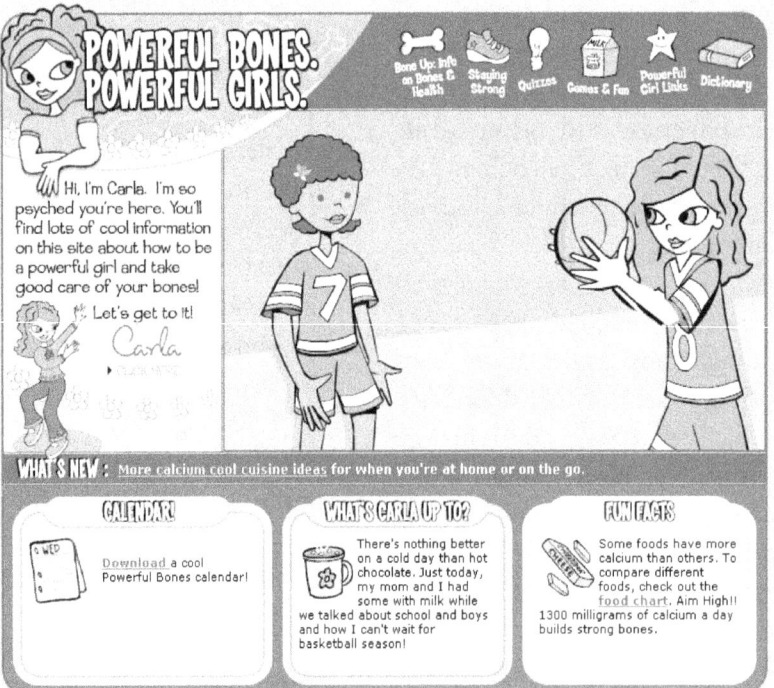

Note: The *National Bone Health Campaign* website educates preadolescent girls about adequate calcium intake and weight-bearing physical activity using interactive games and quizzes.

Source: CDC 2003.

shopping lists, and checklists that include specific action steps for parents. Paid print advertisements were placed in women's magazines such as Essence, Family Circle, and Ladies' Home Journal. A Web site (http://www.cdc.gov/powerfulbones/parents) has been launched to reinforce these key messages.

Partners

Several organizations that work directly with girls have tailored the NBHC materials to their needs. The Girl Scouts developed troop activity cards, a videotape, and a bone health patch, and Girls Inc. created activity guides and facilitator manuals. The National Association of School Nurses developed materials for use in schools. In addition, the NBHC partners with several local, State, and Federal agencies and nonprofit organizations.

Results, Evaluation, and Challenges

The focus of evaluation of the campaign to date has been on tracking "process measures" that gauge the extent to which people are being exposed to new materials and messages. As of spring 2004, the campaign had more than 122 million print media mentions and more than 3.1 million Web site visits. The plan going forward is to expand the target age of girls to 18 in order to reinforce messages initially introduced to younger girls.

Culture and Health:

Living Healthy: The Asian American Osteoporosis Education Initiative of the National Asian Women's Health Organization

This initiative illustrates the compelling need to understand each community's resources, leadership, and culture before designing and implementing a community-based health intervention.

Background

Most post-menopausal Asian women are at high risk for developing osteoporosis due to low calcium diets, low body weight, and small bones. Asian Americans often suffer from lactose intolerance, making it difficult to digest calcium-rich dairy foods. There are more than 30 distinct Asian-American ethnic groups with varying levels of English proficiency, cultural integration, and economic status. Many Asian Americans face economic and social hardships and require health intervention programs tailored to their linguistic and cultural needs. The lack of such programs, as well as language barriers, low literacy, financial constraints, and other concerns, leave Asian-American women with little incentive to seek health information and services (National Asian Women's Health Organization 1997).

The Intervention

The National Asian Women's Health Organization (NAWHO) has attempted to address these widespread, complex barriers to osteoporosis information through its community-driven education project *Living Healthy: The Asian American Osteoporosis Education Initiative*. NAWHO created a guide, "Living Healthy: The Asian American Women's Osteoporosis Education Implementation Kit," which offers a model program for health and social service agencies to plan, implement, and evaluate educational seminars on osteoporosis for Asian-American women.

NAWHO's program aims to raise awareness of osteoporosis among pre- and post-menopausal Asian-American women and to empower them to engage in positive lifestyle behaviors that promote bone health. The "Living Healthy" kit offers a mix of topics, exercises, cultural perspectives, and examples to enable organizations to tailor workshop agendas to the needs of ethnically diverse Asian groups. The kit includes three major sections:

- *Section One: Osteoporosis Messages.* This section provides key messages in osteoporosis prevention for Asian-American women, combining scientific fact (using materials developed by the National Institutes of Health (NIH) Osteoporosis and Related Bone Diseases~ National Resource Center) with culturally specific content.
- *Section Two: Conveying the Message.* This section includes step-by-step instructions for planning and implementing the education seminar, such as partnership-building, agenda development, program promotion, participant recruitment, logistics preparation, use of Asian language interpreters, and evaluation and follow-up.
- *Section Three: Resources.* This section lists several resources, including contact information for obtaining more information on osteoporosis; a review of health and cultural beliefs shared by many Asian cultures as well as barriers to outreach, education, and screening; and guidelines for working with language interpreters.

Partners

NAWHO worked closely with the NIH Osteoporosis and Related Bone Diseases ~ National Resource Center in developing this campaign. NAWHO also collaborated with three community-based organizations—the Asian American Senior Citizens Service Center, the Lao Family Community of Stockton, and the Southeast Asian Community Center—to test the "Living Healthy" kit with Asian-American women in three California sites. Criteria for selecting community-based partners included knowledge of Asian-American health needs, access to post-menopausal Asian-American women, and adequate infrastructure and programmatic capacity in the local community.

Results, Evaluation, and Challenges

NAWHO has evaluated the impact of the forums and workshops through surveys and interviews of the participants. This evaluation suggests that use of the "Living Healthy" kit has had positive results. For example, the community forums have increased overall knowledge about osteoporosis (i.e., understanding what the disease is), enhanced specific knowledge about the disease (such as screening and exercise as prevention strategies), and strengthened behavioral intentions (such as talking to the doctor and increasing calcium intake).

The evaluation also highlighted specific challenges and barriers for Asian-American women, many of which are being addressed by the "Living Healthy" program:

- *Illiteracy among target population.* Many participants had limited reading and writing capabilities in their native language, which created challenges in completing evaluation forms. To resolve this barrier, evaluations were structured as simple true/false questions that could be read out loud to the participants. In addition, outreach efforts were extended to younger women who were educated to teach their mothers and other elderly relatives about osteoporosis.
- *Duration of presentation and audience.* Feedback suggested that the seminars should be shorter for older participants (those over age 75). Based on this feedback, an abbreviated 90-minute presentation was developed for this audience, rather than the normal 4-hour format.

- *Importance of delivery.* Delivery style can make a difference in terms of how well information is understood. For example, many participants failed to understand the key messages when they were delivered by a well-known doctor who couched his remarks in difficult-to-grasp medical terms.
- *Lactose intolerance among Asian Americans.* To address this issue, the "Living Healthy" kit provides information on alternative high-calcium foods that Asian-American women can include in their diets, such as tofu, bok choy, sea weed, and soybeans.

State Policies and Health Promotion:

Michigan Department of Community Health Osteoporosis Program

This example illustrates the importance of partnerships across multiple community sectors in implementing comprehensive health interventions and demonstrates how a State health department can promote bone health.

Background

The Michigan Osteoporosis Strategic Plan, released in 1999, included 18 recommendations that were part of a detailed plan to reduce the human and economic burden of osteoporosis; the plan called for a variety of activities to be directed at improving the bone health of Michigan residents of all ages (Michigan Department of Community Health 1999). As a result of the strategic planning process, the Michigan Legislature dedicated State funds in 1999 to create the Michigan Osteoporosis Program. The program was launched under the leadership of the Department of Community Health and the guidance of the Michigan Osteoporosis Strategic Plan Advisory Committee. The importance of this

program is underscored by a 2000 economic assessment that found that Michigan citizens suffered 38,614 osteoporosis-related fractures that year, with total related medical care costs being $410 million (Burge et al. 2000).

Intervention

The Michigan Public Health Institute, a nonprofit organization under contract with the Michigan Department of Community Health, manages the program's initiatives, which are focused on reducing the prevalence of osteoporosis and osteoporosis-related fractures through consumer awareness and education programs, environmental interventions, and provider support, including education and tools. The initiative also includes assessment and evaluation components. Examples of specific interventions are described below.

In-School Education: A key recommendation in the Strategic Plan was to incorporate lessons about bone health into the existing Michigan Model for Comprehensive School Health Education Curriculum. Initiatives were designed to help youth achieve peak bone mass and lay the groundwork for continuing healthy behaviors into adulthood. Educational lessons for children in grades two and three were developed in 2000 and pilot-tested in 2001. A parent component was created to complement the information presented to students.

Community Screening: Michigan established a community screening initiative that combines a written risk assessment, individualized education, and a bone mineral density (BMD) screening test for those at risk for osteoporosis. Those individuals identified as having low bone mass are referred for further medical evaluation, and follow-up telephone calls are placed to check on the outcome from these referrals. Over 3,000 individuals completed a risk assessment and received education between 2000 and 2002. Almost two-thirds of them were identified as being at risk for osteoporosis and therefore received a BMD screening test and follow-up referrals if indicated.

Fall Prevention Program: Through a 3-year grant from the CDC, the Injury Prevention Section of the Department of Community Health is developing, implementing, and evaluating hospital-based geriatric fall prevention clinics at two Michigan hospitals. Patients who come to the emergency departments of these hospitals because of a fall or fall injury will be screened using a validated fall risk assessment tool. Eligible patients will be referred to the clinics, which will provide a comprehensive set of interventions to reduce the risk of future falls. These interventions include counseling and education of patients and families; provision of a fall-related home hazard assessment; a review of medications; lessons in Tai Chi; and referrals to other Medicare-reimbursable hospital services, including vision testing, physical therapy (for gait, balance, and muscle strengthening), treatment of chronic and acute conditions that can lead to falls, and BMD testing. A final component of the project is the development of training courses for providers (nurses, physicians, physical therapists, and occupational therapists) on how to improve their skills in identifying and managing adults over age 65 with fall injuries.

Health Department Education: In October 2001, Michigan began integrating osteoporosis education and risk-reduction initiatives into existing health department programs, such as the Breast and Cervical Cancer Control Program, WIC, and Senior Screening.

Partners

Partnerships became critical in late 2002 when State funding for the osteoporosis program was eliminated due to a budget crisis. Fortunately, by that time the program had alternative sources of funding that allowed several smaller initiatives to move forward, including the development of the fall prevention program and State quality assurance standards for bone densitometry providers.

Another project that was done in partnership with other organizations was the Partnership for Better Bones Project, a two-pronged initiative that includes both professional training and community education designed to make health care professionals and the general public more aware of osteoporosis and its risk factors. Educators from existing networks are trained and receive program materials to implement a standardized osteoporosis education program, "Better Bones, Brighter Futures."

Results, Evaluation, and Challenges

From the beginning, the program included an extensive evaluation component. Baseline data were collected to determine where education, prevention, and treatment efforts should be targeted. In 2000 and 2001, a statewide random telephone survey of 1,108 adults (age 18 and older) and 1,101 women (age 50 and older) was conducted using a survey instrument that included questions on osteoporosis knowledge and attitudes, risk factors, functional limitations, and self-reported prevalence. The survey was repeated in 2003 and will be regularly repeated in the future in an effort to allow evaluation of the overall program's efficacy.

The effectiveness of individual components of the overall initiative is also being evaluated. For example, the school health program, which included pilot lessons in three school districts, used intervention and control groups to assess the educational impact. Each group took a pre- and post-education test, the results of which suggest that the education had a meaningful impact. A post-lesson survey with parents indicated students had made behavior changes related to eating foods high in calcium and increasing weight-bearing physical activity. The impact of the fall prevention program will be tested through a controlled group study. Patients who meet the eligibility criteria for referral to the fall prevention clinic will be randomly assigned to intervention and control groups. Both groups will be followed for 1 year, with an assessment of risk factors and documentation of subsequent falls and fall injuries taking place at 6 months and 12 months after entry into the study. The evaluation will also assess quality-of-life issues for older adults and their caregivers, along with changes in health professionals' knowledge and behavior regarding fall risk assessment and management.

Perhaps the biggest challenge facing the Michigan Osteoporosis Program came when the State government, faced with budgetary problems, decided to eliminate funding for the initiative. Thanks to strong partnerships, the program has been able to continue even in the absence of financial support from the State.

Health Messages for Older Adults:

Project Healthy Bones
New Jersey Department of Health and Senior Services

The program demonstrates opportunities for health promotion messages and activities among older citizens, as well as the use of peer leaders as advocates for bone health.

Background
The New Jersey Department of Health and Senior Services (NJDHSS) began osteoporosis prevention activities in 1991 under a grant from the CDC. These efforts continue to this day, as the State still suffers tremendously from the impact of osteoporosis. There were over 36,000 osteoporosis-related fractures in New Jersey in 2000, leading to total medical expenses of $469 million and total nursing home costs of $137 million (Burge and Worley 2001).

NJDHSS's initial efforts focused on educational programs throughout the State, but it quickly became apparent that education alone was not enough. Based on scientific research showing that osteoporosis and osteoporosis-related disability can be prevented or slowed by balance and strength training exercises, diet, appropriate medications, and a safe environment, *Project Healthy Bones* was developed This project was directed toward older women and men who are at risk for or have osteoporosis.

Intervention
The objectives of *Project Healthy Bones* are to:
- Train peer advocates as leaders for *Project Healthy Bones*;
- Educate older adults on the importance of exercise, nutrition, safety, drug therapy, and lifestyle factors relating to osteoporosis; and
- Improve strength, balance, and flexibility in older adults, using weight-training exercises (Figure 12-2).

Project Healthy Bones includes both education and exercise components. The 24-week curriculum provides information on exercise, nutrition, safety, drug therapy, and lifestyle factors related to osteoporosis. Classes are interactive, with peer leaders facilitating information exchange.

The peer leaders are older adults who guide and support group participants as they exercise and learn. Peer leaders understand the beliefs, limitations, and concerns of the participants and work in pairs to provide both class instruction and individualized assistance. *Project Healthy Bones* includes exercises that target the body's larger muscle groups to improve strength, balance, and flexibility. Participants receive weight cuffs with 1-pound pellets that allow for individualized progression.

More than 1,700 older New Jerseyans currently participate in the program as either a peer leader or class member in 125 sites throughout the State. Waiting lists exist in most counties, as classes often elect to continue to meet after completing the 24-week cycle.

Partners

Project Healthy Bones is a partnership of NJDHSS, the New Jersey Association of Retired and Senior Volunteer Program Directors, Inc. (RSVP), and the Saint Barnabas Health Care System. NJDHSS administers *Project Healthy Bones*, acting as liaison among the three partners, developing policies for program operation and managing program funds. NJDHSS also develops and distributes peer leader and participant manuals and other educational materials.

RSVP's primary focus is local project administration, including recruiting volunteer peer leaders, linking at-risk older adults with classes in or near their communities, securing sponsors and sites for classes, and ensuring that classes operate smoothly on a daily basis.

The third partner in Project Healthy Bones includes two departments of the Saint Barnabas Health Care System. The Saint Barnabas Osteoporosis and Metabolic Bone Disease Center

Strength Training for Older Adults

New Jersey's *Project Healthy Bones* was developed based on research at Tufts University investigating the use of strength training exercises to improve bone density in older adults. This and other research resulted in several educational programs for enhancing strength training. One example is "Growing Stronger: Strength Training for Older Adults" (Seguin et al. 2002). This self-instructional workbook on strength training includes exercise instructions, a progression logbook, safety advice, and information on additional resources.

Another example is the "Strong Women Tool Kit: A National Fitness Program for Women" (Nelson and Seguin 2002). This tool kit for program leaders of strength training programs for women includes recommendations on physical space and equipment for classes, screening of participants, tracking participants' progress, and use of leadership techniques to encourage class members. Like the "Growing Stronger" book, the material is evidence-based.

Additional information regarding strength training is available on the CDC Web site. "Growing Stronger: Strength Training for Older Adults" can be found at http://www.cdc.gov/nccdphp/dnpa/physical/growing_stronger.

(OMBDC) functions as the program's technical advisor, maintaining and updating educational materials. OMBDC staff educate peer leaders about osteoporosis and Project Healthy Bones curriculum. The Saint Barnabas Center for Health and Wellness provides exercise training to peer leaders. Trainers are certified exercise

Figure 12-2. Weight Training Exercises Can Improve Strength, Balance, and Flexibility in Older Adults

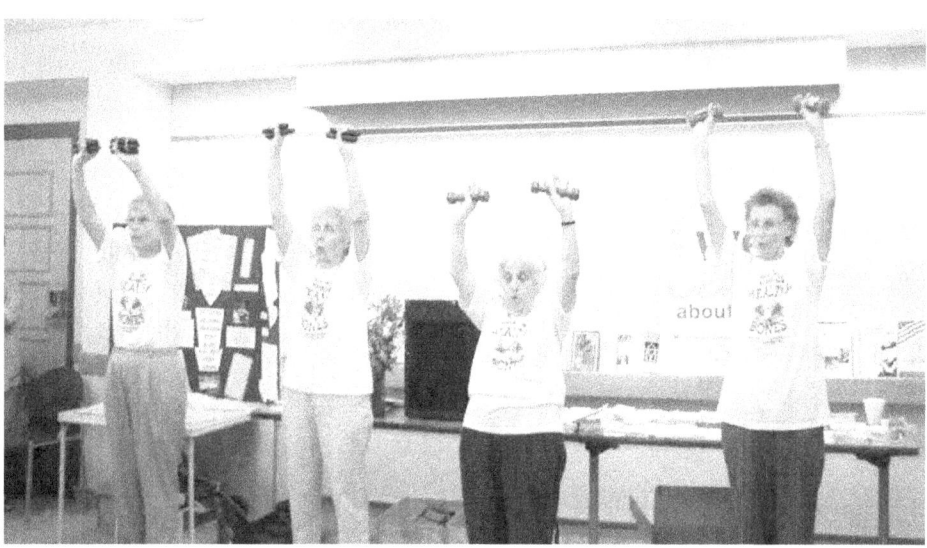

Note: Community exercise programs for older adults are based on evidence that osteoporosis and related disability can be prevented or slowed by balance and strength training exercises, diet, appropriate medications, and a safe environment.

Source: NJDHSS 2000.

physiologists who possess extensive experience with older adults.

Results, Evaluation, and Challenges

The impact of *Project Healthy Bones* is being evaluated through exercise tracking forms. Preliminary data suggest that the programs are making a difference. In 2001, a program review based on 217 forms revealed that 90 percent of the participants who completed at least 12 weeks of the program increased the amount of weight lifted, and 68 percent increased their calcium intake (NJDHSS 2000). Looking ahead, a more rigorous evaluation that examines the program's impact on strength, balance, and individual behavior change is warranted. Such information can be used as feedback to guide program revision and development.

Building Community Capacity and Group Support in Bone Health:

North Carolina

North Carolina was one of the first States to develop a program oriented at osteoporosis. While the State is involved in a variety of initiatives, two are profiled below. The first is a "train-the-trainer" model to build community capacity to address osteoporosis, and the second is a support-group program that helps individuals cope with the effects of osteoporosis.

Background

Low bone density and osteoporosis pose a threat to at least 1,300,000 North Carolinians age 50 and over. Each year more than 13,000 residents are hospitalized for osteoporosis-related fractures, resulting in over $145 million in direct medical costs from hip fractures alone. In addition, there are costs associated with the non-hospital treatment of fractures (wrist and spine being the most prevalent) and other health problems caused by osteoporosis. By 2020, it is projected that the number of North Carolinians with osteoporosis will exceed 400,000, while an additional million individuals will have low bone density (Borisov et al. 2002).

The Osteoporosis Coalition of North Carolina was established in 1996 to promote education and support for prevention, diagnosis, and treatment of osteoporosis; to reduce its prevalence, severity, and economic consequences; and to advocate for public and private support to achieve these goals. In 1997, the State legislature created the Osteoporosis Task Force to assess surveillance, create awareness, and develop a State plan.

Interventions and Partners

Train-the-Trainer Program: The Bone Health/Body Health (BH/BH) Initiative seeks to teach community leaders how to train others about bone health. More specifically, goals for the program include:

- Identify and train community leaders, both volunteer and professional, in techniques for communicating information about osteoporosis prevention, diagnosis, and treatment;
- Train community leaders in how to motivate and teach others the same skills; and
- Provide all training materials and educational support necessary for the community leaders to conduct their efforts effectively.

The BH/BH project targeted health professionals, administrators, and other community leaders in seven counties. The curriculum emphasized workshops on osteoporosis and health communication, with participants completing assignments between workshops. In addition, participants received a training manual, "Carrying Bone Health/Body Health to Your Community" (NCDPH 2001), "Making Health Communication Programs Work" (NCI 1989), a National Cancer Institute document, and a collection of excerpts drawn from the 2000 edition of TST Associates' "Media Relations and Promotion Training Handbook" (TST 2002).

The BH/BH program was conducted as a partnership with the North Carolina Division of Public Health, Osteoporosis Program, and the Regional Area Agency on Aging, Health Promotion and Disease Prevention Program. In addition, multiple community groups and individuals provided training, educational resources, and local venues for educating the communities.

Support Group Program: Public health staff developed a support group curriculum and a support group leader's handbook in 1997 (Condelli 2000). This effort led to the establishment of support groups in a wide variety of geographical settings by a diverse group of leaders.

During 2000–2001, there were 17 active osteoporosis support groups throughout the State, with groups holding meetings every 2 or 3 months. Groups are most active in urban areas, as limited State funding has largely prevented the establishment of groups in more rural areas. Topics for the meetings have included fall prevention, stress management, long-term care, diet, emergency preparedness, exercise, and self-esteem. Group leaders receive up-to-date information through the NOF's quarterly publication, "The Osteoporosis Report" (NOF 2002). In each session, participants are encouraged to share their thoughts and experiences in coping with the effects of osteoporosis. In addition, pharmacists, exercise physiologists, physicians, nurses, nutritionists, wellness coordinators, physical therapists, and others give informational presentations and answer questions from participants.

Results, Evaluation, and Challenges

While no formal evaluation of the programs has been conducted, process measures have been used to track the number of participants in group presentations and free bone density screenings, the number of exhibits displayed at churches, hospitals, and senior centers, and the kinds of media used for advertising programs. In addition, the support group participants have written about their own perceptions of osteoporosis. These vignettes will be compiled in a storybook and used as a resource for future programs. Future plans also include establishing support groups in new counties, providing technical assistance to established groups, and developing an organizational structure that allows groups to receive updated information on osteoporosis and to communicate with "sister" support groups.

Evaluating Community Health Programs:

Missouri *Take Our Trail* Physical Activity Program

This example illustrates the importance of developing a well-planned evaluation of the effectiveness of an intervention program and of establishing linkages with local community groups, both of which are critical to the success of community bone health programs.

Background

In 1997, Missouri State survey data showed that 65 percent of the State's population did not engage in adequate levels of physical activity to meet public health recommendations. To address this health problem, the State health department helped to fund the construction of walking trails in two communities through the Department of Transportation (DOT) (Brownson et al. 1996). A year later, in response to requests from other communities to build trails, the State asked for evidence to determine if further investment would be worthwhile.

Although there had not been a formal evaluation of trail use, anecdotal reports indicated that the trails were underutilized because of safety concerns and lack of amenities such as playground equipment and clean restrooms. The State provided funds to the health department to conduct the *Take Our Trail* campaign, which was designed to enhance trail activities and to conduct an awareness campaign in one of the communities with a year-old trail. If community members were not more physically active after this awareness effort, the State indicated that it would probably not fund additional trails.

Intervention

The *Take Our Trail* campaign was conducted for 3 months and led by the health department and a community health coalition. A variety of initiatives were aimed at increasing awareness of the trail and of the value of physical activity. The campaign kicked off with a 3-mile Family Fun Walk. For the duration of the campaign, signs were placed in busy areas throughout the community to promote the trail. A brochure was developed and provided to all programs in the local health department for distribution to clients, clinics, physician offices, church leaders, and the coalition. The brochure included information on walking and physical activity, safety, the trail, and contact names for walking clubs.

The local television station created a public service announcement to promote the trail and the importance of regular physical activity. The public transportation system placed signs inside buses, encouraging riders to "Take Our Trail." The community coalition helped develop walking clubs in work sites, churches, and social organizations. To address concerns about safety issues, local law enforcement officials patrolled the trail, and local business, city government, and churches raised money to add lights, along with other amenities such as benches, mile markers, painted lanes, and a water fountain.

Partners

The *Take Our Trail* campaign and its evaluation included multiple stakeholders. Participating government agencies included the local public health department, the city government, the Department of Transportation, Department of Parks and Recreation, and the Department of Education. Several local businesses and nonprofit organizations supported the campaign through donated goods, services, and publicity. Many volunteers also helped to build and support use of the trail, including walking, jogging, and cycling clubs; nearby employers; and community members who donated land, money, or other resources.

Results, Evaluation, and Challenges

Since the outcomes of the awareness campaign would directly influence future State budget policy, an extensive campaign evaluation was planned, including process measures that could help to replicate the campaign in the future, along with short- and long-term "outcomes" measures to gauge whether behaviors or intended behaviors changed.

Four primary evaluation questions were identified: 1) What activities were actually conducted as part of the *Take Our Trail* campaign? 2) Did trail use increase as a result of the *Take Our Trail* campaign? 3) Who used the trail, both before and after the campaign? 4) To what extent do trails increase physical activity levels of community members?

Since there were two communities with trails in place, the evaluation was designed as a quasi-experimental trial. Conducting the *Take Our Trail* campaign in one community but not the other allowed an assessment of whether trail use appeared to increase due to the campaign. A third geographically distinct community with similar sociodemographics and no walking trail or campaign was used as an additional comparison group. Data collection included electronic counter monitoring of trail usage; interviews with trail users and other key stakeholders in the community; event logs to capture activities at the trail such as formation of walking clubs, trail enhancements, and related events; media review to identify campaign announcements and news coverage; and community surveys immediately before and a year after the campaign.

The 3-month walking trail counter results indicated increased trail usage in the *Take Our Trail* community. The *Take Our Trail* community had a 35 percent increase in trail use between a month before and a month after the campaign, compared with a 10 percent increase experienced by the community without the campaign. Interviews revealed that individuals in the campaign community felt safer while walking than did those in the community with a trail and no campaign.

More than 60 percent of trail users in both communities indicated an increase in walking since the building of the trail. All types of people used the trail. Those who walked were more likely to be women, older adults, athletes recovering from injuries, and individuals with medical conditions that require a low-impact activity. Many of these groups are people at high risk for osteoporosis. The 1-year follow-up phone survey indicated a 5 percent increase in the number of individuals meeting the physical activity recommendations in the *Take Our Trail* community, compared to a 2 percent increase in the other community with a trail and a 1 percent decrease in the community without a trail. While this level of increase may seem small, it could result in meaningful changes if similar increases were to occur for the next few years.

There have been some challenges for the program. Some organizations and community leaders felt "left out of the loop" despite efforts to achieve broad community support. In addition, evaluation efforts also proved to be challenging, particularly labor-intensive surveying of busy community leaders. In the future, the use of focus groups might be a more efficient way to collect similar information.

Despite these challenges, based on this evaluation and other evidence, the Task Force on Community Preventive Services strongly recommends that communities invest in increasing access to places for physical activity, combined with informational outreach activities to promote use of such places. This approach is advocated as an effective way for communities to increase physical activity levels among the population at large (USDHHS 2002) (see Table 12-1).

Using a Multimedia Approach in a National Campaign:

Milk Matters Campaign
The National Institute of Child Health and Human Development

This example illustrates the use of multiple communication channels to communicate health messages in a national campaign.

Background

Based on 1) strong scientific evidence showing that adequate calcium intake during childhood is necessary for healthy bones throughout a lifetime, 2) consensus among scientific and public health communities on optimal calcium intake, and 3) data indicating that young people were not consuming sufficient amounts of calcium, the National Institute of Child Health and Human Development (NICHD) began the *Milk Matters* public health campaign in 1997. The campaign was directed toward all segments of the population and particularly young people.

Intervention

The long-range goal of the *Milk Matters* campaign is to encourage consumption of recommended daily amounts of calcium, with an emphasis on the importance of lowfat milk and dairy products as good sources of calcium. The more immediate goal is to increase awareness about the importance of calcium in the diets of young children and adolescents, which is seen as a critical step in the process of behavior change.

The campaign used multiple approaches to increase public awareness. Examples include:

- "A Crash Course on Calcium" is an in-school program, which included a video, featuring Olympic Gold medalists Amy Van Dyken and Kristi Yamaguchi, along with a teacher's guide, poster, and brochure. The course was designed to teach teens about bone health, calcium, and how getting enough calcium can help prevent injury now and osteoporosis later in life.

- "Milk Matters with Buddy Brush" is a coloring book for children age 4–8 that teaches the importance of milk for building strong teeth and bones. More than 1.7 million copies were distributed to dentists and health educators around the country.

- "Milk Matters for Your Child's Healthy Mouth" is a booklet about milk and calcium for parents. Its goal is to let parents know that calcium is important for a healthy mouth and to suggest ways to include calcium-rich foods such as milk and dairy products in their child's diet. The booklet is distributed to parents through WIC and Head Start programs, to State dental directors, and at meetings for health care professionals.

- "Bone Up on Bone Loss!" is a one-page brochure for health care professionals to distribute to parents and children that emphasizes the importance of weight-bearing exercise and calcium on building strong bones.
- Two other brochures were developed for parents, along with a brochure for health professionals. Available in both English and Spanish, these three resources have been distributed to health professionals at a number of meetings.

The *Milk Matters* Web site is designed to be an interactive, comprehensive resource for the public that can be viewed in English or Spanish (http://www.nichd.nih.gov/milk). Users can read *Milk Matters* publications online or order them online at no charge. Among other things, the Web site provides in-depth information about foods that are good sources of calcium, facts on lactose intolerance, and scientific abstracts on calcium research. The latest addition to the Web site is the "Kids and Teens" page, which includes puzzles and coloring pages for younger audiences and video games for older children.

Partners

Early in the campaign, NICHD established partnerships with several organizations that could help the campaign reach its primary audience. The campaign also collaborated with several of these organizations in developing its educational resources, including the American Academy of Orthopedic Surgeons (AAOS), the Milk Processor Education Program (MilkPEP), the National Dairy Council (NDC), and the National Institute of Dental and Craniofacial Research (NIDCR).

Results, Evaluation, and Challenges

Evaluation of the *Milk Matters* campaign has focused primarily on collecting information to improve the program, not on assessing its impact with respect to increasing awareness and consumption of calcium. Bounce-back card enclosures are included with outgoing orders for campaign materials. Recipients use these cards to indicate, for example, which materials they requested, how they used the materials, how they learned about the campaign, and if they are a health professional, parent, or teacher. Analysis of this information has influenced *Milk Matters* in several ways. For example, it pointed out the need to reach a Spanish-speaking audience and the need for publications that are easy to read. This feedback led to the development of several new publications, including a coloring book for children.

The *Milk Matters* campaign posed new marketing challenges to NICHD, and these challenges increased the importance of reaching out to new partners. As noted, NICHD worked closely with commercial partners to develop educational materials. At the same time NIHCD also partnered with other non-commercial organizations, such as professional societies, in order to avoid the perception that it was endorsing these commercial entities.

Building on Success

The case examples included in this chapter provide critical observations that can serve as building blocks for population-based interventions:

- Since scientific evidence is an important

aspect of effective decision-making (Eisenberg 2002), it is critical that any population-based campaign be based upon credible evidence suggesting that the proposed approach is likely to be effective in meeting its stated goals. In addition, ongoing, rigorous evaluation activities should test whether the interventions succeed in meeting these objectives.

- Basic education about bone health is an important aspect of population-based interventions. Almost every example cited in this chapter noted that most people do not know that calcium and physical activity are critical to protecting bone health, that fragile bones are not an inevitable aspect of aging, and that the peak time to build bone mass is during childhood and adolescence. Unlike the situation for some other health risk factors, such as smoking or driving under the influence of alcohol, most people remain unaware of the factors that increase or decrease the risks of poor bone health.

- Including health care providers as partners in population-based interventions accomplishes several useful functions, as illustrated in the Elder Floridian Foundation activities and the Michigan Osteoporosis Program. Health providers themselves need education on bone health and its assessment, as well as on population approaches to prevention. Health providers are recipients of referrals from community screening programs, so they need to understand and support these programs. Their support enhances the credibility of these interventions.

- Useful prevention messages on bone health are available for every age group.

Examples include drinking milk for preschoolers (*Milk Matters* campaign), building powerful bones for preadolescent girls (*National Bone Health Campaign*), or weight-lifting for older adults (*Project Healthy Bones*). Opportunities abound for tailoring bone health messages to populations at greatest risk.

- Age is not the only variable affecting the design of population interventions. The *Living Healthy: The Asian American Women's Osteoporosis Education Initiative* illustrates the need to address cultural and community concerns. It is significant that a national Asian-American health organization was not satisfied to take its own knowledge of Asian culture into the field. Instead, NAWHO partnered with Asian-American community-based organizations that were even better informed about local Asian ethnic groups and cultures.

- A number of evidence-based tools can be used in building population interventions for bone health. As noted previously, effective interventions exist for addressing specific bone health risk factors, such as tobacco use or lack of physical activity (the *Take Our Trail* campaign). Strategies such as social marketing have also proved to be useful across multiple health topics and are likely to work in addressing bone health as well.

- Health policy and environmental changes are important tools in health promotion, as illustrated in the section on tobacco prevention and in the Michigan Osteoporosis Program and the *Take Our Trail* program.

- Building partnerships is usually essential

to intervention success. The right partners provide credibility and resources, access to networks and communities, collaboration with other health campaigns and programs, advocacy for health policies, staffing for special projects, and multiple other advantages. For bone health, building strong partnerships, especially at the community level, may be as critical as determining the best population interventions.

- Local culture and circumstances are also part of the decision-making process. Policy may be influenced by a community's choice of interventions, efficiency in using limited resources, and equity in health status, especially with respect to disadvantaged populations.

There are additional factors to consider in developing and implementing population-based bone health interventions. While some evidence-based interventions exist, many more are needed. As new interventions are developed, it will be necessary to design evaluation plans, or even a formal research design, to assess their effectiveness. Since the ultimate outcome of these interventions may not occur for a long period of time (e.g., especially for interventions among younger adults and children), it will be necessary to develop and validate proxy measures to assess effectiveness. For older citizens, however, measuring reductions in osteoporotic fragility fractures can allow for the direct assessment of health outcomes.

Another concern relates to financial support, both for assessing new interventions and for conducting new interventions at a population level. Several of the examples cited in this chapter highlight the difficulty of maintaining financial support for these programs. An economic analysis of the benefits of preventing bone disease may help make the case for support.

Despite these concerns, there is reason for hope. Education and public awareness campaigns may be the most easily understood aspect of population-based interventions and thus may provide the best opportunities for success. While education is essential, it usually cannot change the behavior of the population on its own. Thus, there is also a need for a change in cultural attitudes and in formal policies to support positive behavior changes. Social marketing can assist in creating these types of changes. The good news is that because the essential components of prevention in bone health—good nutrition and physical activity—are also important to many other aspects of health, there is an opportunity for the development of synergistic public health programs to address multiple diseases including not only osteoporosis, but also obesity, diabetes, and heart disease. This multi-pronged emphasis on cultural changes has proven effective in restricting smoking in public settings, increasing use of seat belts in moving vehicles, and making use of designated drivers an accepted social practice.

Though much remains to be learned, enough is known about bone health to move forward with population-based interventions, so that bone disease can become a rare event rather than an everyday occurrence.

National Bone Disease Organizations as Partners in Population-Based Interventions

The national bone disease organizations can be important partners in population-based interventions to promote bone health. As national nonprofit organizations, they play key roles in educating the public and health care professionals about the prevention and treatment of bone diseases and can serve as resources for many of the public and private organizations working at the community and State levels toward improving bone health. There are four leading national bone disease organizations, each with distinct missions, but all working collaboratively to promote bone health. The American Society for Bone and Mineral Research promotes excellence in bone and mineral research and the translation of basic science to clinical practice. The three other organizations—the National Os-

teoporosis Foundation, the Osteogenesis Imperfecta Foundation, and the Paget Foundation for Paget's Disease of Bone and Related Disorders—promote education, awareness, research, and support for patients and health care professionals related to their specific diseases.

In addition to promoting public and professional awareness, the national bone disease organizations are powerful advocates for research funding and public policy through the Federal government to improve the prevention and treatment of bone diseases. They coordinate their advocacy efforts through their participation in the National Coalition for Osteoporosis and Related Bone Diseases, also known as the Bone Coalition. The Bone Coalition's accomplishments in improving bone health have been in the areas of research, policy, legislation, funding, and national guidelines and standards.

For More Information:

American Society for Bone and Mineral Research
2025 M Street, NW, Suite 800
Washington, DC 20036-3309
Phone: (202) 367-1161
Fax: (202) 367-2161
Toll-Free: (800) 981-2663
http://www.asbmr.org

National Osteoporosis Foundation
1232 22nd Street, NW
Washington, DC 20037-1292
Phone: (202) 223-2226
http://www.nof.org

Osteogenesis Imperfecta Foundation
804 West Diamond Avenue, Suite 210
Gaithersburg, MD 20878
Phone: (301) 947-0083
Fax: (301) 947-0456
Toll-Free: (800) 981-2663
http://www.oif.org

The Paget Foundation
120 Wall Street, Suite 1602
New York, NY 10005-4001
Phone: (212) 509-5335
Fax: (212) 509-8492
Toll-Free: (800) 23-PAGET
http://www.paget.org

The National Institutes of Health Osteoporosis and Related Bone Diseases~National Resource Center:

A Resource for Population-Based Interventions

A valuable resource for population-based interventions is the National Institutes of Health Osteoporosis and Related Bone Diseases~National Resource Center (NIH ORBD~NRC). The National Resource Center was established in 1994 to provide patients, health professionals, and the public with an important link to resources and information on metabolic bone diseases, including osteoporosis, Paget's disease of the bone, osteogenesis imperfecta, and hyperparathyroidism. The National Resource Center is operated by the National Osteoporosis Foundation, in collaboration with The Paget Foundation and the Osteogenesis Imperfecta Foundation. It is supported by the National Institute of Arthritis and Musculoskeletal and Skin Diseases (NIAMS) of the National Institutes of Health, with contributions from other Federal offices.

The National Resource Center offers a range of services to provide links to resources and information on metabolic bone diseases that are geared to both professionals and the public. An in-house database contains references to print materials, organizations, and programs. A cumulative index of metabolic bone diseases literature contains the latest clinical research and studies, and customized bibliographies can be developed from this index. New materials have been developed to fill important gaps in information for specific populations, including those who do not speak English, low literacy populations, and the visually impaired.

For more information:
National Institutes of Health Osteoporosis and Related Bone Diseases ~National Resource Center
1232 22nd Street, NW
Washington, DC 20037-1292
Phone: (202) 223-0344
Toll Free: (800) 624-BONE
Fax: (202) 293-2356
TTY: (202) 466-4315
http://www.osteo.org

Key Questions for Future Research

While many population-based interventions have been found to be effective in promoting specific healthy behaviors, such as smoking cessation and promoting physical activity, relatively little is known about how best to tailor these approaches to promoting bone health. Key, unanswered research questions appear below:

- What population-based bone health interventions are most effective in reducing the long-term incidence and burden of osteoporosis and other bone diseases?
- What combinations of health messages are most effective for a bone health campaign, including those messages that have been used in other health campaigns?
- Given the long-term nature of population-based bone health interventions, what are valid "proxy" measures that can be used to assess them when targeted at younger adults and children?
- What are the most effective means of educating the public and providers about the importance of bone health and about basic preventive measures?
- What are the best methods for encouraging providers to take a more active role in promoting bone health with their patients?

- What are the most effective population-based interventions in schools, businesses, health care systems, and communities to increase physical activity to recommended levels throughout the lifespan?
- What are the most effective population-based interventions to increase calcium and vitamin D consumption to recommended levels throughout the lifespan?

- What population-based interventions are most effective for improving bone health in racial and ethnic minorities?
- What are the most effective social marketing interventions to promote bone health?
- What are the best measures of bone health to be used for surveillance?
- What environmental modifications are most effective in preventing fractures?

References

Andreason A. Marketing social change: Changing behavior to promote health, social development, and the environment. San Francisco (CA): Jossey Bass Publishers; 1995.

Bonaiuti D, Shea B, Iovine R, Negrini S, Robinson V, Kemper HC, Wells G, Tugwell P, Cranney A. Exercise for preventing and treating osteoporosis in postmenopausal women. Cochrane Database Syst Rev. 2002 (3):CD000333.

Borisov NN, Balda E, King AB. The cost of osteoporosis in North Carolina: Projections for 2000-2005. Technical report. Mason (OH): Procter & Gamble Pharmaceuticals; 2002.

Briss PA, Zaza S, Pappaioanou M, Fielding J, Wright-De Aguero L, Truman BI, Hopkins DP, Mullen PD, Thompson RS, Woolf SH, et al. Developing an evidence-based Guide to Community Preventive Services—methods. The Task Force on Community Preventive Services. Am J Prev Med. 2000 Jan;18(1 Suppl):35-43.

Brownson RC, Smith CA, Pratt M, Mack NE, Jackson-Thompson J, Dean CG, Dabney S, Wilkerson JC. Preventing cardiovascular disease through community-based risk reduction: The Bootheel Heart Health Project. Am J Public Health. 1996 Feb;86(2):206-13.

Burge, RT, Worley, DJ, King, AB. The cost of osteoporosis in Michigan: Projections for 2000-2025. Cincinnati (OH): Procter & Gamble Pharmaceuticals; 2000 Sep. 8 p. Available from: Michigan Public Health Institute, Okemos, MI.

Burge, RT, Worley, D. The cost of osteoporosis in New Jersey: Projections for 2000-2005. Technical Report. Mason (OH): Procter & Gamble Pharmaceuticals; 2001 Feb.

Canadian Task Force on the Periodic Health Examination. Canadian Guide to Clinical, Preventive Health Care. Ottawa, Canada: Canada Communications Group; 1994. 1009 p.

Carter ND, Kannus P, Khan KM. Exercise in the prevention of falls in older people: A systematic literature review examining the rationale and the evidence. Sports Med. 2001; 31(6):427-38.

Centers for Disease Control and Prevention. Best practices for comprehensive tobacco control programs—August 1999. Atlanta (GA): U.S. Department of Health and Human Services, Centers for Disease Control and Prevention, National Center for Chronic Disease Prevention and Health Promotion, Office on Smoking and Health; 1999. 87 p.

Centers for Disease Control and Prevention. Strategies for reducing exposure to environmental tobacco smoke, increasing tobacco-use cessation, and reducing initiation in communities and health-care systems. A report on recommendations of the Task Force on Community Preventive Services. MMWR 2000;49(No. RR-12):1-20.

Centers for Disease Control and Prevention. Increasing physical activity. A report on recommendations of the Task Force on Community Preventive Services.

MMWR Recomm Rep. 2001 Oct 26;50(RR-18):1-14.

Centers for Disease Control and Prevention. Powerful Bones. Powerful Girls. The National Bone Health Campaign™ Web site [homepage on the Internet]. Atlanta: U.S. Department of Health and Human Services' Office of Women's Health, Centers for Disease Control and Prevention, and National Osteoporosis Foundation; 2003. Available from: http://www.cdc.gov/powerfulbones/.

Centers for Disease Control and Prevention Youth Media Campaign Web site [homepage on the Internet]. Atlanta (GA): Centers for Disease Control and Prevention;[cited 2004 Apr 14]. Available from: http://www.cdc.gov/youthcampaign/.

Committee on assuring the health of the public in the 21st century. The future of the public's health in the 21st century [monograph on the Internet]. Internet ed. Washington: The National Academies Press; c2003 [cited 2003 Apr 21]. Chapter 7: Media; p. 315-362. Available from http://books.nap.edu/books/030908704X/html/315.html.

Condelli, E., B.S.W. Osteoporosis support group leader handbook. Raleigh (NC): North Carolina Department of Health and Human Services, Division of Public Health/Older Adult Health Branch, Osteoporosis Program; 2000.

Eisenberg JM. Globalize the evidence, localize the decision: evidence-based medicine and international diversity. Health Aff (Millwood). 2002 May-Jun;21:166-8.

Fiore MC, Bailey WC, Cohen SJ, Dorfman SF, Goldstein MG, Gritz ER, Heyman RB, Jaen CR, Kottke TE, Lando HA, et al. Treating tobacco use and dependence: Clinical practice guideline. Rockville (MD): U.S. Department of Health and Human Services, Public Health Service; 2000.

Guide to Community Preventive Services Web site [homepage on the Internet]. Atlanta (GA): Task Force on Community Preventive Services supported by the Centers for Disease Control and Prevention; c2001-03 [cited 2003 Apr 21]. Available from http://www.thecommunityguide.org/.

Karlsson M. Has exercise an antifracture efficacy in women? Scand J Med Sci Sports. 2004 Feb;14(1):2-15.

Keller LO, Schaffer MA, Lia-Hoagberg B, Strohschein S. Assessment, program planning and evaluation in population-based public health practice. Journal of Public Health Management and Practice 2002 Sep;8(5):30-44.

Lee IM, Hsieh CC, Paffenbarger RS Jr. Exercise intensity and longevity in men. The Harvard Alumni Health Study. JAMA. 1995 Apr 19;273(15):1179-84.

Lyles A. Direct marketing of pharmaceuticals to consumers. Annu Rev Public Health. 2002;23:73-91. Epub 2001 Oct 25.

McGinnis JM, Foege WH. Actual causes of death in the United States. JAMA. 1993 Nov 10;270(18):2207-12.

McKee, Neill. Social mobilization & social marketing in developing communities: Lessons for communicators. Penang, Malaysia: Southbound; 1992. 220 p.

Michigan Department of Community Health. Michigan osteoporosis strategic plan: Final report of the Michigan Osteoporosis Planning Group. Lansing (MI): Michigan Department of Community Health; 1999. 44 p.

National Asian Women's Health Organization. Expanding options: a reproductive and sexual health survey of Asian American women. San Francisco (CA): National Asian Women's Health Organization; 1997.

National Cancer Institute. Making health communication programs work. Bethesda (MD): U.S. Department of Health and Human Services, National Institute of Health, National Cancer Institute; 1989 Apr. NIH Pub. No. 89-1493.

National Cancer Institute. Population-based smoking cessation: Proceedings of a conference on what works to influence cessation in the general population. Smoking and Tobacco Control Monograph No. 12. Bethesda (MD): U.S. Department of Health and Human Services, National Institute of Health, National Cancer Institute; 2000 Nov. 233 p.

Available from: NIH; Pub. No. 00-4892.

National Cholesterol Education Program [home page on Internet]. Bethesda (MD): National Heart, Lung, and Blood Institute; c2003 [cited 2003 Sep 22]. Available from: http://www.nhlbi.nih.gov/about/ncep/.

National Osteoporosis Foundation. The osteoporosis report. Washington (DC): NOF; Quarterly 2002.

Nelson ME, Fiatarone MA, Morganti CM, Trice I, Greenberg RA, Evans WJ. Effects of high-intensity strength training on multiple risk factors for osteoporotic fractures: A randomized controlled trial. JAMA. 1994 Dec 28;272(24):1909-14.

Nelson ME and Sequin RE. Strong women tool kit: a national fitness program for women. Boston (MA): Tufts University; 2002.

New Jersey Department of Health and Senior Services, Osteoporosis Prevention and Education Program. Report to the Governor and Legislature. Trenton (NJ): New Jersey Department of Health and Senior Services; 2000 Nov.

North Carolina Department of Public Health, Osteoporosis Program. Carrying bone health body health to your community 2001, a three part workshop. Raleigh (NC): NCDPH; Spring 2001.

Paffenbarger RS Jr, Hyde RT, Wing AL, Lee IM, Jung DL, Kampert JB. The association of changes in physical-activity level and other lifestyle characteristics with mortality among men. N Engl J Med. 1993 Feb 25;328(8):538-45.

Potter LD, Duke JC, Nolin MJ, Judkins D, Huhman M. Evaluation of the CDC VERB Campaign: Findings from the Youth Media Campaign Longitudinal Survey, 2002-2003. Report prepared for the U.S. Centers for Disease Control and Prevention; 2004 (Contract Number 200199900020).

Preventive Services Task Force (US). Guide to clinical preventive services: Report of the US Preventive Services Task Force, 2nd ed. Baltimore (MD): Williams and Wilkins; 1996. 953 p.

Robertson MC, Campbell AJ, Gardner MM, Devlin N. Preventing injuries in older people by preventing falls: A meta-analysis of individual-level data. J Am Geriatr Soc. 2002 May;50(5):905-11.

Rosenthal MB, Berndt ER, Donohue JM, Frank RG, Epstein AM. Promotion of prescription drugs to consumers. N Engl J Med. 2002 Feb 14;346(7):498-505.

Seguin RE, Epping JN, Buchner DM, Bloch R, and Nelson ME. Growing stronger: Strength training for older adults. Boston (MA): Tufts University; 2002.

Siegel, M; Donor, L. Marketing Public Health: Strategies to Promote Social Change. Gaithersburg (MD): Aspen Publishers; 1998. 530 p.

Social Marketing Collaborative, Turning Point National Program. Social marketing resource guide [monograph on the Internet]. Internet ed., Turning Point National Program Office; 2002 Apr [cited 2003 Apr 23]. [94 p.]. Available from http://www. turningpoint program. org/Pages/social _marketing_101.pdf.

Task Force on Community Preventive Services. Recommendations regarding interventions to reduce tobacco use and exposure to environmental tobacco smoke. Am J Prev Med. 2001 Feb;20(2S):10-15.

Task Force on Community Preventive Services. Recommendations to increase physical activity in communities. Am J Prev Med. 2002;22(4S):67-72.

Truman BI, Smith-Akin CK, Hinman AR, Gebbie KM, Brownson R, Novick LF,

Lawrence RS, Pappaioanou M, Fielding J, Evans CA Jr., et al. Developing the Guide to Community Preventive Services—Overview and Rationale. Am J Prev Med. 2000 Jan; 18(1 Suppl):18-26.

TST Associates. Media relations and promotion training handbook. Durham (NC); 2002.

U.S. Department of Health and Human Services. Powerful Bones. Powerful Girls. The National Bone Health Campaign™. Report of the National Bone Health Campaign. Research Compendium [Washington]: 2001 Aug. Available from: http://www.cdc.gov/nccdphp/dnpa/bonehealth/index.htm.

U.S. Department of Health and Human Services. Physical Activity Evaluation Handbook. Atlanta: U.S. Department of Health and Human Services, Centers for Disease Control and Prevention; 2002. 70 p. Available from http://www.cdc.gov/nccdphp/dnpa/physical/handbook/index.htm.

Weissman JS, Blumenthal D, Silk AJ, Zapert K, Newman M, Leitman R. Consumers' reports on the health effects of direct-to-consumer drug advertising. Health Affairs Web Exclusive [journal on the Internet]. c2003 Feb 26 [cited 2003 Apr 23]. [14 p.]. Available from http://content.healthaffairs.org/cgi/content/full/hlthaff.w3.82v1/DC1.

Wilkes MS, Bell RA, Kravitz RL. Direct-to-consumer prescription drug advertising: Trends, impact, and implications. Health Aff (Millwood). 2000 Mar-Apr; 19(2):110-28.

Zaza S, Lawrence RS, Mahan CS, Fullilove M, Fleming D, Isham G, Pappaioanou M. Scope and organization of the Guide to Community Preventive Services. Am J Prev Med. 2000 Jan; 18(1 Suppl): 27-34.

Part Six

CHALLENGES AND OPPORTUNITIES: A VISION FOR THE FUTURE

The final chapter summarizes the key themes of the report, highlights those opportunities that have been identified for promoting bone health, and lays out a vision for how these opportunities can be realized so that bone health can be improved today and far into the future. The key to success will be for public and private stakeholders—including individual consumers; advocacy groups; health care professionals; health systems; academic medical centers; researchers; health plans and insurers; public health departments; and all levels of government—to join forces in developing a collaborative national action plan for promoting timely prevention, assessment, diagnosis, and treatment of bone disease throughout life. To that end, these stakeholders need to work together to broaden the public's and providers' understanding of the importance of bone health and its relevance to general health and well-being and to ensure that existing and future preventive, diagnostic, and treatment measures for bone diseases and disorders are made available to all Americans.

Chapter 13

A VISION FOR THE FUTURE: A FRAMEWORK FOR ACTION TO PROMOTE BONE HEALTH

The major messages of this Surgeon General's report are as follows: 1) that bone health is essential to the general health and well-being of all Americans; 2) that great progress has been made in the last several decades in understanding and promoting bone health and in preventing, diagnosing, and treating bone disease; 3) that most individuals have the opportunity to make lifestyle choices that can result in stronger, healthier bones throughout life; and 4) that health care professionals, health systems, communities, and a variety of other stakeholders have critical roles to play in supporting individuals in making appropriate choices and in promoting timely preventive, diagnostic, and therapeutic interventions in those who have or who are at risk of developing bone disease.

However, these messages are not yet widely understood. As a result, the bone health status of Americans remains in jeopardy today, and without concerted action it will get worse in the future. Far too few Americans follow the dietary and physical activity guidelines that can help promote bone (and overall) health. Health care professionals can do a better job in paying attention to the bone health of their patients. Many individuals do not receive timely diagnostic tests and preventive and

therapeutic measures that can serve to minimize the impact of bone disease. The net result is unnecessary pain, suffering, and complications that can imperil overall health and well-being, along with financial and social costs that diminish the quality of life for individuals and burden both individuals and society at large.

Improving the bone health and well-being of Americans requires actions at all levels of society, including individuals and neighborhoods, local communities, health systems, cities, States, and the Nation as a whole. A coordinated effort can overcome the barriers—be they educational, social, systemic, policy-related, or financial—that have created a population whose bone health status is at risk.

A Framework for Action

This Surgeon General's report looks upon the Nation's at-risk bone health status as an opportunity to do better. **A national action plan for bone health** can benefit all Americans. This plan can be aimed at improving overall health and quality of life by enhancing the underlying bone health of all individuals, including men, racial and ethnic minorities, the uninsured, and the underinsured. Everyone has a role to play in improving and promoting bone health, including families and individuals, health care professionals, hospitals and rehabilitation centers, academic medical centers, the research community, health systems, managed care organizations and insurance companies, public and private purchasers, private industry, community-based organizations, State and local public health departments, voluntary health organizations, professional associations, policymakers, and agencies at all levels of government. These stakeholders can work together to broaden the public's and providers' understanding of the importance of bone health and its relevance to general health and well-being and to promote policies and programs to ensure that existing and future preventive, assessment, diagnostic, and treatment measures for bone diseases and disorders are made available on a timely basis to all Americans. This approach can serve as the primary vehicle for improving bone health in this country.

Key Action Steps

❐ **Increase awareness of the impact of osteoporosis and related bone diseases and how they can be prevented and treated throughout the lifespan.**

While much valuable work is already underway, more needs to be done to change the perception that osteoporosis is an inevitable part of aging. On the contrary, like heart disease, it needs to be thought of as a preventable chronic disease, the roots of which begin at a fairly young age even though symptoms may not manifest until later in life. Like heart disease and other chronic conditions, there needs to be a better understanding of how much can be done throughout life to prevent its eventual onset.

❐ **Change the paradigm of preventing and treating fractures.**

Fractures, especially in the elderly, need to be thought of by both the public and practitioners as a sentinel event that probably signals the presence of a frail skeleton and an increased risk of future fractures. Much as a first heart attack is thought of as an opportunity to intervene to prevent future heart attacks, an individual's first fracture must be seized upon as an opportunity to intervene to prevent future fractures. Suffering one fracture is more than enough for any individual, and therefore treating fractures should go beyond the orthopedic aspect of setting and fixing the bone. Rather, fractures should be considered a red flag for the potential for bone disease and therefore should be a catalyst for further assessment, diagnosis, prevention, and treatment of bone disease. Patients who suffer non-spine fractures represent one of the easiest high-risk groups to identify and target for intervention, since most fracture patients seek medical care for their injury. Health care practitioners and the public at large must recognize that fractures caused by weakened bones do not always manifest as broken arms, broken wrists, or other easy-to-recognize problems. Rather, they can occur "silently" in the spine with the collapse of spinal vertebrae. Individual patients may not recognize them as fractures, but rather may come into the office complaining of back pain or discomfort. Today these warning signs are too often dismissed by individuals and health professionals. As a result, too many patients end up suffering multiple fractures before anyone considers the possibility of bone disease. Individuals, especially elderly individuals, must recognize that recurrent back pain could be a signal of a bone-related problem, and practitioners that attend to individuals with back pain must consider the possibility of a spine compression fracture and hence the need for further assessment of the potential for metabolic bone disease.

❐ **Continue to build the science base on the prevention and treatment of bone diseases.**

Further work is needed in the area of basic research, clinical and epidemiological research, health system-based research, and population-based research, including community intervention trials. Specific research questions in each of these areas are discussed in relevant chapters of this report. A broad message of this report is that the Nation is not doing equally well in all areas of research and prevention. While extensive work is being done in the area of basic research, the translation of this research to clinical practice often lags behind. Clinical and epidemiological research and evaluation enjoy significant support as well. More needs to be done, especially with respect to research related to men and racial and ethnic minorities and how best to translate basic and clinical research findings into everyday practice. While much of this basic, clinical, and epidemiological research will be focused on osteoporosis, it is important to remember that research breakthroughs in osteoporosis (e.g., the development of bisphosphonates) are already paying dividends for the treatment of other bone diseases, and these benefits will likely continue in the future. More health system- and population-based research in the area of bone health is needed as well. One of the biggest voids is in the area of population-based research on behavior change, where little is known about how to get people to adopt bone-healthy behaviors. Fortunately, many of the behaviors that promote bone health also promote other aspects of health, including cardiovascular health. The goal going forward should be to integrate bone and musculoskeletal health into larger studies that are evaluating these behavioral issues in other disease areas. Within the area of health systems-based research, much more needs to be known about the most efficient and effective ways

to use the various risk assessment, diagnostic, and therapeutic tools available in bone health today. As noted, insights from basic and clinical research need to find their way into everyday practice. There are two components to this issue. First, within a given disease area, many insights from basic and clinical research are never applied in practice. For example, research might show that a particular drug, administered in a particular dose, is effective in treating a specific population. Once these findings are published, practitioners often do not know how to use this population-based information when assessing and treating individual patients. They may not know if a specific patient's situation applies and, if so, how long to use the drug in question. Second, in some situations insights from research into the prevention of other chronic diseases will have applications in the prevention of bone disease. These insights frequently do not become known to health care professionals responsible for bone health. Much more needs to be done to address both of these problems. Work should focus on stimulating the translation and application of basic research into clinical research and to promote the use of basic and clinical research findings in everyday practice. The research community should be encouraged to play a larger role in translating their findings into usable knowledge that helps a health care professional.

❐ **Support the integration of health messages and programs on physical activity and nutrition relating to other chronic diseases.**

As noted earlier, many of the behaviors that prevent bone disease are also critical for preventing other diseases and chronic conditions, including asthma, diabetes, obesity, heart disease, and stroke. Thus, it is absolutely essential that information directed toward the public and physicians about the behaviors that optimize health be integrated. These integrated educational messages need to promote all aspects of health for individuals in various stages of life, including infancy, childhood, adolescence, young adults, middle-aged adults, and the elderly. For the most part, the critical messages in each of these disease areas will be the same. The key is to maintain a healthy weight and diet, avoid smoking, and engage in regular physical activity. For example, the bone health community could join forces with other organizations promoting healthy lifestyles and the prevention of chronic diseases, such as the National Cancer Institute's *5 A Day for Better Health* campaign to advocate consumption of fruits and vegetables and the American Heart Association's efforts to promote cardiovascular health through physical activity, diet, and smoking cessation. The goal should be to ensure that their messages emphasize the bone-health benefits of whatever is being promoted, be it following an appropriate diet, exercising on a regular basis, or other bone-healthy behaviors. These integrated messages will help both the public and practitioners to understand that there is not a different "recipe" for keeping different parts of the body healthy, and that therefore it is not an all-consuming task to do what is needed to maintain one's health. Rather, the message will be a much more positive one—that following healthy behaviors is relatively easy to do and that focusing on a few critical elements such as nutrition and physical activity can go a long way toward achieving overall health and well-being.

❏ **Act now, as we know more than enough.**
While there will always be a need for more research and a greater understanding of bone health and bone disease, more than enough is known today to get started on any of a variety of critical actions that are needed to enhance the bone health status of Americans.

The Roles of Key Stakeholders

Many fruitful activities are already underway in the area of bone health. Advocacy groups, medical and science organizations, and others have been working diligently to promote better bone health for all Americans, including underserved populations. This Surgeon General's report can be a catalyst to build upon, broaden, and expand these efforts. To that end, this report calls for public and private stakeholders in the area of bone health to join forces in the development of a national action plan. The goal of this effort would be to forge consensus on the different action steps that are needed and to determine which stakeholders are best equipped to take responsibility for their execution. Because every stakeholder has an important role to play, this comprehensive effort should include a wide variety of organizations, including those representing families and individuals, health care professionals, hospitals and rehabilitation centers, skilled nursing facilities, academic medical centers, the research community, health systems, managed care organizations and insurance companies, public and private purchasers, private industry, community-based organizations, State and local public health departments, voluntary health organizations, professional associations, policymakers, and agencies at all levels of government. Some of the most important action steps for the key stakeholders are highlighted below:

Individuals and Families

Because many individuals may not realize that they are at risk of bone disease and may not take action (e.g., begin engaging in physical activity) until they are motivated to do so, individuals and families need to:

- Educate themselves on the importance of bone health and to recognize that bone health is a lifelong issue and that osteoporosis is not just a women's disease.

- Set the stage during infancy, childhood, and adolescence for their children to have healthy bones throughout their lives.
- Encourage their middle-aged and elderly parents to take actions to maintain healthy bones and to prevent bone disease and fractures later in life.
- Recognize that, regardless of their age, gender, or racial and ethnic background, they are at risk of getting bone disease and therefore should consider making a lifelong commitment to doing what is necessary (e.g., getting adequate nutrition and physical activity) to maintain strong bones. Doctors cannot do this for their individual patients, although health care professionals clearly have a role in encouraging their patients to adopt bone-healthy behaviors.

Health Care Professionals

All health care professionals, including physicians, nurses, nurse practitioners, physician assistants, dietitians/nutritionists, physical and occupational therapists, social workers, dentists, optometrists, and pharmacists can play a critical role in promoting the bone health of their patients. They need to recognize the potential for bone disease in men and racial and ethnic minorities. While the underlying risk in these population groups may be lower than for White women, the potential for bone disease is still real, particularly in the elderly and the poor.

Primary care providers have an especially critical role to play. They need to:

- Pay close attention to bone health issues when conducting wellness visits and treating people with other illnesses.
- Emphasize the basics of good bone health during their interactions with patients,

including appropriate nutrition and levels of physical activity.

- Recognize red flags and risk factors that might signal the potential for osteoporosis and other bone diseases and take necessary action or refer at-risk patients to other providers for the appropriate work-up.

Health care professionals working in emergency departments and orthopedic practices also have an important role. They must:

- Recognize that many bone fractures signal the potential for metabolic bone disease.
- Go beyond fixing patients' bones by referring them, when appropriate, to another health care professional for further assessment of the potential for bone disease.

Finally, regardless of the setting, consideration should be given to increasing the role of mid-level providers as a way of promoting bone health and minimizing the impact of bone diseases.

Health Systems

Health systems, including hospitals, organized delivery systems, and health plans and insurers, can do much to promote bone health in the populations they serve, including:

- Help individuals practice bone-healthy behaviors.
- Assist health care professionals in promoting such behaviors in all patients and in identifying and treating bone disease in a timely manner. For example, these organizations can help practitioners to identify and implement tools that aid in the diagnosis and treatment of bone disease and can point them to credible sources of information on prevention, assessment, diagnosis, and treatment.
- Implement a comprehensive, systems-based approach to promoting bone health (assuming they have a large enough population of at-risk individuals

to justify it). This approach may include: reminder systems that alert providers of the need for certain services in individual patients; systematic quality measurement and improvement; disease management programs focused on bone health; and/or the setting of appropriate financial incentives for providers and individuals.

- Consider adoption of coverage policies that provide payment for appropriate, evidence-based preventive, diagnostic, and therapeutic services within the area of bone health.

Health Care Purchasers

Health care purchasers, including public and private employers that buy health coverage on behalf of their employees, can use their power both individually and collectively to influence bone health. More specifically, they can do the following:

- Like health plans and insurers, consider adoption of coverage policies that allow for the appropriate provision of evidence-based preventive, diagnostic, and therapeutic services to all who need them.
- Use their purchasing clout to encourage providers to adopt policies and programs that promote bone health and overall health.
- Develop on-site physical activity and nutrition programs.

Communities and Community-Based Organizations

Communities consist of multiple components, including individuals, faith-based and other community organizations, employers, and government agencies. Working together these organizations can:

- Develop a forum in which the public can discuss bone health status and the bur-

den of bone disease and fractures in their community.

- Assess the resources currently available for improving the bone health status of the community, including public education and treatment.
- Evaluate, and if necessary refine, current policies and programs for enhancing the bone health status of the community.
- Promote daily physical activity in schools at all grade levels.
- Make available user-friendly facilities for physical activity for all age groups, such as walking trails and gymnasiums.

Government

Governments at every level—local, State, and Federal—have a vital leadership role to play in promoting bone health. To play this role effectively, elected policymakers and other government leaders need to recognize the long-term financial and social costs of the status quo (less-than-optimal bone health status), and appreciate the potential to reduce these costs and improve quality of life through prevention, early detection, and early treatment. Local public health departments and government agencies—especially those serving the elderly—have an especially important role to play in developing and implementing a public health approach to bone health promotion at the community level. Specific roles that government can play include:

- Promote public education, public awareness campaigns, and treatment services.
- Coordinate actions needed to improve bone health across the public and private sectors. These actions could include the formation of State or local task forces, steering committees, or advisory committees related to bone health, and

the development of strategic plans for improving the bone health status of the population and at-risk groups.

- Support the creation of an environment in which bone-healthy dietary and physical activity options are readily accessible, and needed preventive, diagnostic, and therapeutic services are readily available and affordable to all who need them.
- Promote research on basic bone biology, new approaches to diagnosis and treatment of bone disease, and the translation of research findings into practice.
- Promote research on the effects of community- and population-based interventions on the community and at-risk populations, including their impact on: the prevalence of bone disease and fractures; diet and physical activity; and access to and use of appropriate preventive, diagnostic, and treatment measures.
- Communicate with one another and coordinate activities to ensure that the actions and policies of various levels of government are complementary. The overall goal should be greater harmonization of government activities, thus ensuring more cost-effective and higher-quality services to the public.
- Use the most current, credible evidence when making policy and program decisions related to bone health.

Voluntary Health Organizations

Voluntary health organizations play important roles in promoting bone health. They are often able to reach the public and providers with critical information quickly and with fewer constraints than can government organizations.

More specifically, they can:

- Raise public awareness about specific health problems such as bone disease. By including individuals who have personally been touched by bone disease, these organizations are uniquely positioned to provide important guidance to other sectors of the health system regarding the real-life impact of bone disease on individuals, families, and communities.
- Work with residents in the local community to adopt the lifestyle changes necessary to prevent the onset or progression of bone and other diseases.
- Promote the availability of information and resources related to the prevention, diagnosis, and treatment of bone disease.

Professional Associations

Professional associations play a critical role in promoting bone health. They can:

- Facilitate the training of health professionals needed to address the prevention, diagnosis, and treatment of bone disease.
- Promote changes in the curricula of professional schools and provide continuing education to practicing bone health professionals.
- Develop evidence-based guidelines along with standards of care for bone health. These guidelines help to ensure that individuals who have or are at risk of getting bone disease can benefit from the best practices related to prevention, assessment, diagnosis, and treatment.

Academic Institutions

Academic institutions can be critical facilitators through their two core missions of education and research. With respect to osteoporosis and bone health, they can:

- Develop bone-health specific curricula for the education and training of physicians, nurses, nurse practitioners, physician assistants, dietitians/nutritionists, physical and occupational therapists, social workers, dentists, optometrists, and pharmacists.

- Develop the professional skills needed to become effective members of a health care team that focuses on improving bone health and preventing adverse outcomes. For example, trainees from different disciplines (e.g., medical students and residents, nurse practitioners, physician assistants) could be given the opportunity to rotate through osteoporosis clinics.

- Educate the general public by teaching lifestyles that promote bone health in primary and secondary schools and colleges. Schools can play a role in promoting and supporting good dietary habits and regular physical activity, beginning in childhood.

- Advance research on bone health. To date, such research has focused primarily on laboratory studies and clinical trials. Some academic institutions have active research programs on epidemiology, health care delivery, and outcomes as well. These should be expanded to include research on prevention strategies and on men and racial and ethnic minorities.

Industry

Industry also has an important role to play in promoting bone health. They can:

- Reduce the consequences of poor bone health through the development and promotion of drugs, devices, and other diagnostic and treatment technologies.

- Provide information to health care professionals and the public on the appropriate use of pharmaceutical agents to prevent and treat bone disease. This information needs to be part of a comprehensive approach to promoting bone health that includes education on appropriate diet and physical activity.

- Provide disease-management services that focus on managing osteoporosis and bone health in at-risk populations.

The Importance of Partnerships Among Stakeholders

While the roles and contributions of the individual stakeholders cited above are undoubtedly important, public-private partnerships will also be critical to the successful development and execution of a **national action plan for bone health**. These partnerships can build and strengthen cross-disciplinary, culturally competent, community-based efforts to promote bone-healthy behaviors and support the early identification and treatment of bone disease. There is no question that the collective and complementary talents of both public and private stakeholders will be vital to achieving the goal of improving the bone health status of all Americans.

Conclusion

Significant strides have been made in understanding bone health and bone disease over the past few decades. Much is known about how to keep bones healthy throughout life and how to prevent and treat bone disease and fractures in those whose bone health deteriorates. Yet too few people—individuals and health professionals alike—make use of this information. As a result, too many people have or are at risk of getting bone disease. The time has come to address this problem, to "get the word out" about the importance of bone health and the serious consequences and significant costs of bone disease and fractures. The time has come for everyone—including individual citizens, solo practitioners, the heads of major public and private sector organizations, and the leaders of governmental agencies—to do his or her part in promoting the bone health of all Americans.

Appendix A

CONGRESSIONAL LANGUAGE CALLING FOR SURGEON GENERAL'S REPORT

November 29, 2001

House Labor Report

Osteoporosis is a major health threat for more than 28 million Americans, 80% of whom are women. In 2001, 10 million individuals have already developed the disease. Osteoporosis is responsible for 1.5 million fractures annually and is second leading cause of nursing home admissions in the U.S. The Committee urges the Surgeon General to consider issuing a Report to the Nation on the status of research and education on osteoporosis and related bone disease and setting forth an action plan to comprehensively address the urgent need to reverse the increasing toll of this disease.

Senate Labor Report

Report on osteoporosis and related bone diseases. More than 30 million Americans suffer from some form of bone disease, including ostcoporosis, Paget's disease and osteogenesis imperfecta. The Committee therefore recommends that the Department commission a Surgeon General's report on osteoporosis and related bone diseases, detailing the burden bone diseases places on society, and highlighting preventive measures to improve and maintain bone health throughout life. The report should also identify best practices for collecting data about the prevalence, morbidity and disability associated with bone diseases among minority populations.

Appendix B

HOW DO WE KNOW WHAT WE KNOW: THE EVIDENCE BEHIND THE EVIDENCE

The approach of this report is to give the best evidence and advice available at this time and also to indicate where more evidence is needed. The report relies on evidence reports, consensus conferences, and governmental recommendations that have been developed through a process that reviews and evaluates all evidence in a structured, unbiased, and comprehensive manner.

It is important for clinicians and consumers to understand the origins of this evidence and advice. In fact, the evidence presented in this report has been collected and analyzed in many different ways. Some common study designs include cross-sectional longitudinal studies and randomized clinical trials. These terms, along with others that are commonly used in research, are defined in the box below.

Research Terms and Study Designs

- **Clinical trial (intervention; controlled trial):** A special kind of experimental study that tests the effectiveness of a substance or behavior (drug, diet, exercise) using consenting human subjects. The conditions of the study—selection of treatment groups, nature of interventions, management during follow-up, etc.—are specified by the investigator for the purpose of making unbiased comparisons.
- **Double-blinded:** Neither the participants nor the researchers know who receives the intervention versus the placebo.
- **Placebo:** An inert or innocuous substance used especially in controlled experiments testing the efficacy of another substance.
- **Randomized:** The study participants have been assigned to receive the active intervention or placebo randomly.

- **Observational study:** A study in which the practice or factor being studied is observed in a group of participants who have voluntarily chosen to follow or not follow this practice, i.e., they are not randomly assigned.
- **Cross-sectional study:** Study participants are observed and measurements are made at one point in time.
- **Longitudinal study:** Study participants are observed and measurements made at multiple points in time.
- **Meta-analysis:** A technique in which results from several studies are combined to produce an estimate of the effect of the factor being studied.

(Fletcher et al. 1988, MedlinePlus 2004.)

The endpoints being measured in the various studies often differ. For example, although fractures due to osteoporosis are a serious threat late in life, they are not common in younger individuals. So most studies of young people focus on how much bone mass is accumulated or how much calcium is retained when the body is put under the influence of a factor such as physical activity, calcium, or vitamin D.

Since fractures are more common in older individuals, they are commonly used as an endpoint of interest in studies of this age cohort and often are studied in older populations. A common approach is to compare two groups of people with different rates of fractures to determine which characteristics of the group with low fracture rates are protective of bone health, and/or which factors in the high-fracture group put them at risk. These "observational studies" make very important contributions by generating hypotheses about risky versus protective behaviors and lifestyle practices. The Study of Osteoporotic Fractures, which began in 1987 (see box below), has followed a group of 9,904 White women age 65 and older over a period of years to collect a variety of information as they age (Cummings et al. 1995). This study is the largest and one of the most important contributors to knowledge about the risk of fracture in older women. See Table 8-1 in Chapter 8 for risk factors that were derived from the Study of Osteoporotic Fractures. In 1997, a similar study, called Mr. OS, was launched to address the gaps in knowledge about osteoporosis and fractures in men.

Observational studies have some biases, including the fact that participants are selecting what they do. As a result, these studies can only determine that certain factors (e.g., behaviors, conditions, nutrients) are associated with lower or higher risks, not that the factor causes the change in risks. To get around this problem, some factors can be tested in an even stronger experimental design call the "double-blinded randomized clinical trial" (sometimes also referred to as "controlled" or "intervention" trials). In these studies, two or more groups of individuals are randomly assigned to receive an active intervention—such as calcium supplements—or a placebo (a pill or procedure that appears the same as the active intervention, but does not contain the active treatment). In this design, neither the participants nor the scientists conducting the study know who is receiving the active substance or the placebo. When the groups are large enough, all the other characteristics of the individuals in the study can be balanced similarly across the groups, thus eliminating, or at least reducing, the chances of various biases. This makes it possible to determine the effect of the intervention much more clearly. For this reason, this type of study has been called the "gold standard" for evidence. Drugs approved by the Food and Drug Administration for the treatment of osteoporosis and the prevention of fractures go through the rigorous testing of randomized clinical trials. Lifestyle factors and behaviors are sometimes tested using this design as well. Sometimes there are gaps in the evidence because large, well-designed studies have not yet been carried out in all different age and ethnic groups and in both men and women. Nevertheless, judgments can be made by expert groups to provide the best possible advice based on consideration of all available evidence. When developing guidelines for individuals about the diagnosis, prevention, or treatment of a disease or condition like osteoporosis and fractures, these experts rate the "strength" of the evidence using a variety of factors such as the design (e.g., was it a randomized controlled clinical trial, an observational study, or a report of a single case?), study size, and characteristics of the study population (e.g., gender, age, severity of illness). Sometimes they combine results from several studies using a technique called "meta-analysis."

It is important to remember that the scientific knowledge that fuels recommendations and public policy is built on the contributions of not only dedicated scientists, but also thousands of volunteers—men, women, and children—who decide to participate.

The Human Side of Research

It is often easy to forget that clinical research depends upon the willing participation of real people. Several important studies in the area of osteoporosis and bone health demonstrate the "human" side of research.

Camp Calcium

Camp Calcium is a unique study supported by the National Institutes of Health and conducted by the Department of Foods and Nutrition at Purdue University. Since 1990, Camp Calcium has brought together teenagers to participate in a 6-week camp in which their dietary intake of calcium is strictly controlled. Researchers also checked participants' waste and blood samples each day. The dietary calcium in the foods was varied to determine how much calcium teenagers can absorb during their most active growing period. Due to the higher incidence of osteoporosis in females, the first six camps (1990, 1993, 1996, 1997, 1999, and 2000) included only girls, with each camp designed to provide insight into a specific factor, as described below:

- Comparison of calcium metabolism in adolescents versus young adults (Wastney et al. 1996).
- Establishment of calcium requirements for teenage girls. The Food and Nutrition Board of the National Academy of Sciences used research from Camp

Calcium in setting such requirements (Wastney et al. 2003).

- Effect of maturation on calcium metabolism in teenage girls.
- Effect of race on calcium metabolism (Bryant et al. 2003).
- Effect of high and low levels of sodium on calcium retention in two races (Palacios et al. 2004).
- Determination of whether higher calcium intakes can negate the negative influences of sodium.

The 2001 camp was the first to include males, with the goal of establishing calcium requirements for teenage boys.

Participants in Camp Calcium hardly think of themselves as participating in a serious and important study. The camp itself is designed to be fun, consisting of mini-sports camps led by Purdue University athletic department staff and athletes, along with field trips, movies, nutrition and health classes, and other educational opportunities. The interaction of the young people with the scientists through the camp may inspire a few to choose a career in science. Participants also get the satisfaction of knowing that they are helping in the development of important scientific findings that will have a significant impact on the health of future generations.

The Study of Osteoporotic Fractures

The SOF study began in 1986, when women over age 65 living in four different communities (Baltimore, MD; Portland, OR; Minneapolis, MN; and the Monongahela Valley outside of Pittsburgh, PA) were invited to participate in a study designed to determine the long-term impact of physical activity on osteoporotic fractures and other more general health measures, including mortality. The study has generated important findings, including recently released data indicating that women who become or stay physically active after age 65 were only half as likely as those who are sedentary to die from cardiovascular disease, cancer, or other causes during a 7-year follow-up period (Gregg et al. 2003).

These findings would not have been possible, however, were it not for the dedication of the nearly 10,000 women who signed up for SOF, many of whom are still alive and actively participating today. For as long as 17 years, the "women of SOF" have attended clinic visits, filled out questionnaires/postcards, and received home visits or phone calls from SOF staff, all with the purpose of allowing researchers to track their health status and activity levels and to conduct blood and other tests. Many who have relocated to other parts of the country still participate by filling out and sending in their questionnaires and/or by scheduling visits to the SOF clinic when they are visiting home.

Many do so out of a sense that what they are doing is important, if not for themselves, then for others. As an 87-year-old who was the 15th person to enter the SOF study noted, "I am happy to be involved in a study that will help others." Many also find participation itself to be a rewarding experience, not only because it inspires them to become more physically active, but also because the clinic visits and other activities make them feel important and appreciated. A 78-year-old participant has had such a good experience with SOF that she has joined two other studies at the same clinic.

The organizers of SOF make a concerted effort to make participants feel appreciated. For example, they provide lunches during clinic visits and give participants a framed certificate documenting their participation. These efforts have paid off, as participants routinely make sacrifices to attend their clinic visits. One participant drives over 150 miles each way to attend. Others routinely come in despite facing a variety of health problems and/or mobility limitations that confine them to a wheelchair or that require them to use a walker. Sons and daughters of participants routinely go to great lengths to help their mothers participate; one son even flew from Chicago to Pittsburgh to pick up his mother in a nursing home and take her to the SOF clinic. Participants make these sacrifices because being in SOF means something to them; one participant even left instructions that her participation in SOF be mentioned in her obituary.

References

Bryant RJ, Wastney ME, Martin BR, Wood O, McCabe GP, Morshidi M, Smith DL, Peacock M, Weaver CM. Racial differences in bone turnover and calcium metabolism in adolescent females. J Clin Endocrinol Metab. 2003 Mar;88(3):1043-7.

Cummings SR, Nevitt MC, Browner WS, Stone K, Fox KM, Ensrud KE, Cauley J, Black D, Vogt TM; Study of Osteoporotic Fractures Research Group. Risk factors for hip fracture in white women. N Engl J Med 1995 Mar 23;332(12):767-73.

Fletcher RH, Fletcher SW, Wagner EH. Clinical epidemiology: the essentials. 2nd edition. Baltimore: Williams & Wilkins, 1988.

Gregg EW, Cauley JA, Stone K, Thompson TJ, Bauer DC, Cummings SR, Ensrud KE; Study of Osteoporotic Fractures Research Group. Relationship of changes in physical activity and mortality among older women. JAMA 2003 May 14;289(18):2379-86.

MedlinePlus Dictionary Web site. [database online]. Bethesda (MD): U.S. National Library of Medicine, National Institutes of Health. [updated 2004 Feb 04; cited 2004 Mar 16]. Available from: http://www.nlm.nih.gov/medlineplus/mplusdictionary.html.

Palacios C, Wigertz K, Martin BR, Jackman L, Pratt JH, Peacock M, McCabe G, Weaver CM. Sodium retention in black and white female adolescents in response to salt intake. J Clin Endocrinol Metab. 2004 Apr;89(4):1858-63.

Wastney ME, Martin BR, Bryant RJ, Weaver CM. Calcium utilization in young women: New insights from modeling. Adv Exp Med Biol. 2003;537:193-205.

Wastney ME, Ng J, Smith D, Martin BR, Peacock M, Weaver CM. Differences in calcium kinetics between adolescent girls and young women. Am J Physiol. 1996 Jul;271(1 Pt 2):R208-16.

Appendix C

RESOURCES AND RELATED LINKS

This section provides the names of resources and links in government and the private sector related to bone health. Links to non-Federal organizations do not constitute an endorsement of any organization by the Federal Government, and none should be inferred.

Federal Government

Agency for Healthcare Research and Quality (AHRQ)
Osteoporosis publications and electronic information
http://www.ahrq.gov/news/pubsix.htm

Centers for Disease Control and Prevention (CDC)
Growing Stronger: Strength Training for Older Adults
http://www.cdc.gov/nccdphp/dnpa/physical/growing_stronger

PATCH—CDC's Planned Approach to Community Health
http://www.cdc.gov/nccdphp/patch/index.htm

Physical Activity and Health: A Report of the Surgeon General
http://www.cdc.gov/nccdphp/sgr/sgr.htm

Powerful Bones, Powerful Girls Web Site
http://www.cdc.gov/powerfulbones/
http:/www.cdc.gov/powerfulbones/parents

Powerful Girls Calendar
http://www.cdc.gov/powerfulbones/games_fun/calendar_2004.pdf

Promoting Better Health for Young People Through Physical Activity and Sports
http://www.cdc.gov/nccdphp/dash/presphysactrpt/index.htm

VERB$_{TM}$. *It's what you do.* Youth Media Campaign
http://www.cdc.gov/youthcampaign/

Wisewoman: Well-Integrated Screening and Evaluation for Women Across the Nation
http://www.cdc.gov/wisewoman

National Heart, Lung, and Blood Institute (NHLBI)
DASH (Dietary Approaches to Stop Hypertension) Eating Plan
http://www.nhlbi.nih.gov/health/public/heart/hbp/dash/

Hearts N' Parks
http://www.nhlbi.nih.gov/health/prof/heart/obesity/hrt_n_pk/index.htm

National Cholesterol Education Program
http://www.nhlbi.nih.gov/about/ncep/

National Institute on Aging (NIA)
Exercise: A Guide from the National Institute on Aging
http://www.nia.nih.gov/exercisebook/index.htm

Exercise: A Video from the National Institute on Aging
http://www.niapublications.org/exercisevideo/index.asp

National Institute of Arthritis and Musculoskeletal and Skin Diseases (NIAMS)
Information Package—Ordering Information
http://www.niams.nih.gov/hi/index.htm#ip

Osteoporosis Prevention, Diagnosis, and Therapy
http://odp.od.nih.gov/consensus/cons/111/111_intro.htm

Osteoporosis: Progress and Promise
http://www.niams.nih.gov/hi/topics/osteoporosis/opbkgr.htm

National Institute of Child Health and Human Development (NICHD)
Milk Matters Educational Campaign
http://156.40.88.3/milk/milk.cfm

National Institute of Diabetes and Digestive and Kidney Diseases (NIDDK)
Sisters Together: Move More, Eat Better
http://www.niddk.nih.gov/health/nutrit/sisters/sisters.htm

National Institutes of Health (NIH)
Clinical Trials
http://www.ClinicalTrials.gov

NIH Osteoporosis and Related Bone Disease~National Resource Center
http://www.osteo.org/default.asp

President's Council on Physical Fitness and Sports
The President's Challenge
http://www.fitness.gov
http://www.presidentschallenge.org

U.S. Administration on Aging

Aging Internet Information Notes: Osteoporosis
http://www.aoa.gov/prof/notes/docs/osteoporosis.doc

U. S. Department of Agriculture (USDA)

Dietary Guidelines for Americans
http://www.usda.gov/cnpp/

School Meals
http://www.fns.usda.gov/cnd

USDA Food and Nutrition Service
http://www.fns.usda.gov

United States National Agricultural Library
http://www.nal.usda.gov

U. S. Department of Education (USDOE)

National Institute on Disability and Rehabilitation Research (NIDRR)
http://www.ed.gov/about/offices/list/osers/nidrr/index.html?src=mr

U.S. Department of Health and Human Services (HHS)

Dietary Guidelines for Americans
http://www.health.gov/dietaryguidelines

HealthierUS Initiative
http://www.healthierus.gov

Healthfinder® Gateway to Reliable Consumer Health Information on the Internet
http://www.healthfinder.gov

Healthy People in Healthy Communities: A Community Planning Guide Using Healthy People 2010
http://www.healthypeople.gov/publications/HealthyCommunities2001

Healthy People 2010 Toolkit
http://www.healthypeople.gov/state/toolkit

National Women's Health Information Center
http://www.4woman.gov

STEPS to a HealthierUS Initiative
http://www.healthierus.gov/steps/index.html

U.S. Food and Drug Administration (FDA)
Guidance on How to Understand and Use the Nutrition Facts Panel on Food Labels
http://www.cfsan.fda.gov/~dms/foodlab.html

U.S. Food and Drug Administration—FDA Consumer Magazine (10/02)
http://www.fda.gov/fdac/features/2002/502_men.html

State Government

Association of State and Territorial Chronic Disease Program Directors

Osteoporosis Council
   http://www.chronicdisease.org/Osteo_Council/osteo_about.htm

Osteoporosis Council: Contact information for state osteoporosis directors/coordinators
   http://www.chronicdisease.org/Osteo_Council/osteo_membership.htm

Osteoporosis State Program Practices That Work
   http://www.chronicdisease.org/whc/Practices_that_Work.pdf

Osteoporosis 2000: A Resource Guide for State Programs
   http://www.chronicdisease.org/Osteo_Council/publications/Resource_Guide.pdf

State Osteoporosis Web Sites

Alabama Department of Public Health
   http://www.adph.org/NUTRITION/default.asp?DeptId=115&TemplateId=2022&TemplateNbr=0

Arizona Osteoporosis Coalition
   http://www.azoc.org
   http://www.fitbones.org

California Department of Health Services, Arthritis and Osteoporosis Unit
   http://www.dhs.ca.gov/osteoporosis

Colorado Department of Public Health and Environment: Osteoporosis Web Site
   http://www.cdphe.state.co.us/pp/Osteoporosis/osteohom.html

Florida Osteoporosis Prevention and Education Program
   http://www.doh.state.fl.us/family/osteo/default.html

Georgia Osteoporosis Initiative
   http://www.gabones.com

Indiana Osteoporosis Prevention Initiative
   http://www.in.gov/isdh/programs/osteo

Kentucky Office of Women's Physical and Mental Health: Osteoporosis
   http://chs.ky.gov/womenshealth/resourcecenter/Resources/osteoporosis.htm

Maryland Department of Health and Mental Hygiene
   http://www.strongerbones.org

Michigan Department of Community Health
http://www.michigan.gov/mdch/0,1607,7-132-2940_2955_2978—,00.html

Mississippi State Department of Health
http://www.msdh.state.ms.us/msdhsite/index.cfm/13,0,225,html

Missouri Department of Health and Senior Services
http://www.dhss.state.mo.us/maop

New Jersey Department of Health and Senior Services
http://www.state.nj.us/health/senior/osteo

New York State Department of Health
http://www.health.state.ny.us/nysdoh/osteo/index.htm

Ohio Department of Health
http://www.odh.state.oh.us/odhprograms/osteo/osteo1.htm

Rhode Island Department of Health
http://www.health.ri.gov/disease/osteoporosis/index.htm

Tennessee Department of Health
http://www2.state.tn.us/health/healthpromotion/osteoporosis.html

Texas Department of Health: Osteoporosis Awareness and Education Program
http://www.tdh.state.tx.us/osteo

Virginia Department of Health
http://www.vahealth.org/nutrition/bones.htm

West Virginia Department of Health and Human Resources
http://www.wvdhhr.org/bph/oehp/hp/osteo/default.htm

Non-Government

American Academy of Orthopaedic Surgeons (AAOS)
http://www.aaos.org

American Academy of Pediatrics (AAP)
Policy Statement on Calcium Requirements of Infants, Children, and Adolescents
http://aappolicy.aappublications.org/policy_statement/index.dtl#C

American Council on Exercise
http://www.acefitness.org

American College of Sports Medicine
http://www.acsm.org

American Dietetic Association (ADA)
http://www.eatright.org

American Society for Bone and Mineral Research (ASBMR)
http://www.asbmr.org

ASBMR Bone Curriculum Web Site
http://depts.washington.edu/bonebio/ASBMRed/ASBMRed.html

Bone Builders
http://www.bonebuilders.org/

BoneKEy-Osteovision®
http://www.bonekey-ibms.org

Foundation for Osteoporosis Research and Education (FORE)
http://www.fore.org/

Growing Stronger: Strength Training for Older Adults
http://nutrition.tufts.edu/research/growingstronger

International Bone and Mineral Society (IBMS)
http://www.ibmsonline.org/

International Osteoporosis Foundation (IOF)
http://www.osteofound.org/

International Society for Clinical Densitometry (ISCD)
http://www.iscd.org/osteoblast/index.cfm

National Dairy Council (NDC)
http://www.nationaldairycouncil.org

National Osteoporosis Foundation (NOF)
http://www.nof.org

National Strength and Conditioning Association
http://www.nsca-lift.org

Osteoporosis and Bone Physiology, University of Washington
http://courses.washington.edu/bonephys

Osteoporosis Education, University of Washington
http://www.osteoed.org/faq/index.html#male
http://www.osteoed.org

Osteogenesis Imperfecta Foundation (OIF)
http://www.oif.org

The Paget Foundation (TPF)
http://www.paget.org

Shape-Up America!
http://www.shapeup.org

U.S. Bone and Joint Decade
http://www.usbjd.org

Abbreviations and Acronyms

AAOS	American Academy of Orthopaedic Surgeons
ACOVE	Assessing Care of Vulnerable Elders
ACS	American Cancer Society
ACSM	American College of Sports Medicine
ACTH	adrenocorticotropic hormone
AD	autosomal dominant
AGS	American Geriatrics Society
AHRQ	Agency for Health Care Research and Quality
AI	adequate intakes
AIAN	American Indian and Alaska Native
AR	autosomal recessive
BH/BH	Bone Health/Body Health
BMD	bone mineral density
BSAP	bone specific alkaline phosphatase
BUA	broadband attenuation
CDC	Centers for Disease Control and Prevention
CEE	conjugated equine estrogens
CMAJ	Canadian Medical Association Journal
CME	continuing medical education
CMS	Centers for Medicare and Medicaid Services
CNS	central nervous system
COPE	computerized physician order entry
CTx	C-terminal collagen crosslinked peptides
DASH	Dietary Approaches To Stop Hypertension
DNA	deoxyribonucleic acid
DOT	Department of Transportation
Dpd	free deoxypyridoline crosslinks
DRG	diagnosis-related group
DTCA	direct-to-consumer advertising
DV	daily value
DXA	dual x-ray absorptiometry
E + P	estrogen-progestin combination
ECF	extracellular fluid
EPESE	Established Populations for Epidemiologic Studies of the Elderly
FDA	Food and Drug Administration
fl oz.	fluid ounce
FNB	Food and Nutrition Board

g/cm²	grams per centimeter squared
GIO	glucocorticoid-induced osteoporosis
gm	gram
GnRH	gonadotrophin-releasing hormone
HEDIS	Health Plan Employer Data and Information Set
HIV	human immunodeficiency virus
HMO	health maintenance organization
HOPE	Health, Osteoporosis, Progestin, Estrogen
HRR	hospital referral regions
HRSA	Health Resources and Services Administration
HT	hormone therapy
IGF-1	insulin-like growth factor-1
IOM	Institute of Medicine
IPA	independent practice association
ISCD	International Society for Clinical Densitometry
IU	international units
kg	kilogram
m-CSF	macrophage colony stimulating factor
mg	milligram
MilkPEP	Milk Processor Education Program
ml	milliliter
MM	multiple myeloma
MMA	Medicare Modernization Act
MPA	medroxyprogesterone
NAWHO	National Asian Women's Health Organization
NBHC	National Bone Health Campaign
NCDPH	North Carolina Department of Public Health
NCEP	National Cholesterol Education Program
NCHS	National Center for Health Statistics
NCI	National Cancer Institute
NCQA	National Committee for Quality Assurance
ND	not determinable
NDC	National Dairy Council
NDDIC	National Digestive Diseases Information Clearinghouse
NGC	National Guideline Clearinghouse
NHANES	National Health and Nutrition Examination Survey
NHDS	National Hospital Discharge Survey
NIA	National Institute on Aging
NICHD	National Institute of Child Health and Human Development
NIDCR	National Institute of Dental and Craniofacial Research

NIH	National Institutes of Health
NIHORBD~NRC	National Institutes of Health, Osteoporosis and Related Bone Diseases~National Resource Center
NJDHSS	New Jersey Department of Health and Senior Services
NOF	National Osteoporosis Foundation
NORA	National Osteoporosis Risk Assessment
NTX	N-telopeptide of type I collagen
OI	osteogenesis imperfecta
OMBDC	Saint Barnabas Osteoporosis and Metabolic Bone Disease Center
OPG	osteoprotegerin
ORAI	Osteoporosis Risk Assessment Instrument
OST	Osteoporosis Self-Assessment Tool
OTA	Office of Technology Assessment
OTA	Orthopaedic Trauma Association
OWH	Office on Women's Health
oz.	ounce
PA	physical activity
PDSA	Plan, Do, Study, Act
pDXA	peripheral dual x-ray absorptiometry
PE	physical education
PEPI	Postmenopausal Estrogen/Progestin Interventions
PICP	carboxyterminal propeptide of type I collagen
PINP	aminoterminal propeptide of type I collagen
pkt	packet
pQCT	peripheral quantitative computed tomography
PROOF	Prevent Recurrence of Osteoporotic Fractures
PTH	parathyroid hormone
PTHrP	parathyroid hormone-related protein
Pyd	free and total pyridinolines
QALY	quality-adjusted life year
QCT	quantitative computed tomography
QOL	quality of life
QUS	quantitative ultrasound
RA	radiographic absorptiometry
RANKL	receptor activator of nuclear factor kappa B ligand
RDA	recommended daily allowance
RPCT	randomized placebo-controlled trial
RSVP	New Jersey Association of Retired and Senior Volunteer Program Directors
SCORE	Simple Calculated Osteoporosis Risk Estimation

SD	standard deviation
SERM	selective estrogen receptor modulator
SHPPS	School Health Policies and Programs Study
SOS	speed of sound
SPF	sun protection factor
SXA	single x-ray absorptiometry
Tbsp	tablespoon
TSH	thyroid stimulating hormone
UL	upper intake levels
USDA	United States Department of Agriculture
USDHHS	United States Department of Health and Human Services
USP	United States Pharmacopoeia
USPSTF	United States Preventive Services Task Force
USRDS	United States Renal Data System
WHI	Women's Health Initiative
WHO	World Health Organization
WIC	Women, Infants, and Children Program
yr	year

List of Tables and Figures

Index

www.ingramcontent.com/pod-product-compliance
Lightning Source LLC
Chambersburg PA
CBHW081429170526
45166CB00008B/2137